U0908781

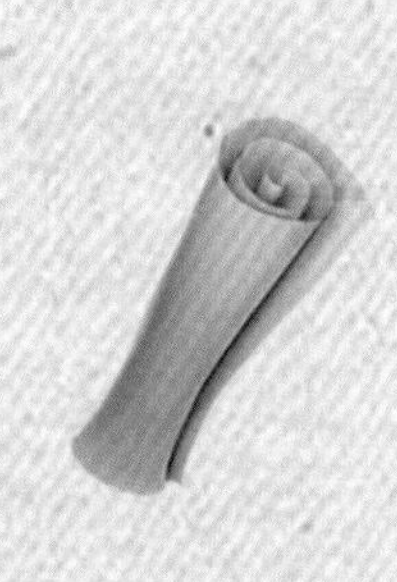

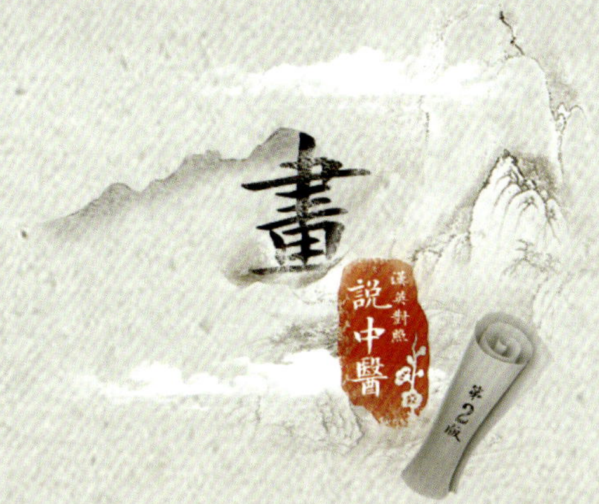

An Illustrated Guide to

Chinese Medicine

Chinese-English | Second Edition | Xu Yi-bing, Xu Wu, Wei Qin

人民卫生出版社
PMPH
PEOPLE'S MEDICAL PUBLISHING HOUSE

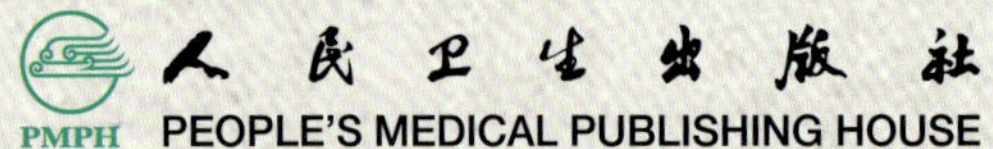

Website: http://www.pmph.com/en

Book Title: An Illustrated Guide to Chinese Medicine (Chinese-English) (Second Edition)
画说中医（汉英对照）（第2版）

Contact address: No. 19, Pan Jia Yuan Nan Li, Chaoyang District, Beijing 100021, P.R. China, phone/fax: 8610 5978 7340, E-mail: pmph@pmph.com

For text and trade sales, as well as review copy inquiries, please contact PMPH at pmph@pmph.com

Disclaimer

This book is for educational and reference purposes only. In view of the possibility of human error or changes in medical science, the author, editor, publisher and any other party involved in the publication of this work do not guarantee that the information contained herein is in any respect accurate or complete. The medicinal therapies and treatment techniques presented in this book are provided for the purpose of reference only. If readers wish to attempt any of the techniques or utilize any of the medicinal therapies contained in this book, the publisher assumes no responsibility for any such actions. It is the responsibility of the readers to understand and adhere to local laws and regulations concerning the practice of these techniques and methods. The authors, editors and publisher disclaim all responsibility for any liability, loss, injury, or damage incurred as a consequence, directly or indirectly, of the use and application of any of the contents of this book.

First published: 2019
ISBN: 978-7-117-28659-6

Cataloguing in Publication Data:
A catalogue record for this book is available from the CIP-Database China.

Printed in The People's Republic of China

責任編輯：曾純
封面設計：趙京津
版式設計：趙京津
Project Editor: Zeng Chun
Cover Designer: Zhao Jing-jin
Book Designer: Zhao Jing-jin

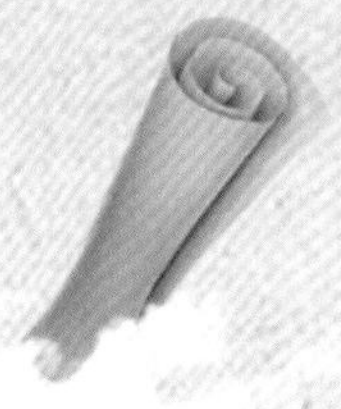

主编 徐宜兵 徐 武 魏 勤

编委 何 葦 黄 葦 樂麗霞

楊 琴 李 琳 雷 姗

包奇昌 楊永壽 吴 健

繪圖 徐 武

翻譯 魏 勤

編輯 Eran Pupkin

Chief Editors **Xu Yi-bing, Xu Wu & Wei Qin**

Contributors **He Wei Huang Wei Le Li-xia**

Yang Qin Li Lin Bao Qi-chang

Yang Yong-shou Wu Jian

Illustrated by Xu Wu

Translated by Wei Qin

Edited by Eran Pupkin

作者简介

徐宜兵，祖籍江西宜黄，1963年8月出生於臨川，現為江西中醫藥高等專科學校三級教授，主任中醫師，人淳樸，研醫理，喜詩文，好書墨，曾榮獲江西省衛生科技創新壹等獎，主編教材或著作10部，發表論文近50篇。為江西省百千萬人才工程人選、江西省高校中青年骨幹教師、江西省撫州市政府特殊津貼專家、江西省高職高專人才培養水準評估專家。

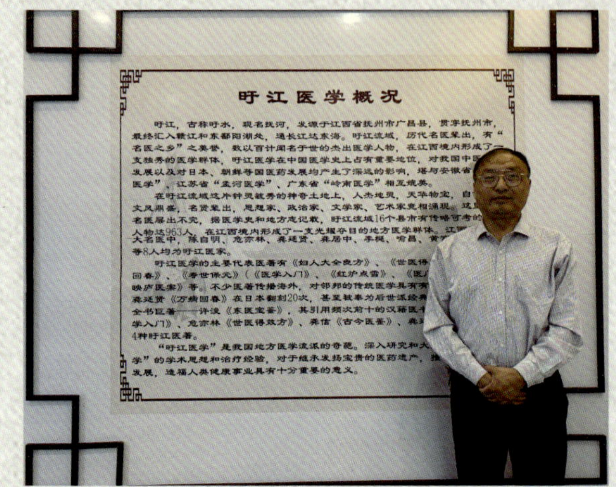

About the Author

Xu Yi-bing, a native of Yihuang County, was born in Linchuan, Jiangxi Province, P. R. China in August 1963. He is a professor of third level in Jiangxi College of Traditional Chinese Medicine and a TCM Chief Physician. He is simple and honest. He studies principles of medical science and loves poetry and writing. His awards include the "First Prize for Scientific and Technical Invention" awarded by Department of Health of Jiangxi Province. He has served as editor of 10 articles and textbooks, written 50 dissertations on various topics. He is selected for New Century Talents Project of Jiangxi Province and is entitled as a Provincial-approved Most Outstanding Teacher of Jiangxi Province. He is an expert enjoying the special government allowance of Fuzhou, Jiangxi Province and an expert for the Talent Cultivation Level Assessment Project for Higher Technical and Vocational Institutions of Jiangxi Province.

序言

勤勞的祖先用智慧創造了古代科學技術的燦爛，
中國古代發明推動了人類進步和社會發展。

中國醫藥學是一個偉大寶庫，
中華民族的繁衍昌盛做出了巨大貢獻。
你想瞭解古老的東方文化的精粹嗎？
你想領略神奇的中醫中藥的奧秘嗎？
請閱讀《畫說中醫》漢英對照版，
它將引領你穿越時空，
回歸文明的發源地，

謹以此書：
獻給大同世界。

Foreword

The wise and industrious Chinese ancestors invented magnificent sciences and technologies, resulting in the forward movement of human progress and social development. Chinese medicine is a tremendous treasure that has made a huge contribution to the increased prosperity of the Chinese nation.

Would you like to have a profound understanding about this essence of ancient East Asian culture?

Would you like to appreciate the mystery of magical Chinese medicine?

We invite you to read *An Illustrated Guide to Chinese Medicine*, it will help you to traverse through space and time, and return to the cradle of civilization. And so, we humbly offer this book to all over the world.

第2版前言

中醫藥是中國優秀的民族文化遺產。

2007年，為喜迎2008年北京夏季奧運會，我們創作編譯了漢英雙語版的《畫說中醫》，首次嘗試以圖畫的形式，配以精煉的中英文雙語描述，淺顯易懂地講述古樸深奧的中醫基礎理論。作為一本較好的入門讀本，《畫說中醫》受到了國內外中醫初學者和中醫愛好者的喜愛。

十二年過去，彈指一揮間。

《中華人民共和國中醫藥法》於2017年正式實施，為提升中醫藥在全球的影響力提供法律保障。中醫藥傳承創新實現突破，養生保健潛力釋放，海外影響日趨擴大，中醫藥振興發展迎來天時、地利、人和的新時機。

我們創新團隊在第一版基礎上完善了體質學說內容，並增加了中醫治未病章節及法規內容，力圖促進中醫藥與外界文化交融，形成互鑒共賞的新格局。圍繞"一帶一路"戰略，推動中醫藥走向世界，使民族瑰寶惠及各國民眾，為共同建設人類命運共同體的重要框架貢獻綿薄之力。

人民衛生出版社在傳播中醫藥工作中有着長期實踐與積累，其中優良的傳統在修訂過程中得到很好的發揚。本書得到江西省中醫藥管理局的熱心指導和幫助，得到江西中醫藥高等專科學校領導的支持，在此表示衷心感謝。本書寫作過程中得到諸多專家的幫助，引用了許多學者的學術資料，在此一併致謝！

徐宜兵

2019年4月8日

於盱江流域南昌滕王閣

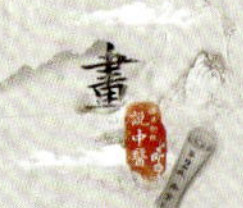

Preface to the 2nd Edition

Twelve years have passed quickly.

Chinese medicine is the excellent cultural heritage of China.

In 2007, we compiled *An Illustrated Guide to Chinese Medicine* for 2008 Beijing Summer Olympics. In this book, we explained the profound Chinese medicine's basic theory by using illustrations with brief simple explanations. As an introductory book, it is popular among beginners and fans of Chinese medicine at home and abroad.

In 2017, Law of the People's Republic of China on Traditional Chinese Medicine was officially implemented to provide legal protection for the improvement of Chinese medicine's global influence. It's now the time for the rejuvenation and development of Chinese medicine as the inheritance and innovation of Chinese medicine achieve a breakthrough, health care releases potential and the global influence has been increasingly expanded.

On the basis of the first edition, our team improved the content of constitutions and added the chapter of preventive treatment of diseases and related laws to promote the cultural integration and form the new pattern of mutual learning. Guided by the "Belt and Road" initiative, we want to promote Chinese medicine to the world so that it can benefit people from all over the world and we can contribute to the important framework of a community of shared future for mankind.

People's Medical Publishing House has a long time practice of spreading Chinese medicine and its fine tradition has been carried forward during the revision and publication of this second edition of the *An Illustrated Guide to Chinese Medicine*. Firstly, we would like to express our appreciation to the Jiangxi Provincial Administration of Chinese Medicine for the guidance and help. Then our faithful appreciation also goes to Jiangxi College of Traditional Chinese Medicine for the support. Ultimately, we owe our heartfelt thanks to the experts who helped me a lot as this book's references are the results of their contemporary researches.

Xu Yi-bing

April 8th, 2019

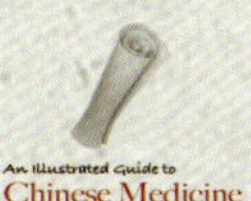

第1版前言

中醫學是中華民族幾千年來同疾病作鬥爭的經驗總結，是中國傳統文化的重要組成部分。在中國古代哲學思想的影響和指導下，通過長期醫療實踐及學科之間的互相滲透，逐步形成並發展成為獨特的醫學理論體系，為中國人民保健事業和中華民族的繁衍昌盛做出了巨大貢獻。如今，這一古老的醫學正煥發出新的光彩，並走向全球為全世界人民的衛生保健事業做出新的貢獻。

中醫基礎理論源遠流長，語言深奧。為了給初學中醫者和中醫愛好者提供一本較好的入門啟蒙讀本，我們嘗試採用圖畫形式，配以簡短的文字描述，使古樸的中醫基礎理論淺而易見地表達出來。

本書的特點是文字通俗流暢，插圖生動有趣，化簡為繁，圖文並茂，直觀形象，新穎實用。力求科學嚴密與親切可讀皆備，專業高雅與通俗易懂共融，莊重嚴謹與生動活潑一體。

本書集知識性、趣味性、資料性為一體，是一部符合現代人閱讀理解特點的中醫科普之作，對中醫愛好者有較大的助益。

本書得到江西省教育廳、江西省衛生廳和江西省中醫藥管理局的熱情關心和支持，書中參考了中国國內大中專教材的內容及當代學者研究成果，在此一併致謝。

用圖畫的形式來注釋中醫基礎理論是新的嘗試，限於編者水準有限，編寫中難免有遺漏和謬誤，敬請讀者批評，以便今後得以提高。

編譯者

2006年12月30日

江西臨川

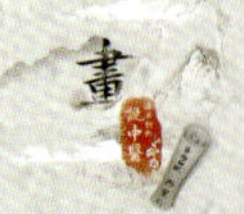

Preface to the 1st Edition

Chinese Medicine is the summary of the rich experiences of the Chinese people, from thousands of years of struggling against diseases. It is an important component of Chinese traditional culture. Chinese medicine, under the guidance of ancient Chinese philosophy, and the long history of the mutual influence of medical practice and medical theory, has formed a unique medical theoretical system and made remarkable contributions to health care and the prosperity of the Chinese nation. Now, the brilliance of ancient Chinese medicine is shining forth and making contributions to the health care of people all around the world.

Chinese medicine's basic theory was established a long time ago and so its language is profound. In order to provide an introductory book for both beginning students and fans of Chinese medicine, we explained this profound Chinese medicine's basic theory by using illustrations with brief simple explanations.

This book uses a smooth language style, the pictures are lively and interesting; the authors have made every effort to combine scientific details and easily understood reading; and to fuse precision and vividness.

This book is informative and interesting, and Chinese medicine lovers will find it a great benefit.

We would like to express our appreciation to the Departments of Education and Health of Jiangxi Province and the Jiangxi Provincial Administration of Chinese Medicine. This book's references are the Chinese medicine textbooks published in Chinese editions for the Chinese medicine students in college level, and also the results of contemporary research.

This book is a new attempt to explain Chinese medicine's basic theory by using illustrations. The authors, translators and editors have done their best to avoid mistakes in this text, but it is hard to avoid completely. All criticisms, corrections of errors and suggestions will be appreciated and considered for future editions.

The authors, translators and editors

December 30, 2006

Linchuan, Jiangxi Province

目録

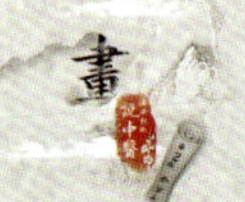

CONTENTS

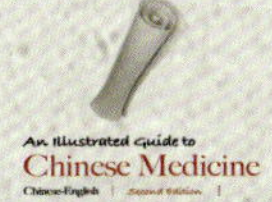

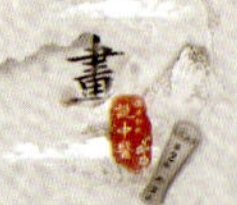

CONTENTS

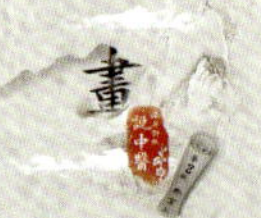

CONTENTS

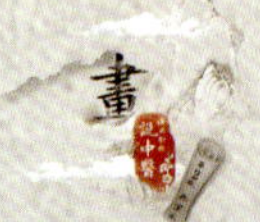

CONTENTS

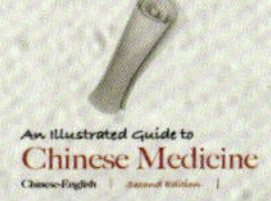

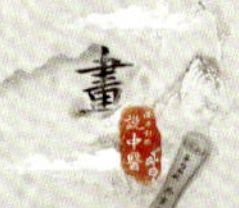

CONTENTS

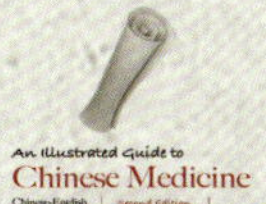

CONTENTS

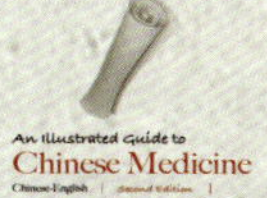

緒論　Introduction

中國醫藥學是一個偉大的寶庫

中國醫藥學集中華民族數千年文化於一身，其獨特理論之博大精深，其臨床經驗之豐富多彩，一枝獨秀屹立在世界傳統醫學之林。

有史記載：著名的中醫藥學家有 10,452 位，方劑有 96,592 首，中草藥有 12,000 多味。

中醫藥現已傳至 180 多個國家和地區，這一古老的醫學正煥發出新的光彩，爲世界人民的衛生保健事業做出新的貢獻。

Chinese Medicine Is a Tremendous Treasure

Thousands of years of Chinese civilization has been concentrated in Chinese medicine. Its broad, profound and unique theory and its rich, varied clinical experience make it outstanding in world medicine.

According to historical records, there have been 10,452 renowned Chinese medicine doctors, 96,592 prescriptions and 12,000 kinds of medicaments.

Chinese medicine has already spread to over 180 regions and countries. This age-old medicine is radiating new splendor and making new contributions to the health care of people all over the world.

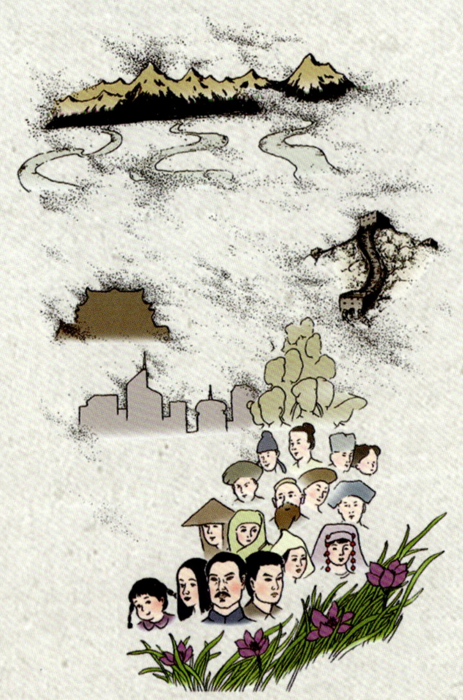

一、醫學模式："生物—心理—社會—環境"醫學模式

Medical Model:"Biology-Psychology-Society-Environment" Medical Model

1. 天人合一觀

中醫學以天地人一體的整體觀念爲指導思想，以人爲中心，從人與自然、社會三者的關係去探討人的生命過程及防治疾病的規律，强調心理因素、體質因素以及社會和環境因素對疾病發生發展和防治的影響。

1. The Concept that Human Beings and Nature Correspond to Each Other

Chinese medicine views the vital process and the regulations of prevention and care of diseases based on the relationships between human, nature and society. It emphasizes the influence of mental factors, constitutional factors, the social and environmental factors on the occurrence, development and prevention of diseases.

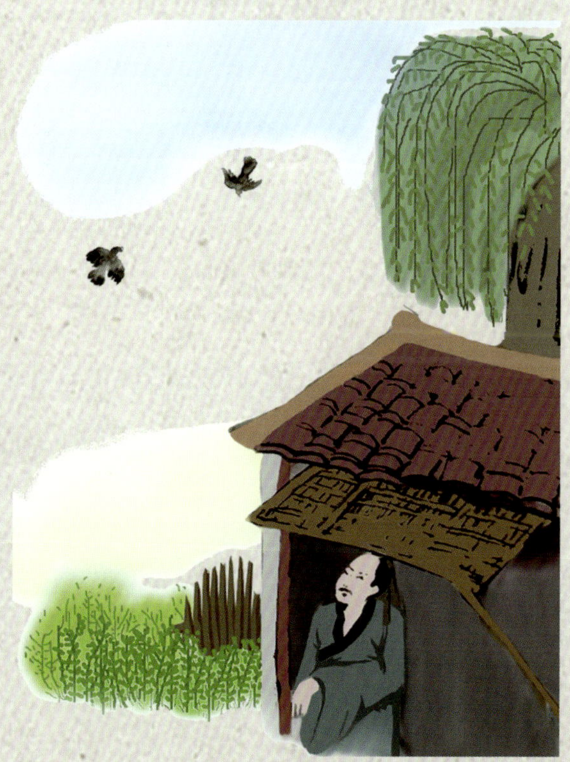

2. 形神合一觀

中醫學將人體的有形肉體和精神心靈連貫成爲一個係統的整體。形神合一觀認爲，形與神俱，不可分離。形是神藏會之處，神是形的生命體現。形與神不能分離，形神相生、形神統一，是生命存在的保證。

2. The Concept that the Body and Spirit Correspond to Each Other

Chinese medicine views the tangible and intangible body as a combined whole. This concept argues that body and spirit cannot individually exist because the spirit hides inside one's body and the body is the external embodiment of spirit. The mutual production and unification of body and spirit assures human survival.

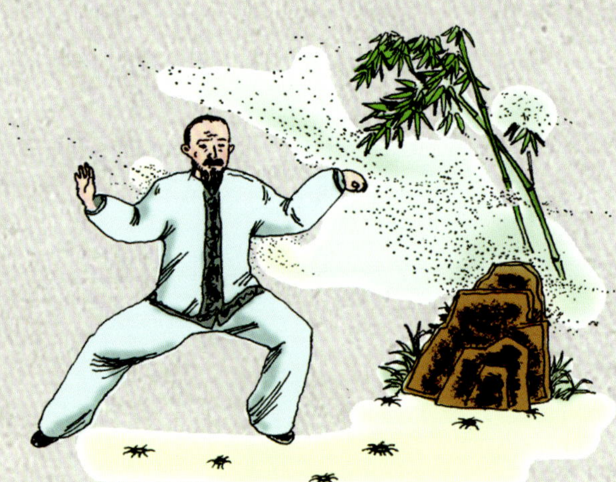

二、四部經典

Four Classic Texts of Chinese Medicine

東方文化博大精深，
中醫典籍浩瀚如海，
在此簡介“四部經典”。

1.《黄帝内經》

成書於春秋戰國時期，是中國醫學史上最古老的、最宏偉的經典著作。

Asia's profound culture has given birth to a vast accumulation of classics. Below, is an introduction to four of the classic texts of Chinese medicine.

1. *Huáng Dì Nèi Jīng*

The Yellow Emperor's Classic of Internal Medicine, the most ancient and the greatest classic of Chinese medicine, was compiled during the Spring-autumn and Warring States periods.

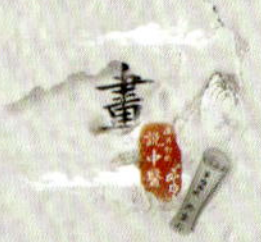

《黄帝内經》是由《素問》九卷和《靈樞》九卷兩大部分組成，各有醫學論述性文章 81 篇。書中許多解剖、生理、病理學的認識大大超越了當時的世界醫學水準。

《黄帝内經》標誌着中醫學理論體係的初步形成。初步確立了中醫學獨特的理論體係，成爲中醫學進一步發展的基礎和源泉。

It consists of two parts—*Basic Questions* (*Sù Wèn*) and *Miraculous Pivot* (*Líng Shū*), each containing nine volumes and 81 chapters. Knowledge of the anatomy, physiology and pathology written in this classic text played a leading role in the medical field at that time.

The Yellow Emperor's Classic of Internal Medicine marks the formation of Chinese medicine and the initial establishment of its unique theoretical system. It provides the foundation and the resources for the further development of Chinese medicine.

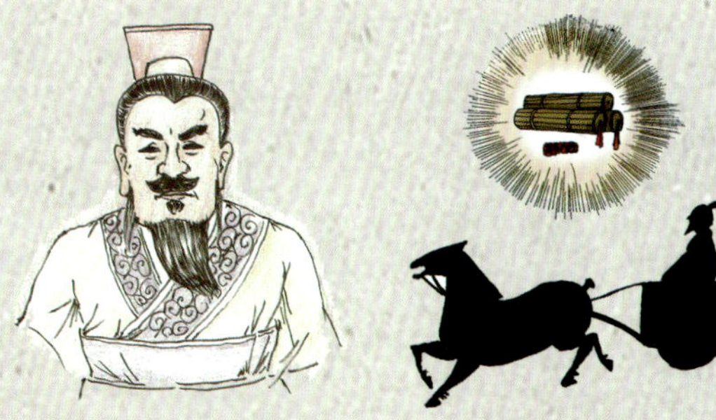

2.《難經》

大約成書西漢時期，相傳係秦越人（扁鵲）所撰。

本書以假設問答，解釋疑難的方式編纂而成，闡述了人體結構、生理、病因、病機、診斷、治則和治法等，是繼《黄帝内經》之後的又一部中醫經典著作。

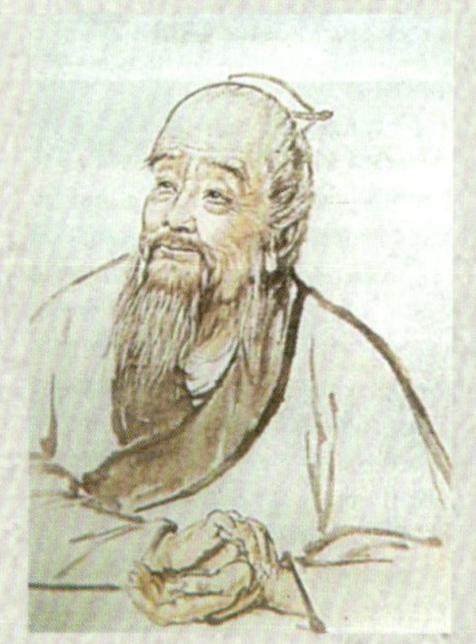

2. *Nàn Jīng*

The *Classic on Medical Problems*, another classic of Chinese medicine, emerged in the West Han Dynasty after the appearance of *the Yellow Emperor's Classic of Internal Medicine*. It is attributed to Bian Que, a famous Chinese physician of the past.

It was compiled in the model of posing and answering questions. The book explained body constitution, physiology, pathogenesis, diagnosis, and the methods and principles of treatment.

3.《傷寒雜病論》

爲東漢末年張仲景所著，分爲《傷寒論》和《金匱要略》。

《傷寒論》載方 113 首，《金匱要略》載方 262 首，除去重複方劑，兩書實載方 269 首，使用藥物達 214 種。

《傷寒雜病論》被譽爲“方書之祖”，它的問世，代表了臨床醫學的發展和辨證論治的確立。

3. *Shāng Hán Zá Bìng Lùn*

In the late East Han Dynasty, Zhang Zhongjing wrote *The Treatise on Febrile and Miscellaneous Diseases* which was later divided into two books: one is *The Treatise on Febrile Diseases* (*Shāng Hán Lùn*), which lists 113 prescriptions; the other is called *The Synopsis of Prescriptions of Golden Cabinet* (*Jīn Guì Yào Lüè*), which contains 262 prescriptions. Not counting duplicates, the two books contain 269 prescriptions in total and refer to 214 kinds of medicinals.

The Treatise on Febrile and Miscellaneous Diseases is praised as "the ancestor of formularies". It represents the development of clinical medicine and the establishment of treatment by differentiation of syndromes.

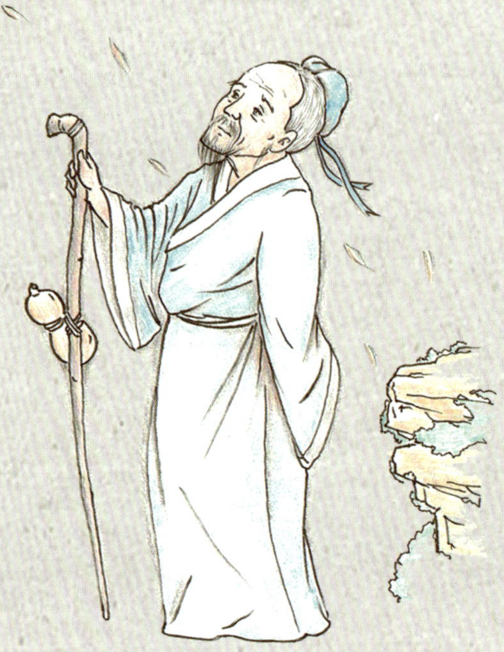

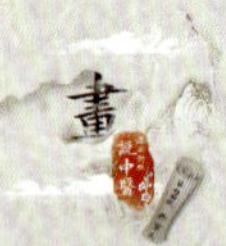

4.《神農本草經》

大約成書於漢代，託名神農所著。是我國現存最早的藥物學專著。全書 3 卷，共收載藥物 365 種。該書奠定了中藥理論體係發展的基礎。書中記述的黃連治痢、常山截瘧、麻黃治喘、海藻治癭瘤、水銀治疥瘡等，是世界藥物學上的最早記載。

4. *Shén Nóng Běn Cǎo Jīng* (*Shen Nong's Herbal Classic*)

The earliest book on medicinals still extant in China, was written in the Han Dynasty by Shen Nong, considered the father of Chinese agriculture. Its three volumes collect together 365 medicinals. The book applies the foundation for development of the theoretical system of Chinese traditional medicine; and it has the earliest records ever that *huáng lián* (Rhizoma Coptidis) cures dysentery, *cháng shān* (Radix Dichroae) cures malaria, *má huáng* (Herba Ephedrae) cures asthma, *hǎi zǎo* (Sargassum) cures goiters and tumors, and *shuǐ yín* (Hydrargyrum) cures itching.

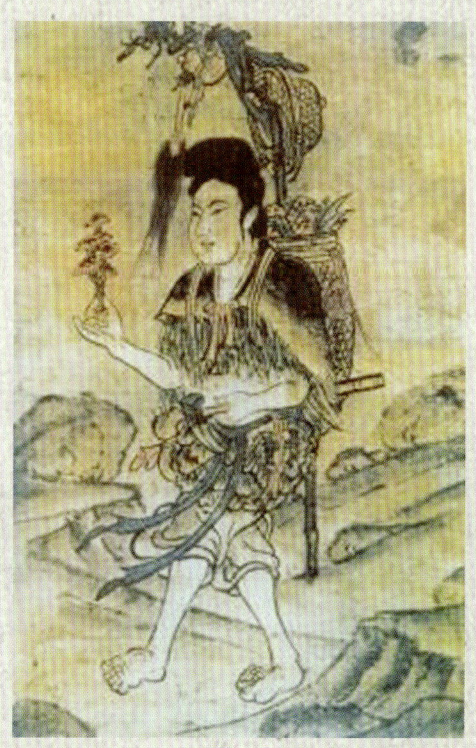

三、世界醫學之最

The Earliest of the World Medicines

中醫藥歷史源遠流長
中醫藥學家群星璀爛

1. 華佗——外科鼻祖

公元 2 世紀時華佗首先使用麻沸散進身全身麻醉，施行剖腹手術，這是世界醫學史上的最早記載。華佗在繼承古代氣功導引的基礎上，模仿五種動物的活動姿態所創製的“五禽戲”，開創了中國醫療體育的先河。

Chinese medicine can be traced back to remote antiquity. In the long course of its development, there are many shining examples of outstanding physicians and pharmacologists.

1. Hua Tuo

The ancestor of Surgery. In 2nd century A.D., he first used *Má Fèi Săn* as general anaesthesia in order to carry out abdominal surgery, which is the earliest record of such anesthesia in the world. On the basis of ancient Chinese qi gong, Hua Tuo developed the "five animal exercises" which imitate five types of different animals' movements. This was the start of Chinese medical exercises.

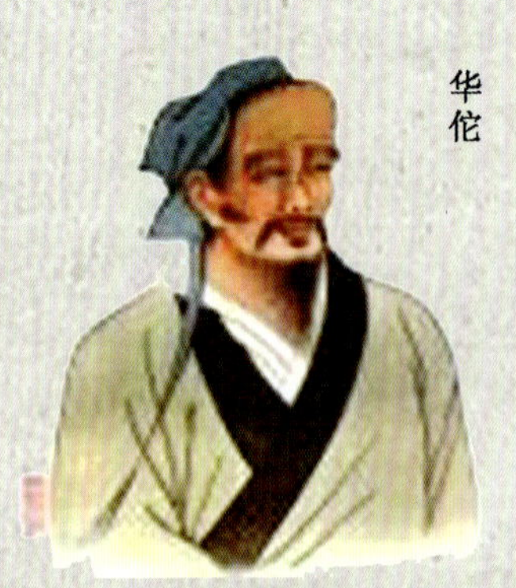

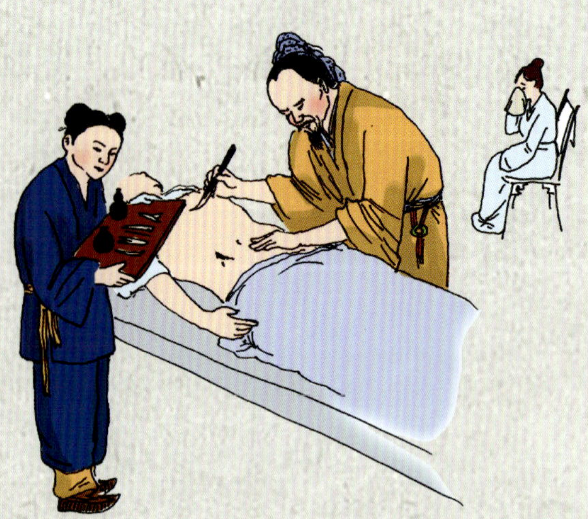

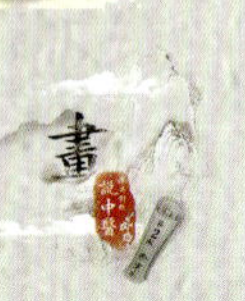

2. 葛洪

晋代人，研究煉丹術，著《抱樸子》詳記了無機物煉製金丹的過程和服用方法，應用了升華、蒸餾等製藥法，成爲現代化學的先驅。

2. Ge Hong

who is in the Jin Dynasty studied methods of pill-making, compiled the *Bào Pǔ Zǐ*, in which he wrote detailed instructions of the use of minerals to make pills and how to take them. In the book, he recorded the methods of sublimation and distillation used to make pills, which made him the pioneer of modern chemistry.

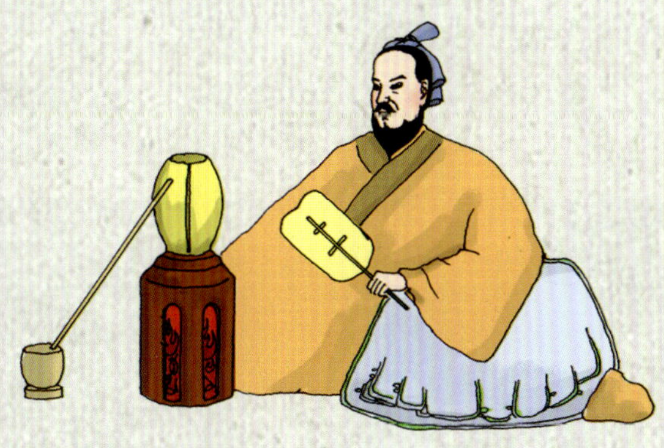

3.《新修本草》

公元 659 年，唐政府組織編寫的《新修本草》，不僅是中國歷史上由政府頒發的第一部藥典，也是世界上最早的國家藥典。

4.《洗冤録》

宋代宋慈的《洗冤録》（公元 1247 年），在法醫學方面有很高的成就，比歐洲最早的法醫學著作《法醫學專書》（意大利人菲德裏於 1602 年所著）還早 350 多年。

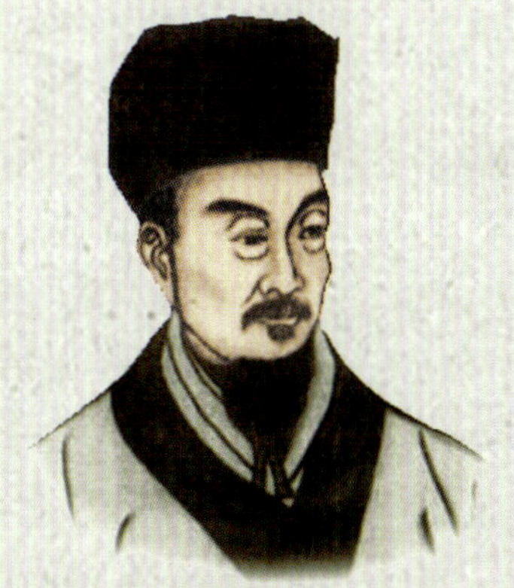

3. ***Xīn Xiū Běn Cǎo***

In 659 A.D., the Tang dynasty government instructed physicians to compile *The Newly-revised Materia Medica*. It is the first pharmacopoeia of its kind to be regulated by the government in the Chinese history, and the earliest state-promulgated pharmacopoeia in the world.

4. ***Xǐ Yuān Lù***

The *Record of Clarifying Injustice* (*Xǐ Yuān Lù*) written by Song Ci in the Song dynasty (1247 A.D.) was a great achievement in the field of legal medicine. It was written 350 years earlier than *the Book on Legal Medicine*, the earliest work of legal medicine in Europe, compiled by an Italian author.

5. 人痘接種法

大約在公元 11 世紀，中國就開始應用“人痘接種法”預防天花，成爲世界醫學免疫學的先驅，爲人工免疫預防接種的發明開創了道路。

5. The Inoculation Method of Preventing Smallpox

Around the 11th century A.D., Chinese people began to use the Inoculation Method of Preventing Smallpox, thus becoming the pioneers of immunology and the inventors of vaccination in the world.

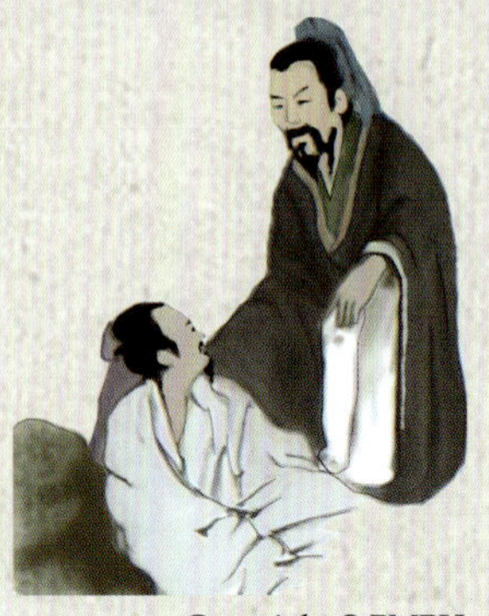

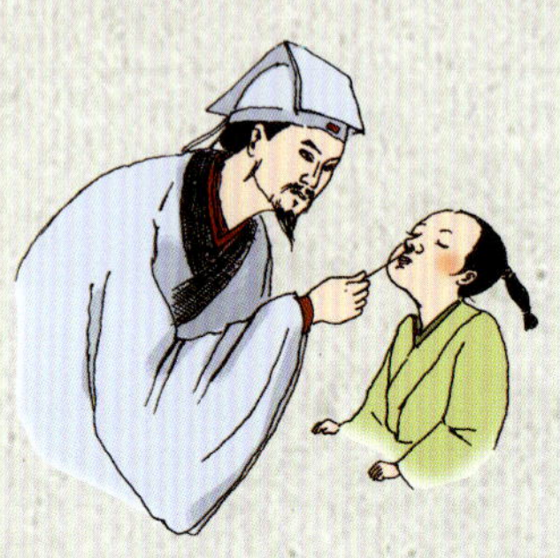

6. 李時珍

16 世紀中葉著名的醫藥學家李時珍編寫了聞名於世的《本草綱目》，該書共 52 卷，收載藥物 1 892 種，繪製藥物圖 1 109 幅，附方 11 096 首。該書豐富了中國藥物學的内容。奠定了植物學的基礎，被譽爲“東方醫藥巨著”，在國内外産生了廣泛而深遠的影響。

6. Li Shi-zhen

A famous ancient physician and pharmacologist, compiled a well-known book, *The Compendium of Materia Medica* (*Běn Cǎo Gāng Mù*). This book consists of 52 volumes with entries about 1,892 medicinal herbs, including 1,109 medicinal pictures and 11,096 prescriptions. *The Compendium of Materia Medica* is honored as the "Greatest Work in East Asian Medicine", and it has a profound effect at home and aboard.

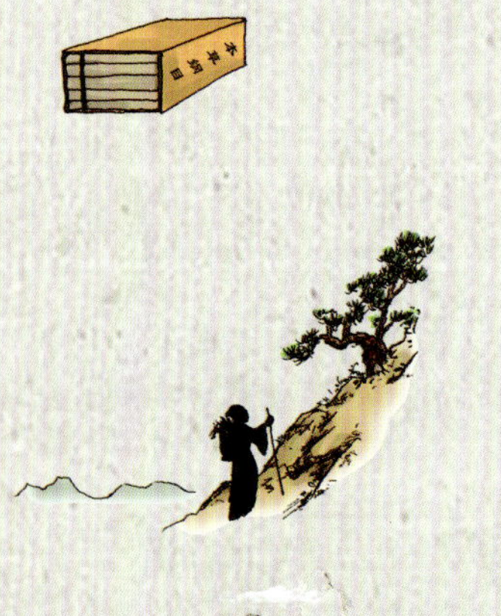

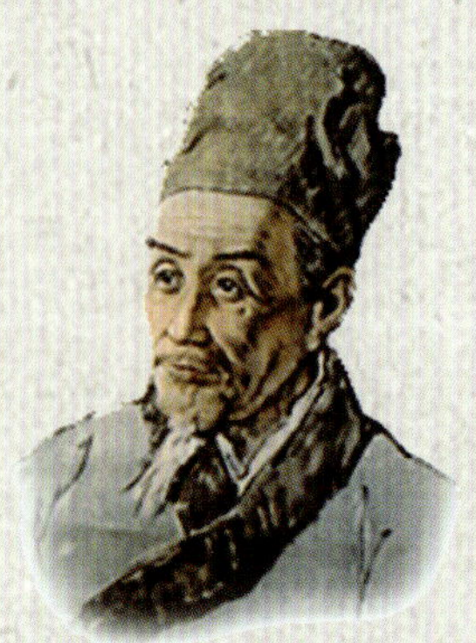

四、中醫學理論的基本特點

中醫學具有獨特的理論體係，整體觀念、恒動觀念、辨證論治是最基本的三大特點。

1. 整體觀念

（1）人體是一個有機整體

各組織器官在生理上相互聯係；在病理上相互影響，臟腑功能失常，可以通過經絡反映於相應的體表組織器官。

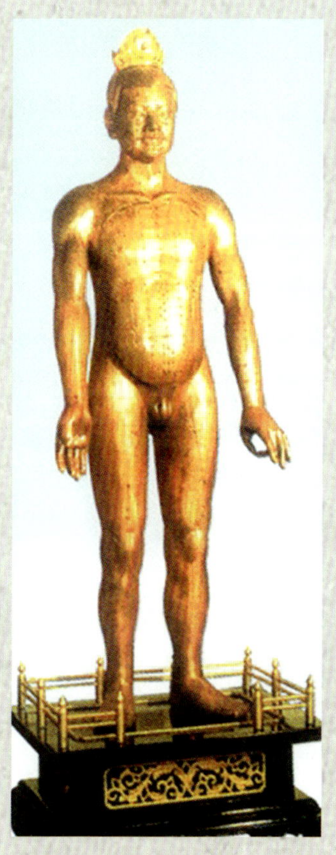

The Basic Characteristics of Chinese Medicine Theory

Chinese medicine has a unique theoretical system which is characterized by the concepts of the holistic body, constant motion, and treatment by differentiation of syndromes. These are three fundamental concepts.

1. The Holistic Concept

(1) The body is an Organic Whole.

In physiology, all of the tissues and organs are closely related with one another. In pathology, the abnormal functions of the viscera can be reflected on the surface by the tissues and organs of body.

（2）人與自然界密切相關

自然界存在着人類賴以生存的必要條件。所以自然界的變化時刻影響着人體。同時，人也時刻在能動地適應和改造自然環境。

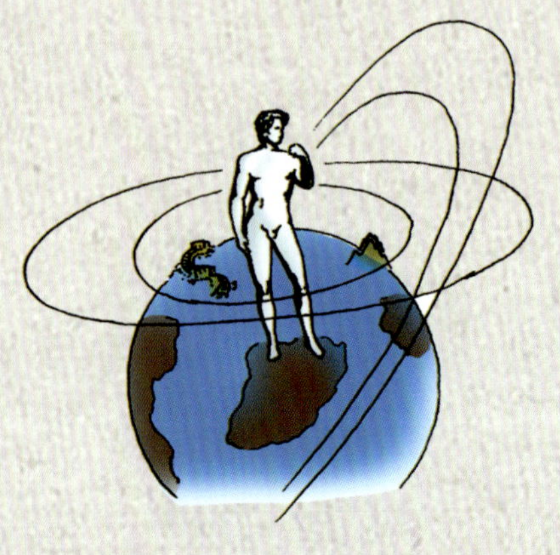

（3）人與社會的關係密切

社會因素（包括精神因素）對人體生理活動和病理變化具有顯著影響。人生活在社會中，人能影響社會，社會環境的變化對人也產生影響。如社會的安定與動亂、社會經濟與文化的發展，以及人的社會地位變動，都可引起人體身心機能的變化。

(2) Interrelationship of the Human and Natural World

Human beings have a close relationship with the natural world where exist the indispensable conditions for human life. As a result, the changes of the natural environment affect the human body. At the same time, human beings adapt well to such changes and also alter the natural environment.

(3) Close Relationship between Human Beings and Society

The social factors also largely influence the physiological activities and pathological changes of the human body. A human person lives in society, and can influence it, meanwhile the changes of the social environment can affect a person. For example, social stability or social ferment, the development of economy and culture, and changes of social status can cause changes of the human body and spirit.

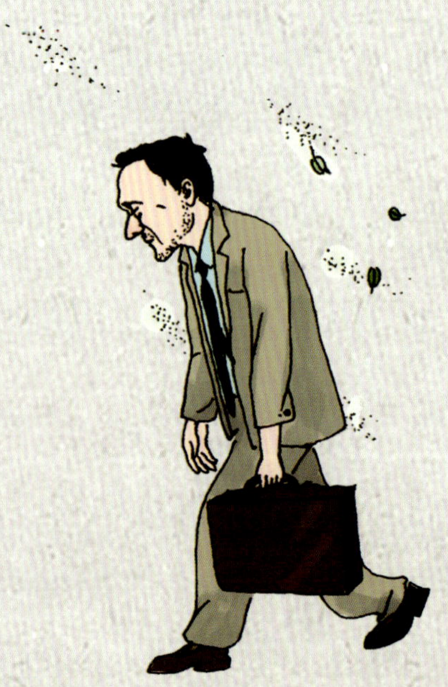

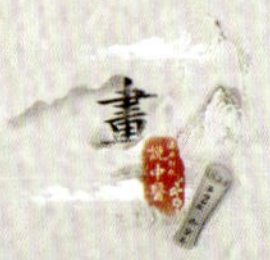

2. 恒動觀念

恒動觀念是指在分析研究生命、健康和疾病等醫學問題時，應持有運動的、變化的、發展的觀點。動而不息是自然界的根本規律，人類的生命具有恒動的特性。中醫學理論認爲人體的生理功能是一個不斷運動變化的平衡協調過程，而生理功能的主要物質基礎氣、血、津液也處於恒動變化之中。五臟六腑的生理功能，都是建立在臟腑之氣的運動變化之上。

中醫學同樣强調以恒動觀念來認識疾病過程及病理變化，在診治疾病時也以恒動觀念爲指導，不斷把握患者出現的新情況、新變化，隨時調整治法及用藥。

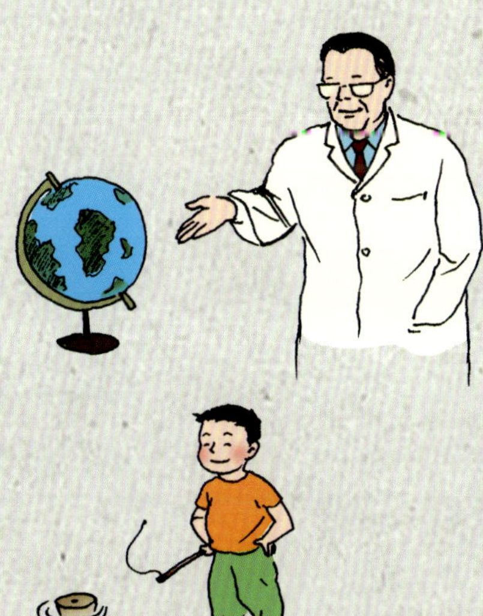

2. The Concept of Constant Motion

The concept of constant motion means that when analyzing and studying medical problems such as life, health and disease, the viewpoints of their motions, changes and development are taken under consideration. Constant motion not only is the basic law in nature, but is also the character of human life.

Chinese medicine theory sees the physiological function of human life as the product of the balance constant motion and change. Qi, blood and body fluids are the main basic materials of physiological functions, therefore they are always in a state of constant motion. The physiological functions of the five Zang-viscera and the six Fu-bowels are based on the motion and changes of the organ. Chinese medicine emphasizes the idea of constant motion in its viewpoint of the disease process and pathological changes. According to the law of constant motion, when treating and diagnosing diseases, the therapeutic methods and medicinals must be adjusted to match new conditions and changes seen in the patient.

3. 辨證論治

辨證論治是中醫學對疾病的一種特殊的研究和處理方法，是中醫學理論體係的主要特點。

病，即疾病。病是指有特定病因、發病形式、病機、發展規律和轉歸的一種完整的病理過程，如感冒、哮喘等。

癥，包括癥狀與體徵。癥是疾病的臨床表現，即病人主觀的異常感覺或某些病態變化，如發熱、咳嗽、頭痛等。而能被覺察到的客觀表現則稱爲體徵，如面黄、目赤、舌紫、脈數等。

證，即證候。證是指疾病發展過程中某一階段的病理概括。它包括疾病的病因、病位、病性和邪正關係，能反應出疾病發展過程中某一階段的病理變化的木質。

3. The Treatment by Differentiation of Syndromes

Treatment by Differentiation of Syndromes is a special method for studying and attending to diseases, and it is the main characteristic of the Chinese medical theoretical system.

Disease means an integrated pathological process which has a given etiology and pathological mechanism, rules of development and prognosis, such as cold, asthma and so forth.

Symptom means both symptoms and physical signs. Symptom refers to the clinical manifestation of disease, which is perceived by patients subjectively, like fever, cough, and headache. The symptom which can be objectively detected is called a physical sign, such as yellowish complexion, red eyes, purple tongue, rapid pulse and so on.

A syndrome, or symptom complex, refers to the pathological generalization of a group of closely related symptoms at a given stage in the course of disease development. It can demonstrate the etiology, location, nature of disease and the relationship between the right and the evil qi. It can reflect the nature of the pathological changes at a certain time of the disease's development.

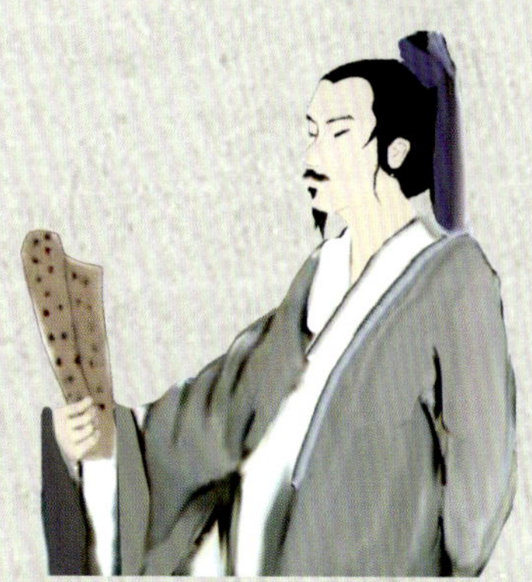

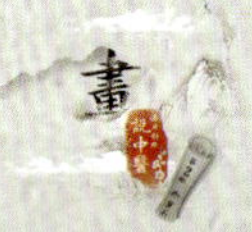

辨證，即辨別證候。

論治，即治療疾病。

辨證是確定治療方法的前提和依據，論治是辨證的目的，通過論治的效果，可以檢驗辨證是否正確。

個體化診療是辨證論治的特點，包括“同病異治”、“異病同治”，這種針對疾病發展過程中不同質的矛盾採用不同方法去解決的法則，這是辨證論治的精髓。

同病異治，同一種疾病，由於發病的時間、地域以及患者機體的反應性不同，或處於不同的發展階段，所以表現的證候不同，因而治法也不一樣。

Syndrome differentiation is to distinguish syndromes from one another, and treatment is curing the diseases.

Syndrome differentiation is both the prerequisite and basis of treatment, while treatment is the goal of syndrome differentiation. Treatment is the proof whether the syndrome differentiation was correct.

Individualization of diagnosis and treatment is a characteristic of the treatment by differentiation of syndromes. This includes both the approaches of different treatments for the same disease and that of different diseases treated by the same therapeutic principle. To treat on the basis of syndrome differentiation is to adopt different problem-solving methods in response to different qualities in the course of disease development.

Different treatments for the same disease: when treating the same disease, because the patient's constitution, climate, season, geographical location and the phase of disease are different, they manifest with different syndromes, therefore different therapeutic methods are used.

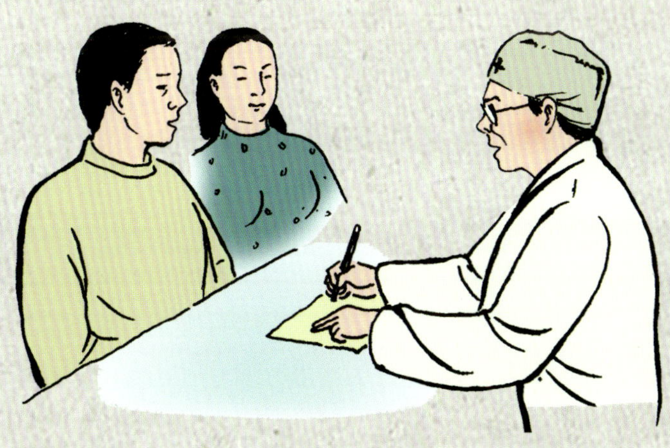

異病同治。不同的疾病，在其發展過程中，出現相同的證候，因而採取同一方法治療。

Different diseases could be treated with the same therapeutic principle. Different diseases may exhibit syndromes with the same characteristics, so one adopts the same therapeutic principle.

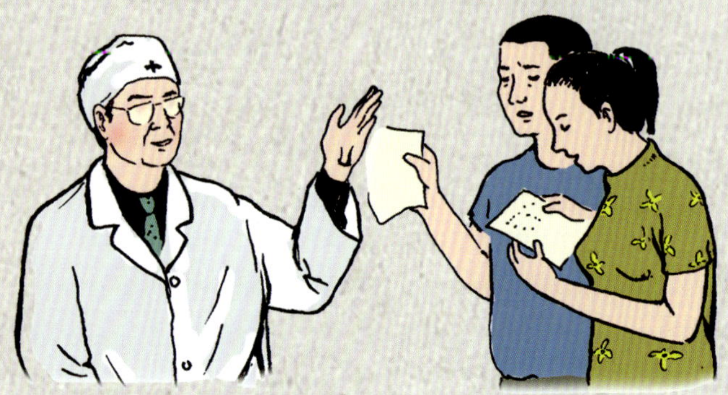

第一章 陰陽五行

Chapter 1 The Theories of Yin & Yang and of the Five Phases

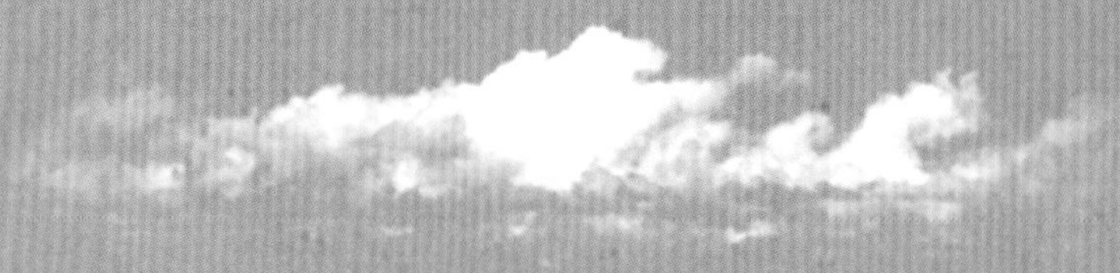

一、陰陽學說

陰陽學說，是研究陰陽的內涵及其運動變化規律，並用以闡述宇宙萬事萬物的發生、發展和變化的一種古代哲學理論。

1. 陰陽的概念和特徵

陰陽是中國古代哲學的一對範疇。最初的含義是指日光的向背，即向日爲陽，背日爲陰。向陽的地方光明、溫暖；背陽的地方黑暗、寒冷，於是古人就以光明與黑暗，溫暖與寒冷分陰陽。

對立
- 互相鬥爭
- 互相製約
- 互相消長

統一
- 交合感應
- 互根互用
- 互相包涵
- 互相轉化

陰陽關係

The Theory of Yin and Yang

1. The Concept and Characteristics of Yin and Yang

Yin and yang is an ancient philosophical theory which explains the laws of motion and change. It can expound the occurrence, development and changes of everything in the universe.

Yin and yang were originally part of Chinese ancient philosophy. Their original meaning was whether a place faces the sun or not. The place exposed to the sun is yang, indicating warmth and brightness, and its opposite side is yin, indicating cold and darkness. Therefore, cold and warmth, darkness and brightness were used to distinguish yin from yang.

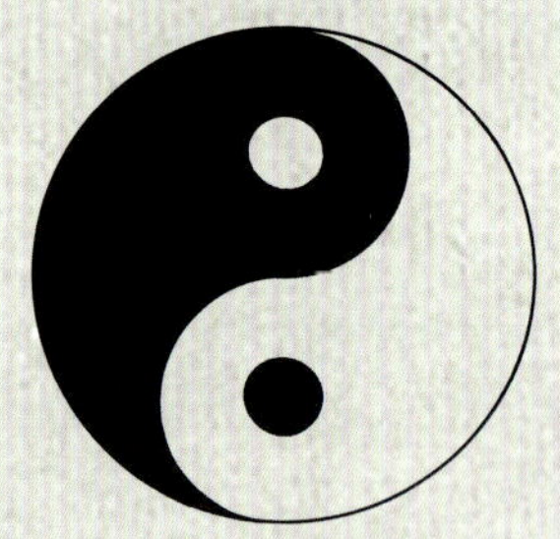

陰陽太極圖

Picture of Yin and Yang (Tai Ji)

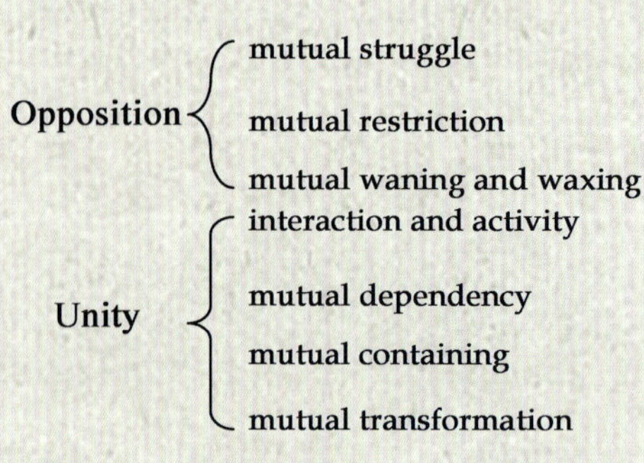

The relationship between yin and yang

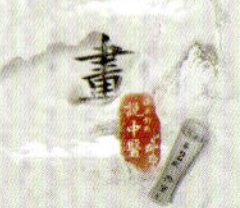

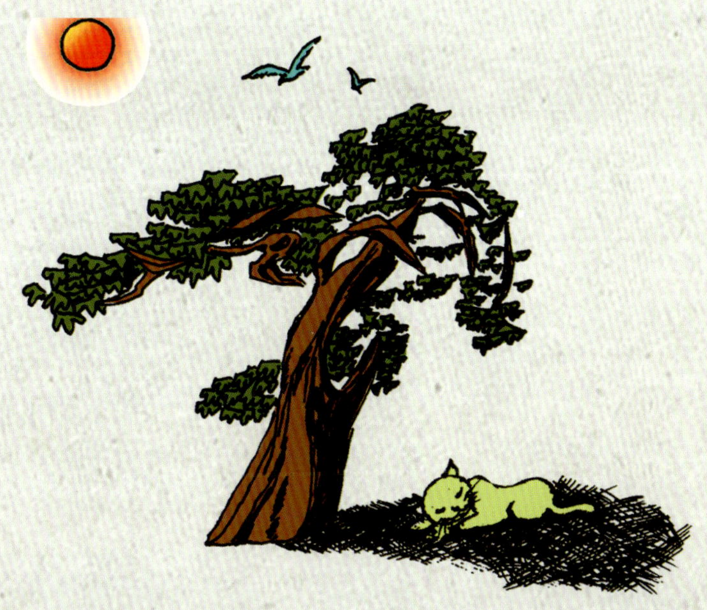

事物的陰陽屬性

陰陽代表相互對立又相互關聯的事物屬性。如水火二者，水爲陰，火爲陽；男女兩性，男爲陽，女爲陰。一般説來，凡是運動的、上升的、外向的、溫熱的、明亮的，都屬於陽；静止的、下降的、内守的、寒冷的、晦暗的都屬於陰。

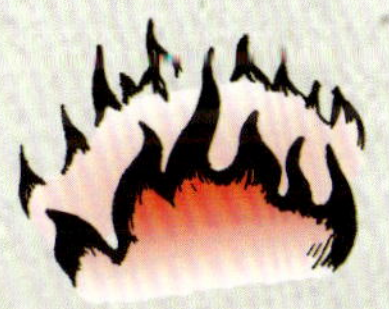

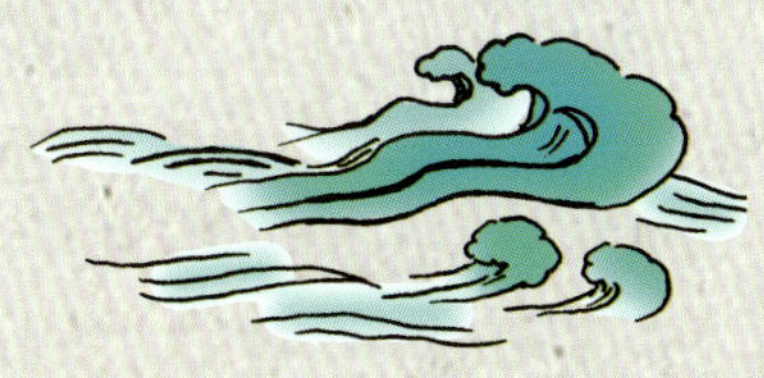

Yin and Yang Property of Things

Yin and yang represents the property of two opposite aspects which are interrelated. For example, water pertains to yin, whereas fire to Yang; male to yang while female to yin. Generally speaking, things or phenomena which are dynamic, rising, active, warm hot, and bright, etc., pertain to the category of yang, while those being static, descending, negative, cold, dim, etc., pertain to that of yin.

陰陽的相對屬性引入醫學領域，則將對於人體具有推動、溫煦、興奮作用的物質和功能統屬於陽；對於人體具有凝聚、滋潤、抑製等作用的物質和功能，統屬於陰。

Relativity of yin-yang property was then used in medical field. As for the human body, matters and functions which are active, warm, exciting pertain to the category of yang while those being agglomerate, moisturizing, depressive belong to the category of yin.

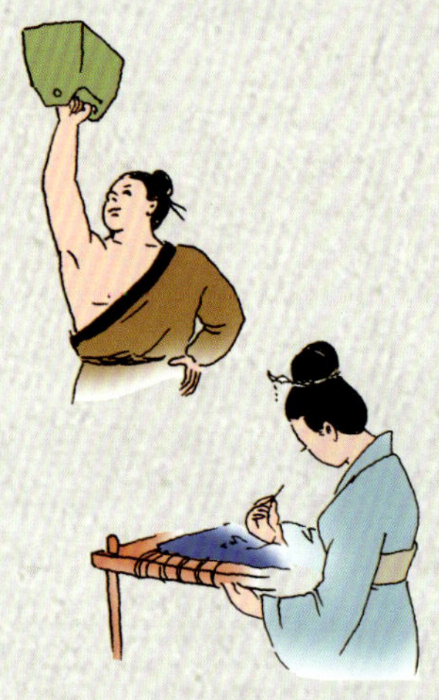

表 1-1 事物和現象的陰陽屬性歸類表

	空間	時間	溫度	濕度	季節	重量	亮度	事物運動	
陽	上、外	白天	溫熱	幹燥	春夏	輕	光亮	上升	動
陰	下、內	黑夜	寒涼	濕潤	秋冬	重	晦暗	下降	靜

Table 1-1 The Classification of Things and Phenomena According to the Property of Yin and Yang

	Direction	Time	Temperature	Humidity	Season
Yang	up and outside	day	warm and hot	dry	spring and summer
Yin	down and inside	night	cool and cold	moist	autumn and winter
	Weight	**Brightness**	**Type of Movement**		
Yang	light	bright	ascending motion		active
Yin	heavy	dark	descending motion		passive

2. 陰陽學説的基本内容

陰陽學説的基本内容，包括對立製約、互根互用、交感互藏、消長平衡，相互轉化五個方面。

2. The Basic Theory of Yin and Yang

The theory of yin and yang encompasses their five aspects, opposition and restriction, mutual dependency, mutual interaction and mutual storage, waning, waxing and their balance, and mutual transformation.

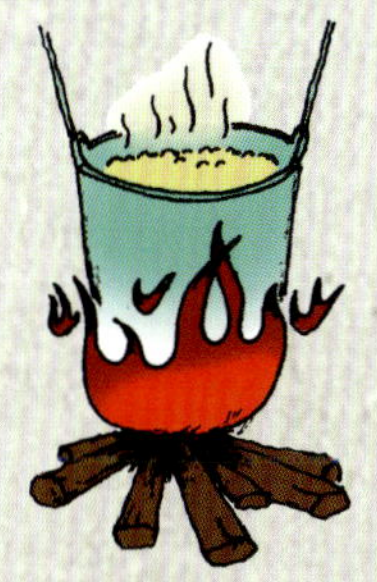

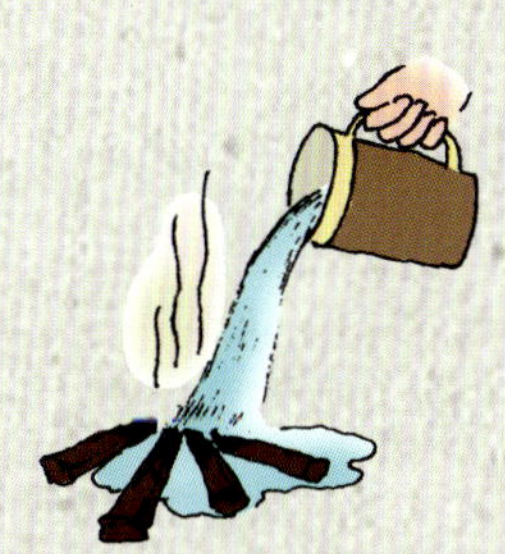

（1）對立製約

陰陽的對立製約，表現於它們之間的相互製約、相互對抗、相互鬥爭，如水能製火，火能克水。陰陽的對立製約，推動着自然界一切事物的發展變化，也貫穿人體生命過程的始終。

（2）互根互用

陰依存於陽，陽依存於陰，雙方均以對方存在爲自己存在的前提。孤陰不生；孤陽不長；陰陽可分不可離。

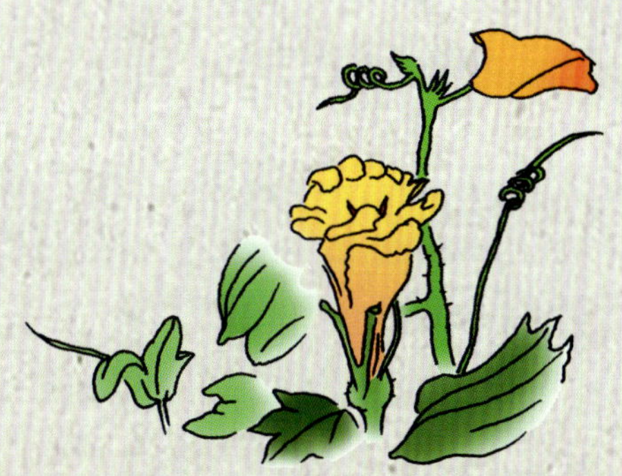

(1) Opposition and Restriction between Yin and Yang

The opposition between yin and yang mainly manifests in their mutual restriction and struggle. For example, water restricts fire, and fire restricts water.

The opposition between yin and yang is visible throughout all of human life, promoting the development and change of everything in the universe.

(2) Mutual Dependency between Yin and Yang

Yin and yang depend on each other, and each needs the other to exist. Without yin, there is no yang, and without yang there is no yin. The two cannot be separated.

（3）陰陽交感

是指陰陽二氣在運動中相互感應並交合的過程。陰陽的相互交感，使對立着的兩種事物或力量，統於一體，於是產生了自然界，產生了萬物，產生了人類。

陰陽互藏，是指相互對立的陰陽雙方的任何一方都包含着另一方，即陰中有陽，陽中有陰。

(3) Mutual Interaction between Yin and Yang

Mutual interaction is a continuing process which is that of the yin qi and yang qi meeting and connecting with each other. The mutual interaction between yin and yang makes two opposite objects or forces into one. As a result of this union, the universe with all its living things and human beings come into being.

Mutual containment between yin and yang refers to any opposite aspects of yin and yang contains the other. For example, yin contains yang and yang contains yin.

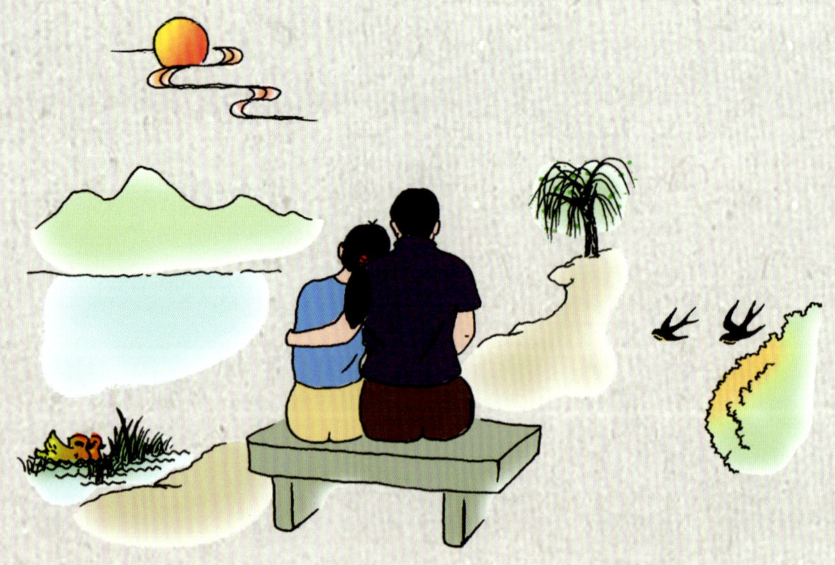

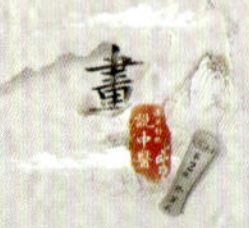

（4）消長平衡

陰陽在不斷消長運動中維持着相對的動態平衡。

運動是絶對的，静止是相對的，消長是絶對的，平衡是相對的。陰陽在絶對的消長之中維護着相對的平衡，在相對的平衡中又存在着絶對的消長。

陰陽消長是陰陽運動的“量變”過程。

(4) Waning and Waxing between Yin and Yang, always in Balance

Yin and yang maintain a dynamic balance relative to each other during the process of waning and waxing.

Because their movements are absolute and constant, whereas their motionlessness is only relative; the movement of waning and waxing is absolute, and that of motionlessness is relative. So, yin and yang maintain a relative balance and relative motionlessness relies on absolute waning and waxing.

The process of the waning and waxing of yin and yang means their relative quantities are changing.

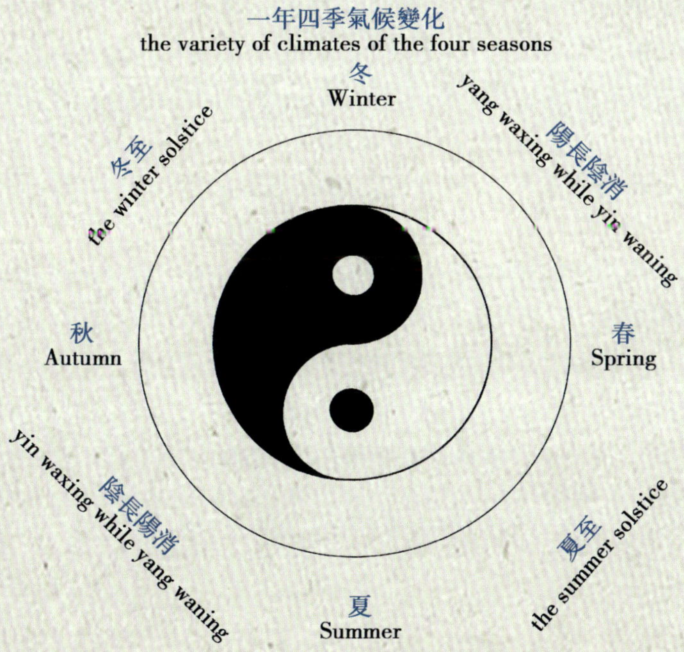

一年四季氣候變化
the variety of climates of the four seasons

冬
Winter

陽長陰消
yang waxing while yin waning

春
Spring

夏至
the summer solstice

夏
Summer

陰長陽消
yin waxing while yang waning

秋
Autumn

冬至
the winter solstice

（5）相互轉化

陰陽雙方在一定條件下，可以各自向其相反的方向轉化。陰可以轉化爲陽，陽也可以轉化爲陰。陰陽轉化，一般都發生在事物的“物極”階段，即“物極必反”。

陰陽相互轉化，必須具備一定的條件。“重陰必陽，重陽必陰”，“寒極生熱，熱極生寒”，陰發展到“重”的階段，就會轉化爲陽，陽發展到“重”的階段就會轉化爲陰（《靈樞》）。寒發展到“極”的階段，就要向熱的方向轉化，熱發展到“極”的階段，也要向寒的方面轉化（《内經》）。

陰陽轉化是“質變”的過程，是在陰陽消長“量變”基礎上的質變。

(5) Mutual Transformation between Yin and Yang

Under certain conditions, yin and yang transform into their opposite aspects. Yin transforms into yang, and yang transforms into yin. When the quantity of yin or yang reaches its peak, it will transforms into its opposite.

Yin and yang transform themselves into each other as they reach the stage of abundance. For example, the *Divine Pivot <Líng Shū>* says: "extreme yin will turn into yang and the extreme yang will turn into yin", and *the Yellow Emperor's Inner Classic <Huáng Dì Nèi Jīng>* says: "The extreme cold gives rise to heat, and extreme heat gives rise to cold".

Mutual transformation between yin and yang is the qualitative change based on the quantitative changes of the waning and waxing of yin and yang.

春
注意：春節過後有寒潮。
Attention please, a cold wave is coming after the Spring Festival.

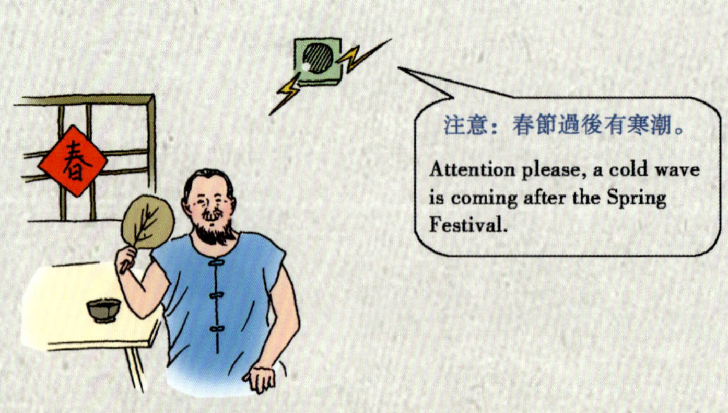

3. 陰陽學説在中醫學中的應用

（1）説明人體的組織結構

人體是一個有機整體，人體内部充滿着陰陽對立統一的現象。人的一切組織結構，即有機聯係，又可以劃分爲相互對立的陰陽兩部分。

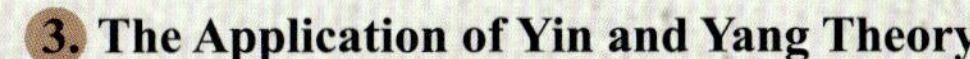

3. The Application of Yin and Yang Theory

(1) Explaining Human Body Tissues and Structure

The human body is regarded as a holistic organism of unity and opposites. The body's structure can be divided into two respective opposites of yin and yang, which are closely related to each other and interact.

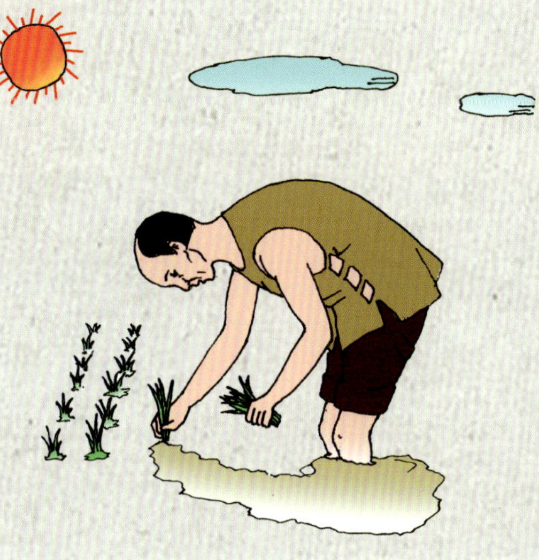

表 1-2　人體組織結構的陰陽屬性歸納表

	人體部位	臟腑組織
陽	上部、體外、背、四肢外側	六腑、絡脈、氣、皮毛
陰	下部、體内、腹、四肢内側	五臟、經脈、血、筋骨

Table 1-2　The Classification of the Tissues and Structures of the Human Body According to the Yin and Yang Properties

	Location	Viscera and Tissues of the Human Body
Yang	upper regions, exterior, back, the outside of limbs	six Fu-bowels, collaterals, qi, skin and hair
Yin	lower regions, interior, abdomen, the inner side of limbs	five Zang-viscera, meridians, blood, tendons and bones

（2）説明人體的生理功能

人的正常生命活動，是陰陽雙方在對立互根基礎上，相互製約，相互促進，從而“陰平陽秘”協調平衡的結果。若人體内陰氣、陽氣不能相互爲用而分離，人的生命活動也就終止了。

(2) Explaining Physiological Function of the Human Body

The human body's normal life activities are based on the two opposite aspects of yin and yang which depend, restrict and support each other. Yin is calm when yang is quiet, hence balance is achieved. If yin qi and yang qi cannot support each other and they separate, life comes to an end.

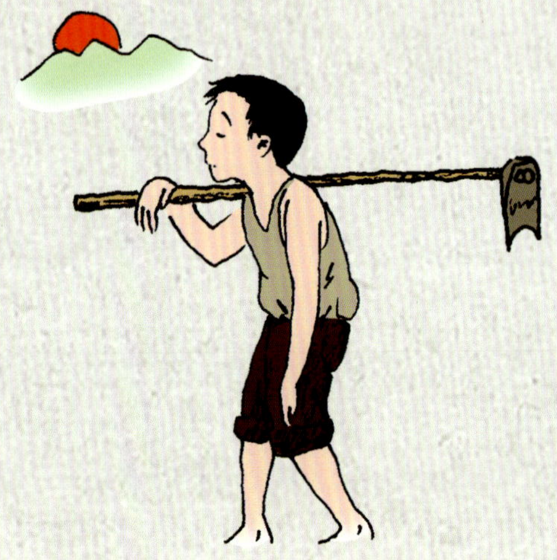

表 1-3　人體生理功能的陰陽屬性歸納表

	生理活動	氣機運動
陽	興奮、亢進、煦、功能活動	升出
陰	抑製、衰退、滋潤、營養物質	降入

Table 1-3　The Classification of the Physiological Function of the Human Body According to the Property of Yin and Yang

	Physiological Movement	Qi Movements and Their Patterns
Yang	lively, warming and active functions	ascending, exiting
Yin	restrained, declining, moistening and nourishing matters	descending, entering

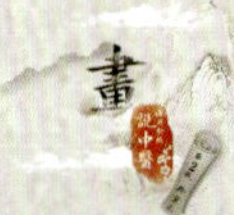

（3）説明人體的病理變化

中醫學常以陰陽學説來説明人體的病理變化。人體的正常生命活動是陰陽保持着對立統一協調的結果。疾病的發生及病理過程，是因某種原因使陰陽失去動態平衡。因此，陰陽失調是疾病發生的基礎。無論疾病的病理變化如何複雜，都不外乎陰陽的偏勝和偏衰。

(3) Explaining Pathological Changes of Human Body

Chinese medicine's yin-yang theory explains the pathological changes of the human body. The human body's normal activities result from maintaining coordination and unity between yin and yang opposites. Pathology and diseases arise when yin and yang lose this balance. So, imbalance between yin and yang is the basis of disease. No matter how complex the pathological changes are, they are no more than the result of the relative predominance or weakness of yin and yang.

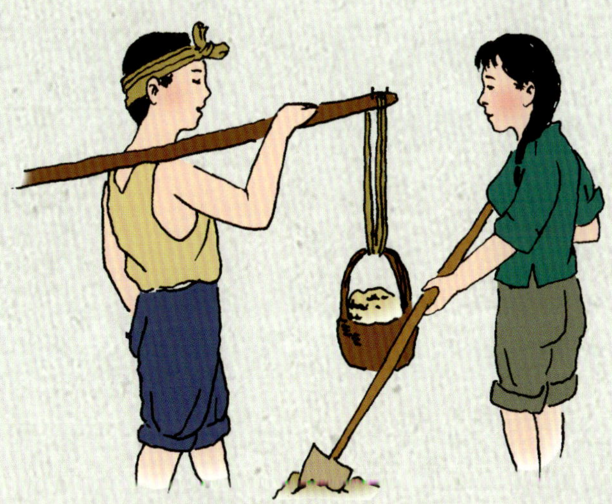

（4）用於疾病診斷

疾病的癥狀與體徵千變萬化，錯綜複雜，但都可用陰陽來加以概括。在臨床診斷中將望聞問切四診收集的各種資料，按照陰陽特徵來辨别疾病癥狀和體徵的

(4) Application to Clinical Diagnosis

Yin and yang are used to classify complex and constantly changing signs and symptoms. In clinic, the four diagnostic methods of observing, listening and smelling, questioning, and palpating are used to collect information about illness. Differentiating syndromes is to distinguish the yin and yang prop-

陰陽屬性，爲辨證提供依據。如色澤鮮明者屬陽，晦暗者屬陰。聲音高亢洪亮者屬陽，低微斷續者屬陰。脈象浮、大、滑、數屬陽，沉、小、澀、遲屬陰等。在臨床辨證中，可用陰陽來概括分析錯綜複雜的證候，將其分爲陰陽二大類，從而抓住了疾病的本質，做到執簡馭繁。

erties of signs and symptoms. For example, a bright and shining complexion indicates yang, while a dark and gloomy complexion indicates yin. A loud and clear voice is yang, while a low voice is yin. Floating, big, slippery, and rapid pulses pertain to yang; deep, small, rough and slow pulses pertain to yin. In clinical syndrome differentiation, even very complex syndromes are analyzed and summarized into only two categories, that is, into yin and yang syndromes. Once the nature of the disease is understood, solving a complex problem is easy.

表 1-4　癥狀、體徵的陰陽屬性歸納表

	望診		聞診		脈診		
	顏色	光澤	語音	呼吸	部位	至數	形勢
陽	赤黃	鮮明	高亢洪亮	聲高氣粗	寸部	數	浮大洪滑
陰	青白黑	晦暗	低微無力	聲低氣怯	尺部	遲	沉小細澀

Table 1-4　The Classification of Symptoms and Physical Signs According to Yin and Yang Property

	Observation		Smelling and Listening		Pulse Feeling		
	color	brightness	voice	respiration	location	rate	type
Yang	red and yellow	bright	loud and strong	loud voice and husky breath	cun	rapid	floating, large slippery, surging
Yin	green, black and white	darkish	low and weak	low voice and weak breath	chi	slow	deep, small thread, rough

表 1-5 病癥的陰陽屬性歸納表

	表裏	寒熱	虛實
陽證	表證	熱證	實證
陰證	裏證	寒證	虛證

Table 1-5 The classification of the Syndrome of Diseases According to Yin and Yang Properties

	Exterior and Interior	Cold and Heat	Deficiency and Excess
Yang Syndrome	exterior syndrome	heat syndrome	excess syndrome
Yin Syndrome	interior syndrome	cold syndrome	deficiency syndrome

（5）用於指導疾病的防治

疾病的發生機理是陰陽失調。因此，調整陰陽，補偏救弊，恢復陰陽的相對平衡，即是治療的基本原則。

(5) Using the Theory of Yin & Yang to Guide the Prevention and Treatment of Diseases

Because diseases emerge from imbalance of yin and yang, the basic therapeutic principle in Chinese medicine is to regulate and restore this balance.

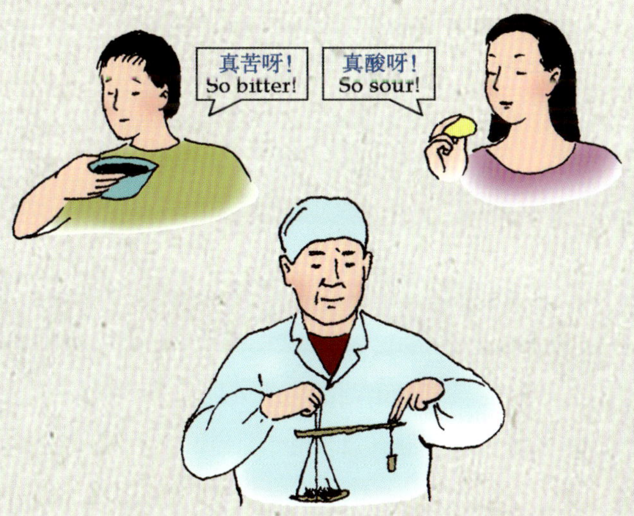

表 1-6　藥物性能的陰陽屬性

	四氣	五味	升降浮沉
陽	溫熱	辛甘（淡）	升浮
陰	涼寒	酸苦鹹	降沉

Table 1-6　The Classification of Herbs Nature according to Yin and Yang Properties

	Four Natures	Five Flavors	Directions and Actions
Yang	warm and hot	acrid, sweet, weak	ascending, floating
Yin	cool and cold	sour, bitter, salty	descending, sinking

臨床用藥，就是要依據藥物性能的陰陽屬性，針對病證的陰陽盛衰情況，選擇相應的藥物，以糾正陰陽的失調狀態。中藥的四氣指寒、熱、溫、涼。寒涼屬陰，溫熱屬陽。寒涼藥物能清熱瀉火，如石膏、黃連；溫熱藥物能散寒溫補，如附子、肉桂。中藥的五味指辛、甘、酸、苦、鹹，其中酸、苦、鹹屬陰，辛、甘屬陽。

Clinical herb application is based on the yin and yang properties of herbs; depending on the predominance or weakness of yin and yang, the appropriate herbs can repair this imbalance. The four natures of herbs are divided as hot and warm which pertain to yang; and cold and cool which pertain to yin. Cold and cool herbs like *shí gāo* (gypsum fibrosum) and *huáng lián* (Coptidis Rhizoma) can clear heat and drain fire while warm and hot herbs like *fù zǐ* (Radix Aconiti Lateralis Praeparata) and *ròu guì* (Cortex Cinnamomi) can scatter coldness, warm and tonify. The five flavors are sour, bitter and salty which pertain to yin and acrid and sweet which pertain to yang.

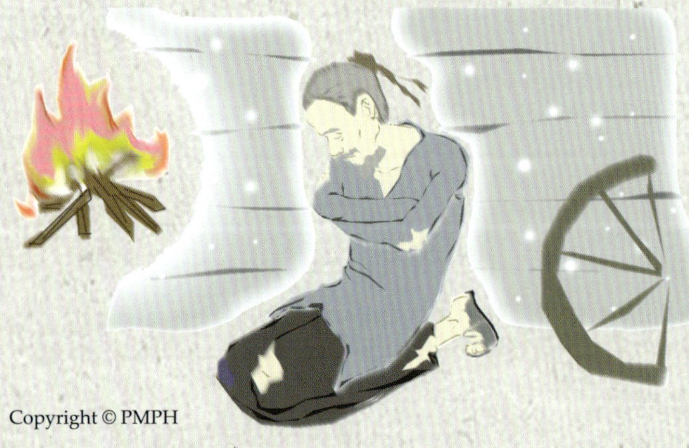

二、五行學説

五行學説是以木、火、土、金、水五種物質的特性及其“相生”和“相克”規律來認識世界，解釋世界和探索宇宙規律的一種世界觀和方法論。

1. 五行的概念、特性及分類

（1）五行的概念

五行是指金、木、水、火、土五種物質及其運動變化。五行學説認爲宇宙世界是由這五種基本物質所構成。古人把五行學説應用於醫學領域，用來説明人體的生理、病理以及人體與外在環境的相互關係，指導着臨床診斷和防治。

The Theory of Five Phases

The five phases: Wood, Fire, Earth, Metal and Water are categories of quality and relationship. They are in a continuing cycle of supporting and restraining each other and they correspond with the laws of the universe.

1. Five Phases: Concept, Characteristics and Classification

(1) The Concept of the Five Phases

The five phases of wood, fire, earth, metal and water are elements of motion and change. Five phases theory holds that the universe is built from five basic substances. The ancient Chinese people used the five phases theory in the medical field to explain the physiology and pathology of the human body. The correlation between the human body and the external environment can guide both the clinical diagnosis and the prevention and treatment of diseases.

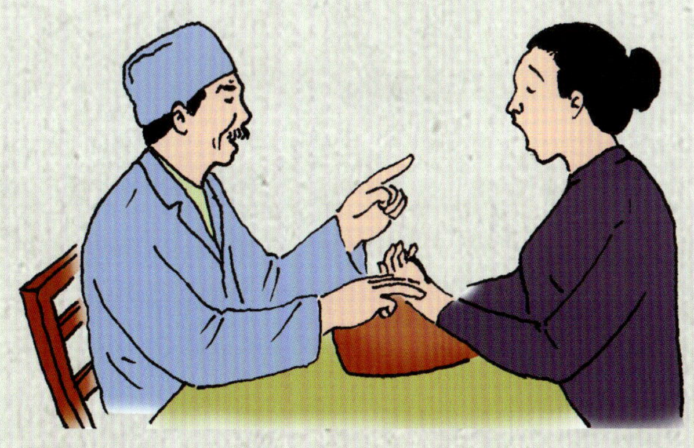

（2）五行的特性

古人通過長期觀察，逐漸形成了五行特性的基本概念。五行各有特性。木具有生長、升發、條達舒暢的特性；火具有溫熱、上升的特性；土具有載物、生化的特性；金具有從革、肅殺的特性；水具有滋潤、向下的特性。

(2) The Features of the Five Phases

After long observation, the ancient Chinese people gradually formed the basic concept of the five phases. Every phase has its respective characteristic, for example, wood represents growth, flourishing, flexibility and extension; fire has the features of heat and flaming upwards; earth represents cultivation; metal has the features of changing, astringency and restraining and water has the features of moisturizing and descending.

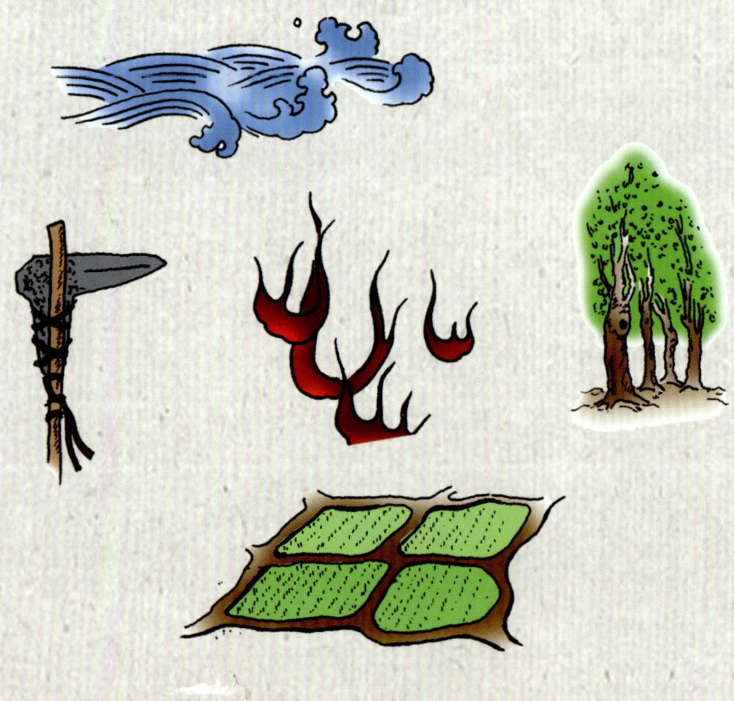

（3）事物屬性的五行歸類

古人運用取象比類法和推演絡繹法將自然界各種事物和現象，以及人體的臟腑組織生理病理現象分別歸屬於木、火、土、金、水五行之中。五行學說以天人相應爲指導思想，以五行爲中心，以空間結構的五方、時間結構的五季、人體結構的五臟爲基本間架，將人體的生命現象與自然界的事物和現象聯係起來，形成了聯係人體内外環境的五行結構係統，用以説明人體以及人與自然環境的統一性。

(3) Attribution of Things according to the Five Phases

The ancient Chinese people classified all the phenomena in nature as well as the viscera, bowels, tissues, physiology and pathology of the human body into the five phases, wood, fire, earth, metal and water, according to the idea of attributing things to similar phenomena. The theory of five phases takes as its guiding principle the concept that human beings and nature correspond to each other. The five phases is its center, its basic structure is the five directions, five seasons and the five Zang viscera of the human body. The theory of five phases combines phenomena of the human body with things in nature; the system of five phases combines the internal and external surroundings of the human body to explain the human body and its unity with the natural environment.

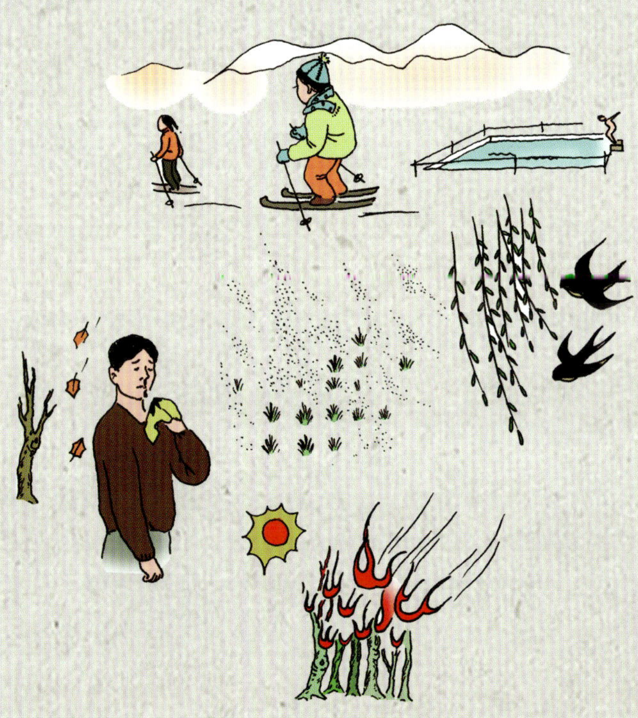

表 1-7　事物屬性的五行歸類

自然界							五行	人體						
五音	五味	五色	五化	五氣	五方	五季		五臟	五腑	五官	五體	五誌	五液	五脈
角	酸	青	生	風	東	春	木	肝	膽	目	筋	怒	淚	弦
徵	苦	赤	長	暑	南	夏	火	心	小腸	舌	脈	喜	汗	洪
宮	甘	黃	化	濕	中	長夏	土	脾	胃	口	肉	思	涎	緩
商	辛	白	收	燥	西	秋	金	肺	大腸	鼻	皮	悲	涕	浮
羽	鹹	黑	藏	寒	北	冬	水	腎	膀胱	耳	骨	恐	唾	沉

Table 1-7　The Property Attribution of the Five Phases

Nature	**Five sounds**	jiǎo	zhǐ	gōng	shāng	yǔ
	Five flavors	sour	bitter	sweet	pungent	salty
	Five colors	green	red	yellow	white	black
	Five transformation	germination	growth	transformation	reaping	storing
	Five climatic agents	wind	summer-heat	dampness	dryness	cold
	Five orientations	east	south	middle	west	north
	Five annual divisions	spring	summer	late-summer	autumn	winter
The five phases		wood	fire	earth	metal	water
The human body	**Five Zang viscera**	liver	heart	spleen	lung	kidney
	Five Fu viscera	gall bladder	small intestine	stomach	large intestine	urinary bladder
	Five sense organs	eye	tongue	mouth	nose	ear
	Five body materials	tendon	vessel	muscle	skin	bone
	Five emotions	anger	joy	pensiveness	grief	fear
	Five fluids	tears	sweat	mucus	nasal discharge	sputum
	Five pulse	wiry	surging	moderate	floating	deep

2. 五行學説的基本內容

五行學説的基本內容包括相生、相克、相乘、相侮四個方面。

（1）相生

是指一行對另一行具有資生、促進和助長的作用。如木可以燃燒，所以説木生火；木燃燒産生灰，所以説火生土；沙土中可淘出金，所以説土生金；金遇高溫會熔化成水，所以説金生水；樹木要水澆灌，所以説水生木。

2. The Basic Content of the Theory of Five Phases

The basic content of the theory of five phases includes the concepts of generation, restriction, over-restriction and reverse restriction.

(1) Generation

refers to the functions of production, promotion and assistance between one phase and another. For example, wood can burn, so wood generates fire. Burned wood turns to ash, therefore fire generates earth. Metal can be found in soil, so earth generates metal. Metal melts with high temperature, so fire generates water. Wood needs watering, so water generates wood.

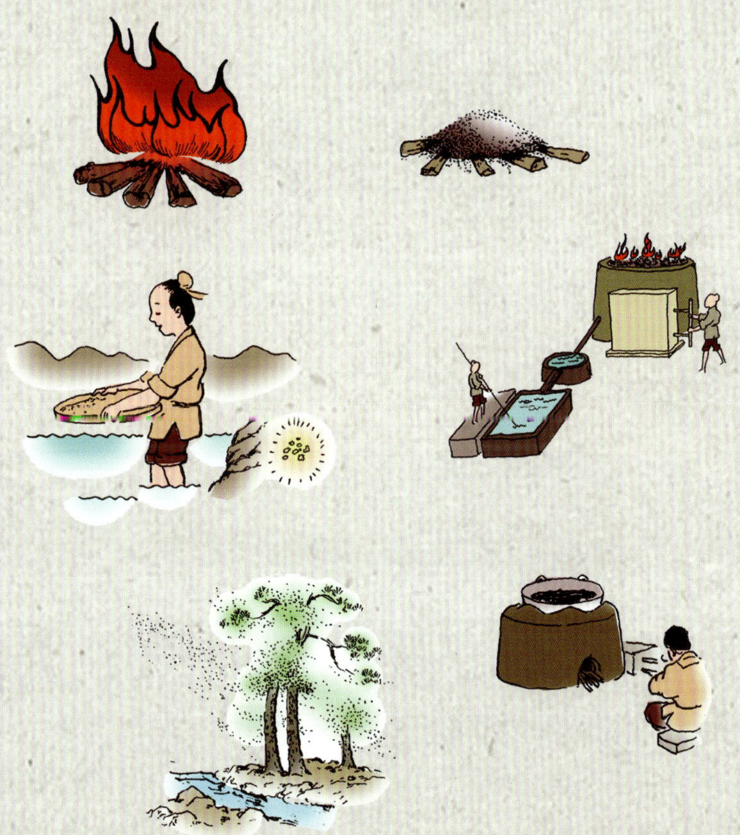

（2）相克

是指一行對另一行具有抑製、製約、克服的作用。木破土而出，所以說木克土；水可以使火熄滅，所以說水克火；金屬刃器可以砍伐樹木，所以說金克木；火能使金屬熔化，所以說火克金；泥土能擋水，所以說土克水。

(2) Restriction

refers to the functions of controlling and inhibition between one phase and another. Wood grows from soil, so wood restricts earth. Water puts out fire, so water restricts fire. Metal tools cut down trees so metal restricts wood. Metal can be melted by fire, therefore fire restricts metal. Soil blocks water, so earth restricts water.

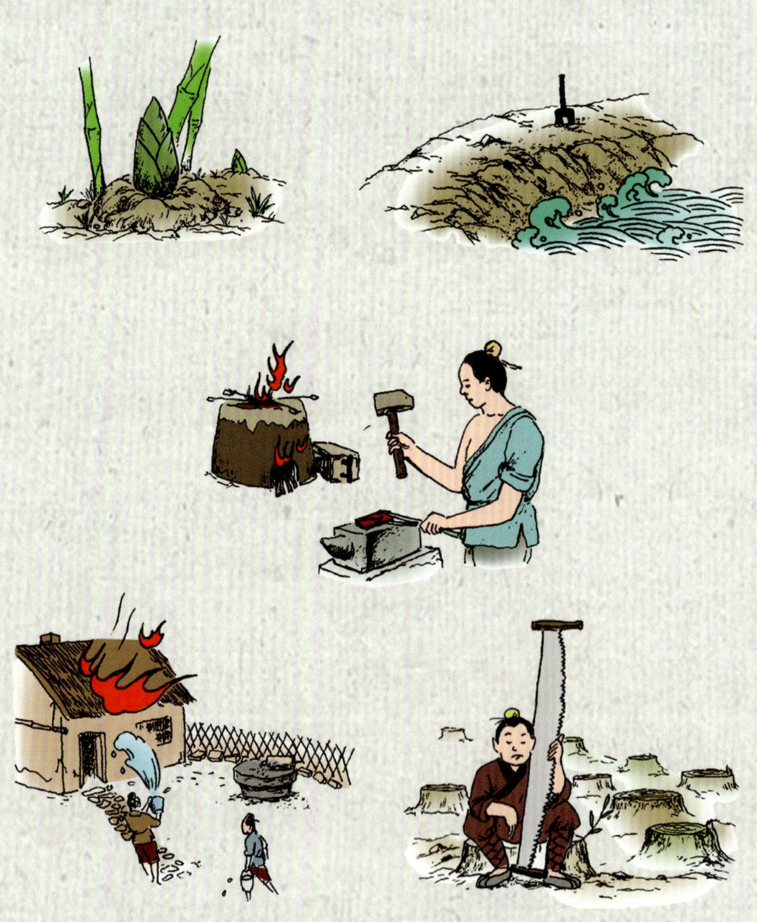

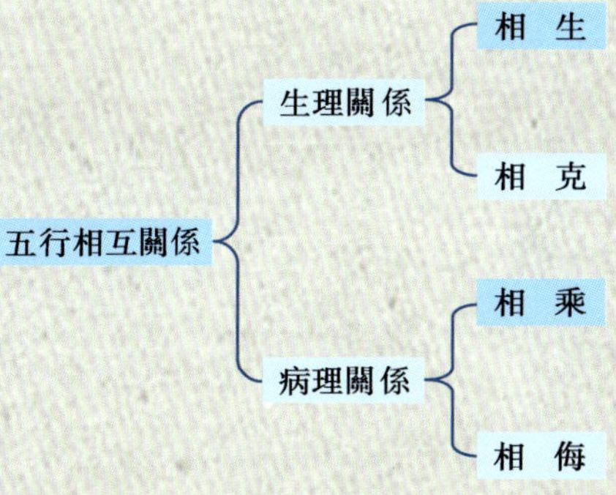

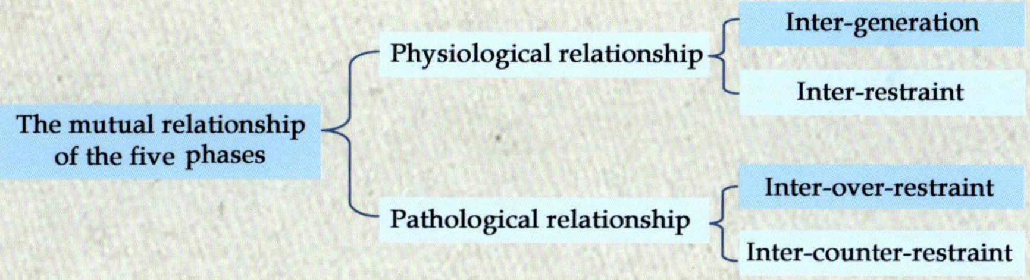

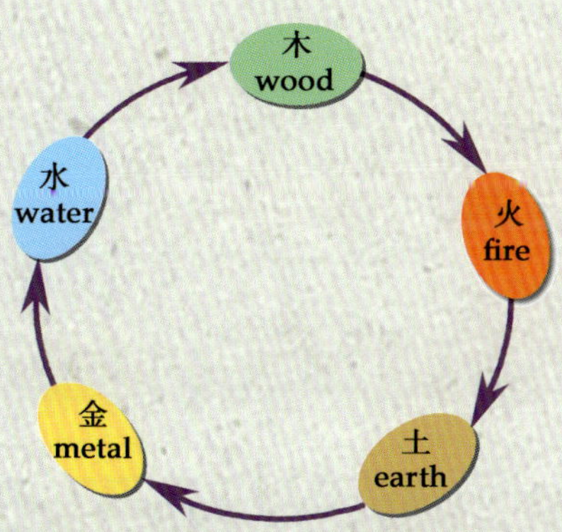

五行相生示意圖

Diagram of the Generating Relationships among the Five Phases

表示相生（⟶Generating）

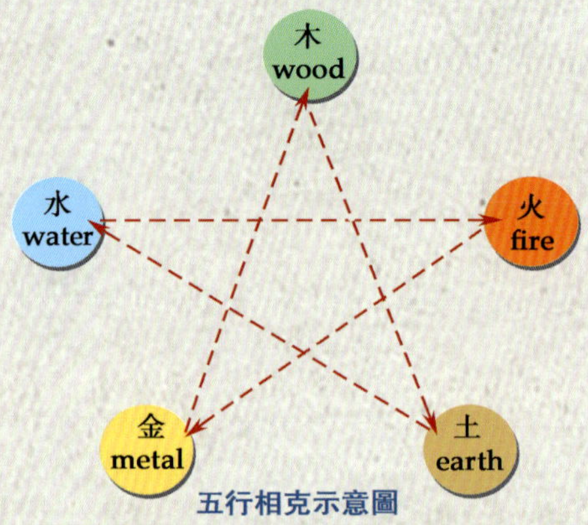

五行相克示意圖

Diagram of the Restrictive Relationships among the Five Phases

表示相克（→Restriction）

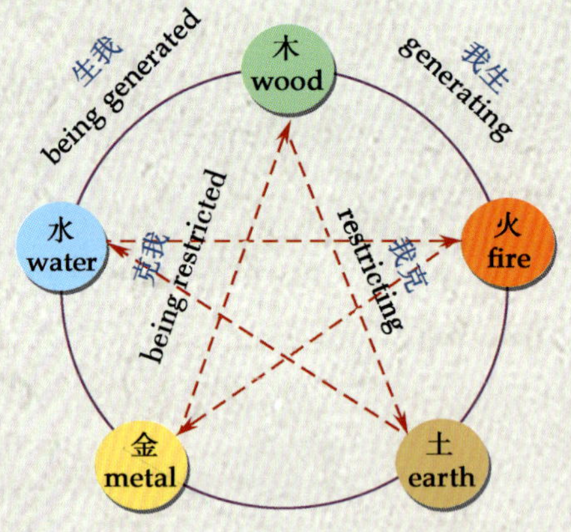

五行生克示意圖

Diagram of Generative and Restrictive Relationships among the Five Phases

表示相生（→Generating）表示相克（→Restriction）

在五行相生相克關係中，任何一行皆有“生我”、“我生”、“我克”、“克我”四個方面的關係同時存在。以木爲例，“生我”者水，“我生”者火，“克我”者金，“我克”者土。

Within the relationship of generation and restriction, each of the phases has four situations: generating, being generated, restricting and being restricted. For example, wood is generated by water and it can generate fire. Meanwhile, it is restricted by metal while it can restrict earth.

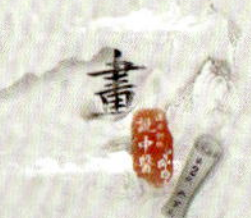

（3）相乘

是指五行中某一行對所勝一行的過度克製。五行相乘的次序與相克相同，即木乘土，土乘水，水乘火，火乘金，金乘木。但相克是五行之間的正常製約關係，而相乘是五行之間的異常製約現象。在人體，相克是生理現象，相乘是病理現象。

(3) Over-restriction

means that one phase excessively restrains another. The sequence of subjugation among the five phases is the same as restriction, for example, wood can over control earth, earth can over control water, water can over control fire, fire can over control metal and metal can over control wood. However, restriction is a relationship under normal conditions, while the over controlling relationship is an abnormal phenomenon. In the human body, restriction is a physiological phenomenon and over controlling is a pathological phenomenon.

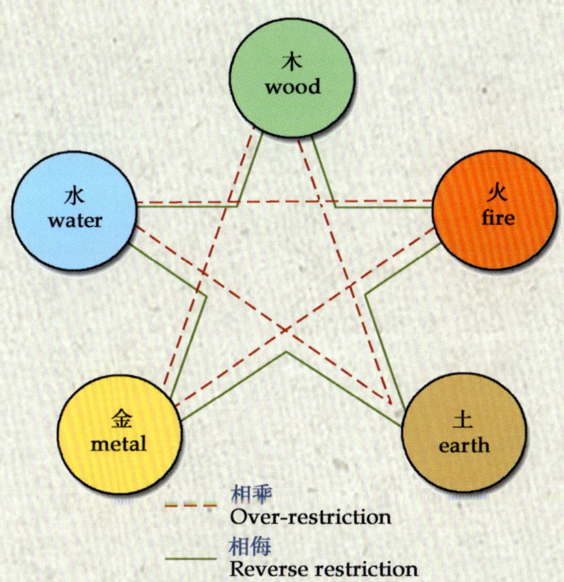

（4）相侮

指五行中的某一行自身偏盛，使原來克它的一行，不僅不能去製約它，反而被它所克製，即反克，又稱反侮。

(4) Reverse restriction

means rebelling against other phases. When one of the five phases is in excess, the phase that should have originally restricted it will instead be restricted by it. Hence the name called reverse-restriction.

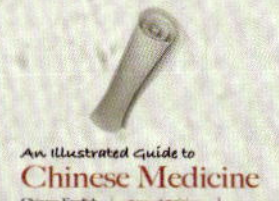

3. 五行學說在中醫學中的應用

（1）說明五臟的生理功能特點

五行學說將人體的臟腑組織分別歸屬於五行，以五行的特性來說明五臟的生理功能。五行學說又用五行間相生和相克規律來說明臟腑之間的生理聯係，如肝（木）的疏泄（情誌條暢），可以克製脾（土）的壅鬱（即調節消化功能）。

3. The Application of the Theory of the Five Phases in Chinese Medicine

(1) Physiological Functions of the Five Viscera

The theory of five phases attributes viscera and tissues respectively to one of the five phases, explaining the physiological functions of the five viscera in accordance with the features of the five phases; the physiological connection between viscera and bowels according to the laws of generation and restriction of the five phases. For example, the conveyance and dispersion of the Liver (wood) which regulates emotional activities, restricts the Spleen's (earth) building up, or regulation of the digestive function.

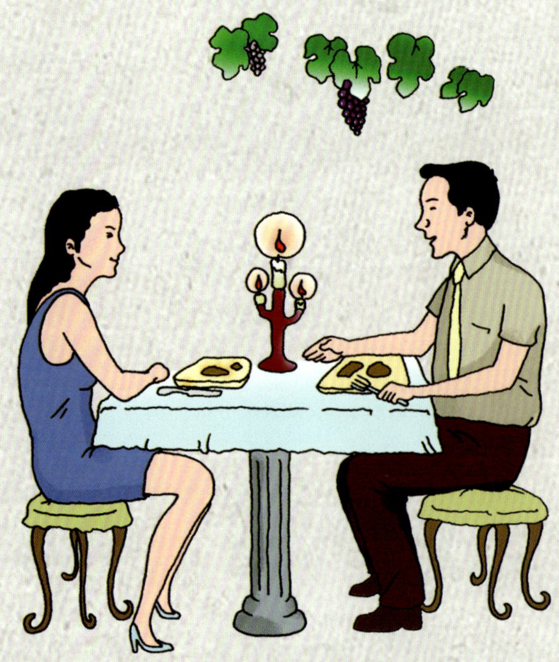

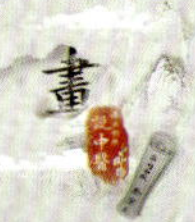

（2）說明五臟病變的相互影響

中醫學運用五行學說的生克乘侮理論，來說明病理狀況下五臟之間的相互影響，即本臟之病可以傳到他臟，他臟之病也可傳至本臟。臟腑之間的傳變，可分爲相生關係的傳變和相克關係的傳變。相生關係的傳變包括“母病及子”和“子病及母”，相克關係的傳變包括“相乘”與“相侮”，如肝病日久，會損傷腎陰，出現腰疼。

(2) Pathological Influences between the Five Viscera

According to the five-phases theory, generating, restriction, over-restriction and reverse restriction, Chinese medicine emphasizes the inner influence within the five viscera during the physiological state. The primary visceral diseases can be transferred to other viscera, and vice-versa. The transformation of disease can be divided into two patterns: transformation of generating relationships and transformation of restriction relationships. The transformation related to the generating relationship includes "the mother disease affecting the child" and "the child disease affecting the mother." The transformation related to the restriction relationship includes two patterns: over-restriction and reverse restriction. For example, long-term Liver disease can injure the nourishment of the Kidney-yin, and give rise to soreness and weakness of the lumbar region.

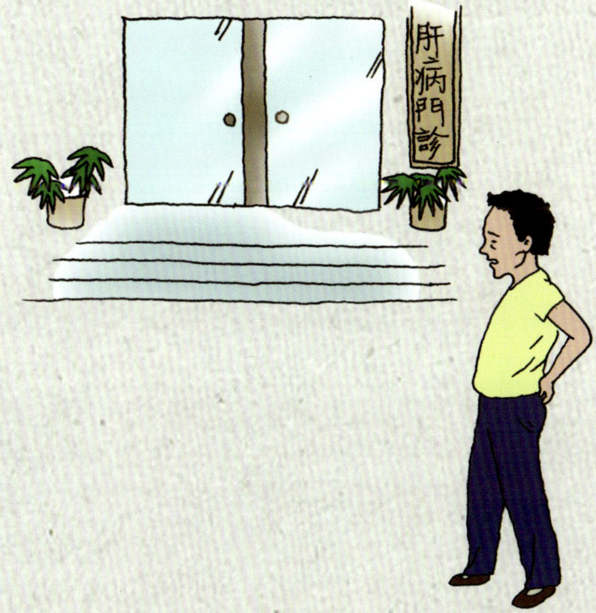

（3）用於疾病的診斷

人體内臟功能活動及其相互關係的異常變化，可以從病人的面色、聲音、口味、脈象等方面反映出來。五臟六腑及五色、五味、五誌等可歸屬於五行。臨床對望、聞、問、切四診所得的資料，可根據五行的配屬關係及其生克乘侮的變化規律，以確定五臟病變及部位，推斷病情進展和判斷疾病的預後。

(3) Using the Diagnosis of Diseases

When the human body is imbalanced, the internal viscera and their inner relationships are reflected in their corresponding aspects of facial color, voice sound, taste sensations and pulse condition. The five Zang-viscera, six Fu-viscera, five colors, five flavors and five emotions, all belong to the five phases. Clinically, all the information gathered from the four diagnostic methods (observation, smelling, listening, questioning, pulse-taking and palpation) are classified according to the properties of the five phases and the principles of generation, restriction, over-restriction and reverse restriction to determine the imbalance of the five Zang-viscera and to understand the development of diseases.

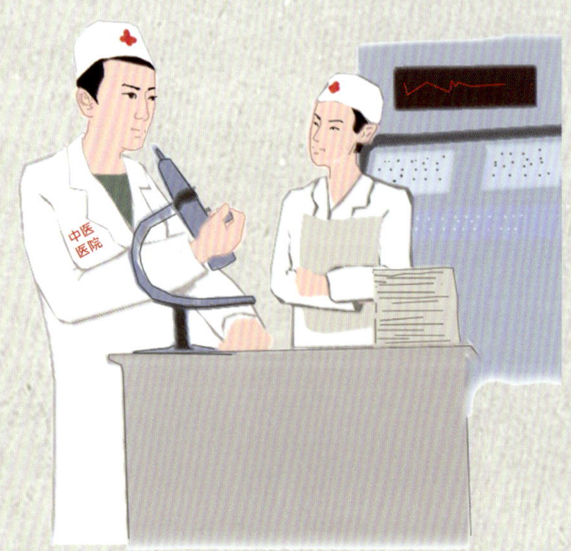

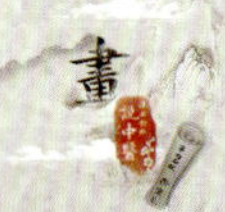

(4) 用於疾病的治療

根據五行的配屬關係，以指導臨床臟腑用藥，如青色，酸味入肝；赤色，苦味入心。並根據五行的生克乘侮規律，來指導控製疾病的傳變，如治療肝病時要先一步健脾，以防肝病傳脾。中醫的許多治則治法也是根據五行相生、相克規律確定的，如培土生金法，滋水涵木法，抑木扶土法等。五行學説還用來指導情誌療法和針灸療法，如以五行生克乘侮規律進行針刺選穴。

(4) Using the Treatment of Diseases

Clinical manifestations match the properties of five phases. For example, blue-green complexion and sour taste in the mouth indicates Liver imbalance; a red face and bitter taste in the mouth indicates Heart imbalance. The principles of generation and restriction of the five phases control the transformation of diseases. For example, if the Liver is imbalanced, strengthening the Spleen and Stomach will prevent the disease transfer to the Spleen. A lot of treatment methods use the principles of generation and restriction of the five phases. For example, reinforcing earth to generate metal, nourishing water to moisten wood, and supporting earth to restrict wood. The treatment of the emotions and acupuncture therapy are based on the theory of the five phases. For example, acupuncture points are selected according to the principles of generation, restriction, over-restriction and reverse restriction.

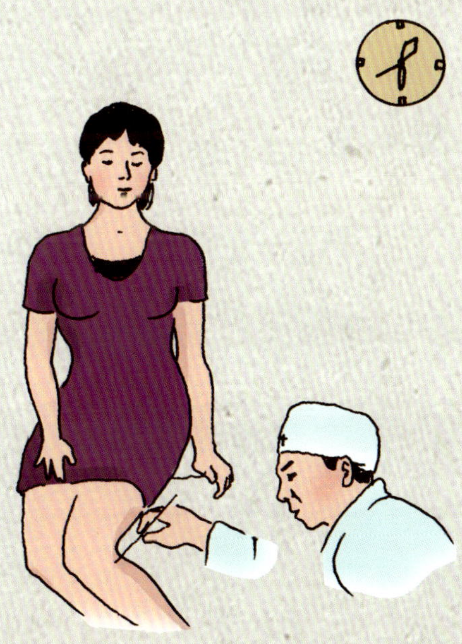

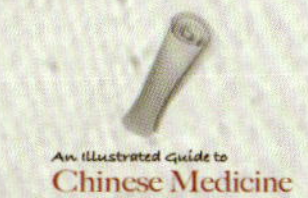

陰陽五行學說在醫學領域中是綜合運用的，至今仍是中醫理論體係的最基本內容。我們應該以現代科學技術進一步研究和發展中醫學的基本理論。

2008 年北京奧運會吉祥物福娃，則是根據五行理論設計而成。

In the medical field the yin-yang and the five phases theory are used together and they are the most basic concepts in Chinese medical theory. We should further study and develop the Chinese medicine basic theory in accordance with modern science and technology.

Fuwa, the official mascots of the Beijing 2008 Olympic Games were designed according to the five phases.

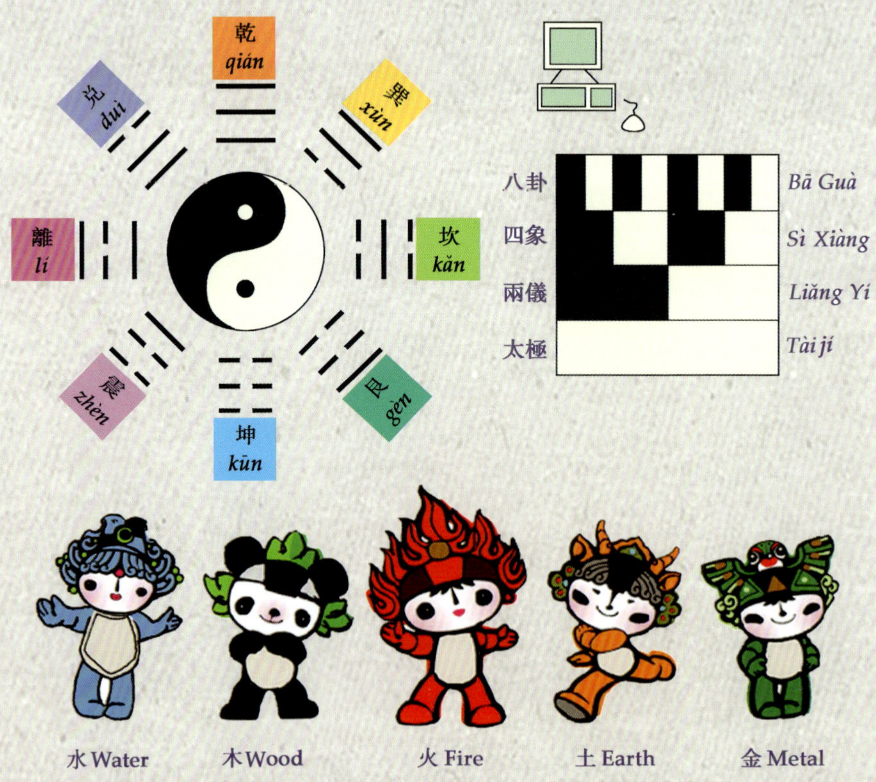

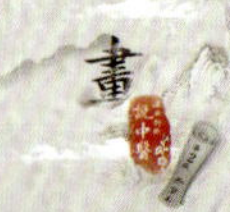

第二章 藏象

Chapter 2 Zang-fu Manifestation (*Zàng Xiàng*)

一、藏象學説概述

The Introduction of the Zang-fu Manifestation Theory

藏象學説，是研究臟腑形體官竅的形態結構、生理功能、病理變化及其與精、氣、津液、神之間的相互關係，以及臟腑之間、臟腑與形體官竅之間、臟腑與自然環境之間的相互關係的學説。藏象學説是中醫理論體係的核心内容。

The Zang-fu manifestation theory is the study of Zang-fu organs and their orifices' structure, physiological functions, pathological changes and relationships with essence, qi, body fluids and spirit. It also discusses the relationships between the organs themselves, and between the Zang-fu organs and the natural environment. This is the core of Chinese medicine theory.

1. 藏象的含義

藏是指藏於體内的内臟，像是内臟表現於外的生理、病理現象。根據人體外在表現來推測内臟的生理、病理情況，是中醫獨特的觀察研究方法。

1. The Concept of the Zang-fu Manifestation

The term "Zang" refers to the Zang-fu organs which are located inside the body. "*Xiàng*" means the external manifestation of their physiology and pathology. Chinese medicine has a unique method to view, study and explain the physiological and pathological activities of Zang-fu organs according to their external manifestations.

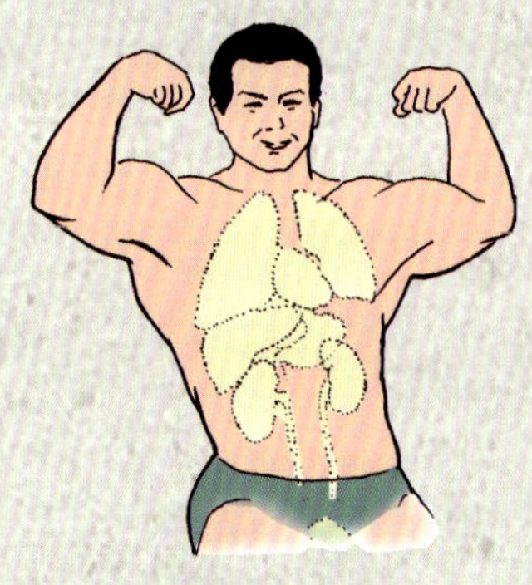

2. 藏象學説的内容

藏象學説以臟腑爲中心。臟腑包括五臟、六腑、奇恒之腑三類。心、肝、脾、肺、腎稱五臟；膽、胃、大腸、小腸、膀胱、三焦爲六腑。腦、髓、骨、脈、膽、女子胞稱爲奇恒之腑。

2. The Content of the Zang-fu Manifestation Theory

The core of the Zang-fu organs manifestation theory is the internal organs of the body. The Zang-fu organs consist of five Zang-organs, six Fu-organs and the extraordinary organs. The five Zang-organs are the Heart, Lung, Spleen, Liver and Kidney. The six Fu-organs are the Gallbladder, Stomach, Small Intestine, Large Intestine, Bladder, and San Jiao. The extraordinary organs are the Brain, Marrow, Bone, Blood vessels, Gallbladder and the Uterus.

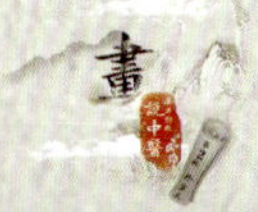

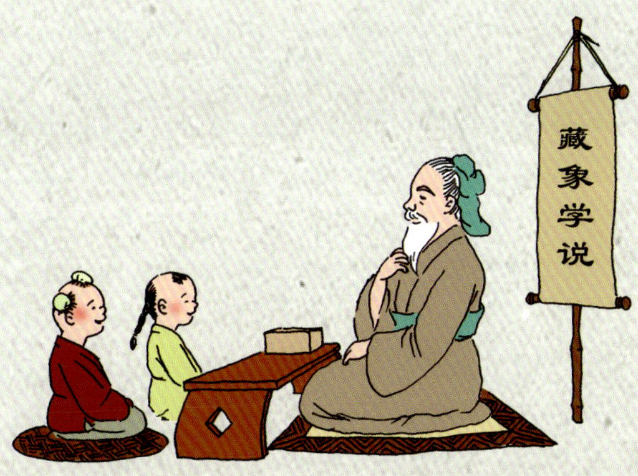

3. 藏象學説的特點

藏象學説主要是基於“有諸內，必形諸外”的觀察研究方法。藏象學説的特點之一，是以五臟爲中心的整體觀。這主要體現在：

（1）是臟腑是一個整體，如腎與膀胱相表裏。

（2）是五臟與形體官竅聯結成爲一個整體。如腎其華在發，開竅於耳及前後陰等。

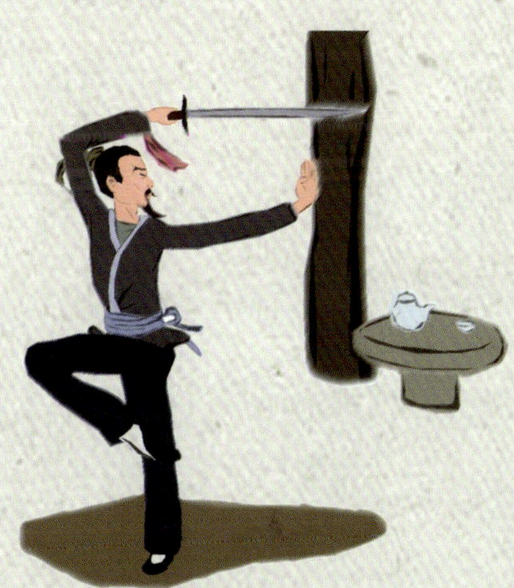

3. The Characteristics of the Zang-fu Manifestation Theory

The Zang-fu organs manifestation theory is primarily based on the idea that external symptoms can reflect the condition of the internal environment. One of the characteristics of the Zang-fu organs manifestation theory places the five Zang-organs at the center of this holistic perspective. This is mainly manifested in the following ideas:

(1) The Zang-organs and the Fu-organs are a whole entity. For example, Kidney and Bladder form an exterior-interior relationship.

(2) The five Zang-organs are connected with the sense organs and orifices, forming an integrated whole. For example, the Kidney manifests in the hair and opens into the ears, and the two lower orifices (genitals and anus).

藏象學説的特點之二，是臟腑不單純是解剖學的概念，而且是一個綜合性的功能單位。

西醫學的臟器是解剖學的概念，而中醫的臟腑是在古代解剖學基礎上演變的人體功能係統的概括。

以脾爲例：西醫是指脾臟，爲淋巴器官；中醫的脾包含了整個消化係統的功能。

Another characteristic of the Zang-fu organs manifestation theory is that Zang-organs and Fu-organs are considered to be not only an anatomical concept but also an integrated unit of functions.

In Western medicine, the concepts of the internal organs are only based on their anatomical aspects, but in Chinese medicine the Zang-fu organs are instead a system of the human body's functions, which idea evolved on the basis of theories of ancient anatomy.

For example, the Spleen in Western medicine is the Spleen-organ, or namely, a lymph gland; on the contrary, in Chinese medicine it indicates the function of the whole digestive system.

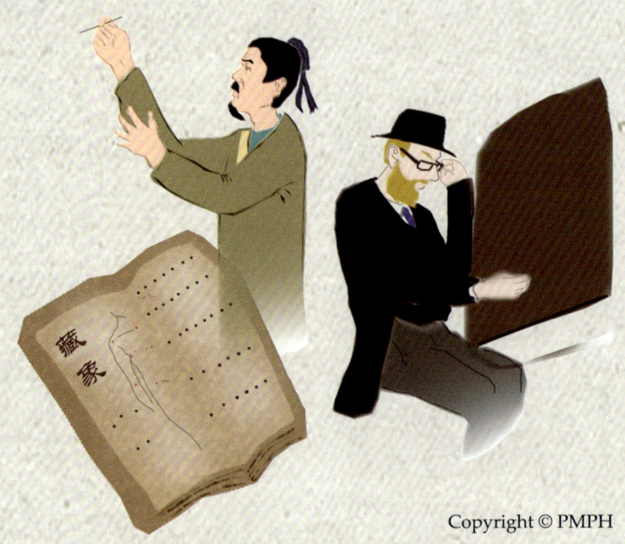

二、五臟

心、肺、肝、脾、腎合稱五臟，五臟的形態結構屬實體性器官，分别位於胸腔和腹腔之中。

五臟的生理功能是主化生和貯藏精、氣、血、津液等精微物質。

1. 心

主要生理功能是主血脈、主藏神。

（1）心的位置

心位於胸中，有心包衛護於外。它主宰人體的生命活動，在五臟六腑中居於首要地位。

Five Zang-organs

The five Zang-organs are the Heart, Lung, Spleen, Liver and Kidney. They have solid structures and are located in the chest and abdominal cavities.

The physiological functions of the five Zang-organs are the transformation, generation and storage of essential substances, like essence, qi, blood and body fluids.

1. The Heart

The main physiological functions of the Heart are to control the blood and vessels, and to store the spirit.

(1) The Location of the Heart

The heart is located in the chest, surrounded by the Pericardium. It controls the life activities of the human body, and it is the most important among the Zang-fu organs.

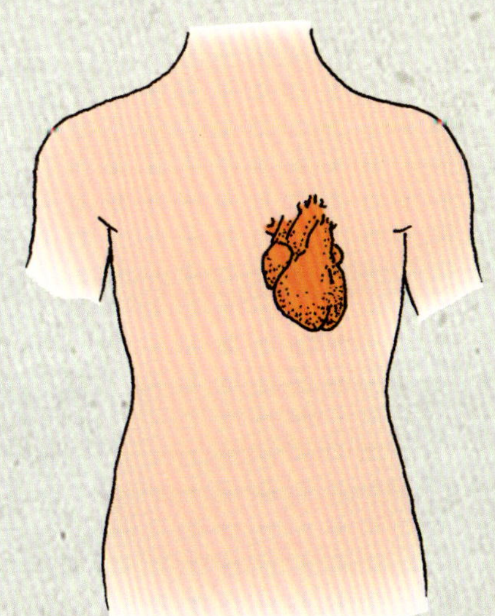

（2）心的比喻

心，《内經》稱之爲“君主之官”、“五臟六腑之大主”。心爲神之居，血之主，脈之宗。

(2) The Heart's Metaphor

The Yellow Emperor's Classic of Internal Medicine <Huáng Dì Nèi Jīng> says: The Heart is "the monarch of all the organs", "the controller of the five Zang-organs and the six Fu-organs." The heart is considered the home of the spirit, the master of the blood, and the governor of the vessels.

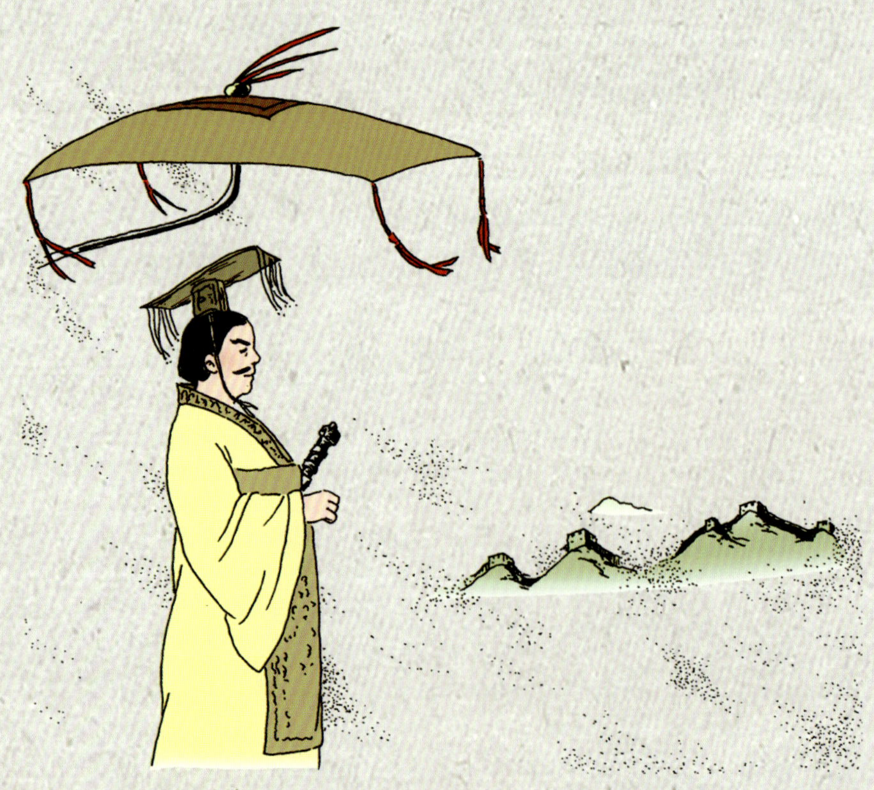

（3）心的生理功能

1）心主血脈

心有推動血液運行全身的作用。心氣充沛、血液充盈、脈道通利是正常血液迴圈必備的三個條件。

(3) Physiological Functions of the Heart

1) Controls the Blood Vessels

The function of the Heart is to circulate the blood through the whole body. In order to circulate the blood normally, the Heart needs sufficient qi, blood, and the vessels should be open.

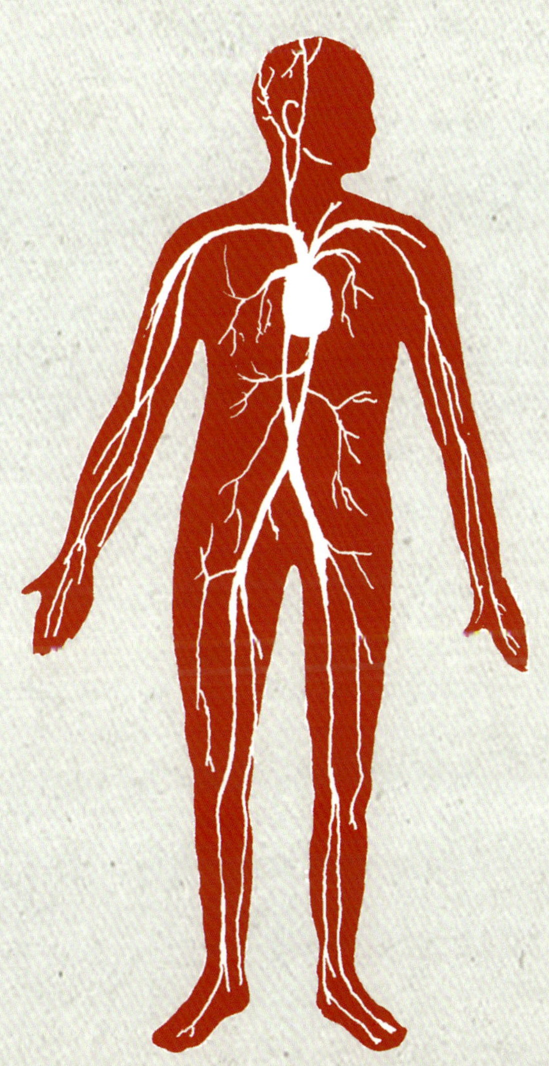

心主血脈功能是否正常，可以從面色、舌色、脈象及胸部感覺四個方面反映出來，心主血液功能正常，則面色紅潤，胸部舒暢，舌色淡紅榮潤，脈緩和有力。

TCM believes that whether or not the function of "the heart dominates the blood vessels" performs normally can manifest from four aspects: the face, the color of the tongue, the pulse condition and the feeling of the chest. If heart-blood flourish, the face will be lustrous and moist, the chest will feel comfortable, the color of the tongue will be red and moist, soft and flexible, and the pulse beat will be smooth and forceful.

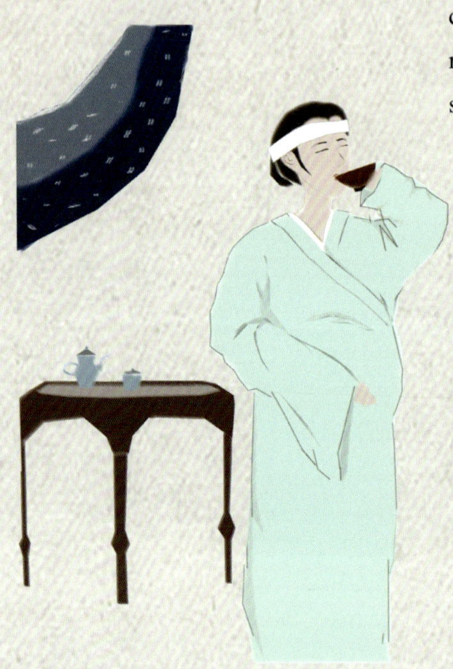

2）主藏神

中醫認爲心主精神、譩識、思維活動。人的精神、譩誌、思維雖是大腦對外界事物的反映，但藏象學説認爲心爲神之主。這是藏象學説的特點所決定的。中醫藏象學説特點是以五臟爲中心的整體觀，因此把大腦的功能分屬於五臟之中。

2) Stores the Spirit

The heart controls the spirit's activities, consciousness, and thinking. Although these activities are the reactions of the brain to the external environment, the Zang-organs manifestation theory holds that the heart controls the mind. This is determined by the characteristics of the Zang-organs manifestation theory. The characteristic of Zang-fu organs manifestation theory is a holistic viewpoint, which argues that the five Zang-organs are central among all the organs in the body. Therefore, the functions of the brain are attributable to the five Zang-organs.

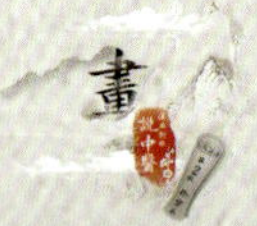

（4）心的生理功能聯係

1）心合小腸

心與小腸以經絡相互絡屬，構成表裏關係。心與小腸疾病可以相互影響。

2）心主神誌與心主血脈息息相關

血液是神態活動的物質基礎。衹有心主血脈的功能正常，心神得以血液的濡養，才能保持良好的精神心理狀態。

3）心，其華在面

心主血脈功能是否正常，可以從面色、舌色、脈象及胸部感覺四個方面反映出來，心主血液功能正常，則面色紅潤，胸部舒暢，舌色淡紅榮潤，脈緩和有力。

(4) The Relationship among the Physiological Functions of the Heart

1) The Heart and the Small Intestine connect with each other, and form an exterior-interior relationship due to their meridians interconnection. Therefore, diseases in the Heart and the Small Intestine affect each other.

2) The concepts that the Heart controls the mind and that the Heart controls the blood vessels are closely related because blood is a basis for the mental and emotional activities. If the Heart's function of controlling the blood vessels is normal, the blood can nourish Heart and mind, and thus the mental state will be normal.

3) The Heart manifests in the face. Its function of controlling the vessels can manifest in the complexion, tongue color, pulse condition and whether a sense of tension is felt in the chest area. If the function of governing the blood is normal, the complexion is red and moist, the chest feels comfortable, the tongue is light red and moist, and the pulse is moderate and has force.

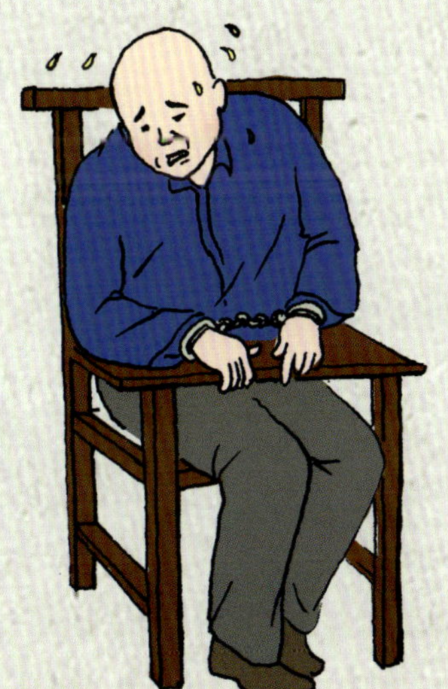

4）汗爲心之液

汗爲津液所化生，津液是血液的重要組成部分，而血又爲心所主，故有“汗血同源”之說。

5）心開竅於舌

舌主味覺和表達語言。心功能正常，則舌質紅活；心氣不足，心血虧虛則舌質淡白；心血瘀阻，則舌質紫暗或有瘀點等。

4) Sweat is a fluid of the Heart; it is transformed from the body fluids which are also an important part of the blood. Because the Heart controls the blood, perspiration and blood share the same source.

5) The Heart opens into the tongue, which controls the ability to sense tastes and to speak. If Heart's function is normal, the tongue texture will be red and moist. Insufficient Heart blood or Heart qi deficiency will manifest in a pale tongue texture, while Heart blood stasis will result in a purple tongue texture or stasis spots.

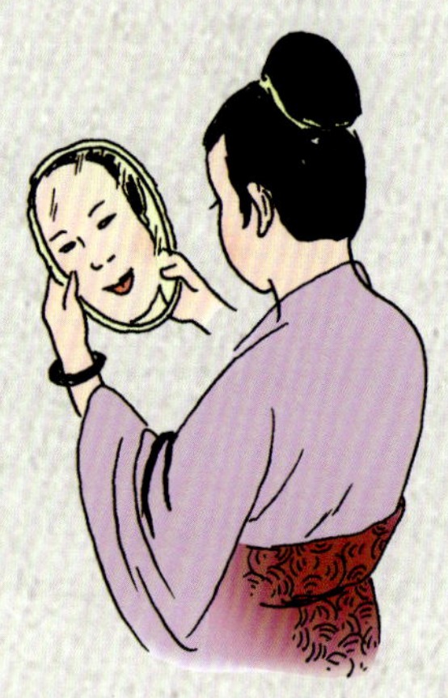

6）喜爲心之誌

人的心情舒暢歡快則氣血和調。一般說來喜對身體有益，但喜樂過度，則傷心神。

6) In five-phase theory, joy is the emotion of the Heart. If a person is in a good mood, the qi and blood will flow freely. In general, joy functions as a normal emotion that is good for the health, but excessive joy can hurt the mind.

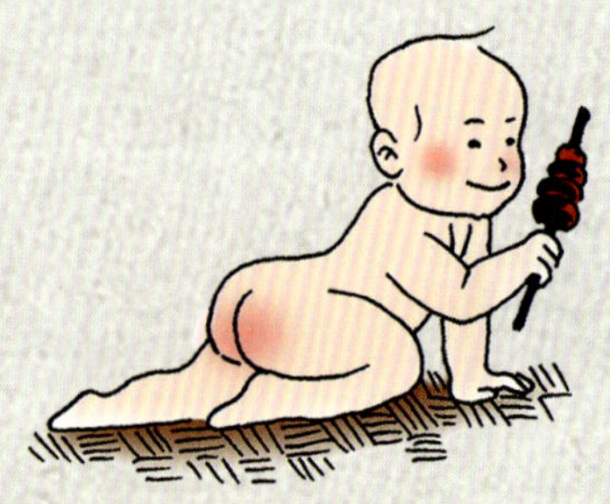

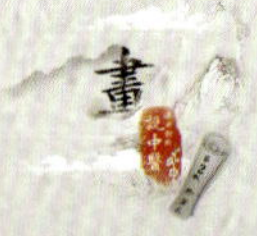

2. 肝

主要生理功能是主疏泄、主藏血。

（1）肝的位置

肝位於右脅内，其經脈布於兩肋。

（2）肝的比喻

《内經》稱肝爲"將軍之官"、"罷極之本"。肝的生理特點是主升發，喜條達。

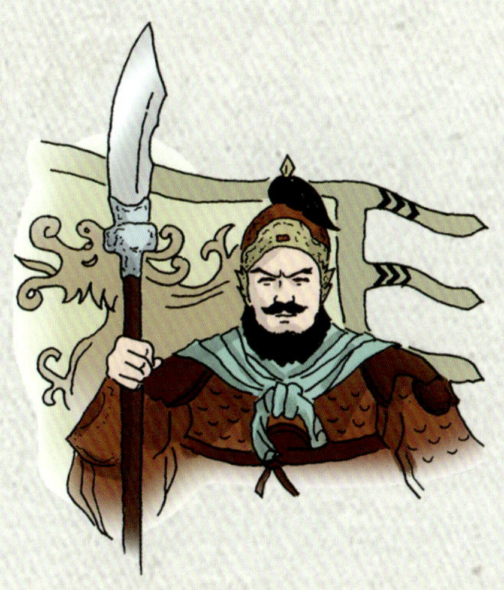

（3）肝的生理功能

1）肝主疏泄

肝主疏泄的生理功能，其一是調暢氣機。如七情失調，可致肝氣鬱結，肝氣上逆等病理變化。

2. The Liver

The main physiological functions of the Liver are to govern free coursing and to store the Blood.

(1) The Location of the Liver

The Liver is located in the right hypochondriac region. Its meridian and vessels are distributed over both sides of the ribs.

(2) The Liver's Metaphor

The Yellow Emperor's Classic of Internal Medicine <Huáng Dì Nèi Jīng> says: The Liver is a general, who governs the contraction and relaxation of the muscles and tendons. The Liver's physiological functions are to govern, ascend and disperse, it likes to promote the free flow of qi.

(3) Physiological Functions of the Liver

1) Liver Controls Dispersion

The Liver's first physiological function is to regulate qi activities. For example, lack of coordination of the seven emotions will induce Liver qi constraint, upward invasion of Liver qi, or other pathological changes.

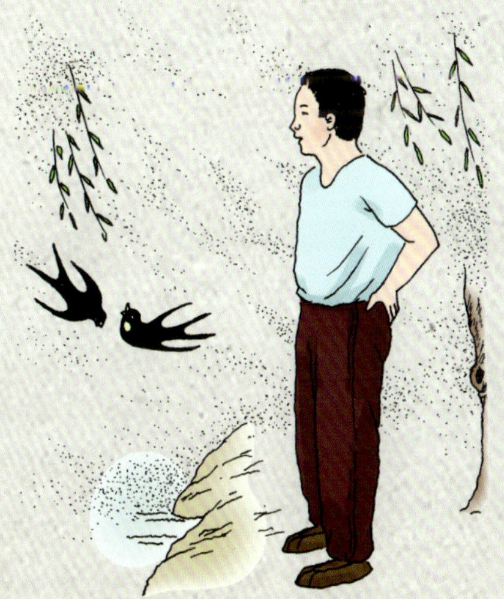

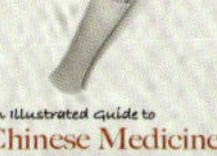

其二是調暢情誌。若肝失疏泄則肝氣鬱結，表現爲憂鬱不樂、多愁善慮；若肝疏泄太過，則表現爲肝氣亢奮，可出現急躁易怒、煩躁不安等。

Secondly, it regulates the emotions: the failure of the Liver to govern free coursing can cause Liver qi constraint and manifest in poor mood. Hyperactivity of the Liver in the government of free coursing causes hyperactivity of the Liver qi, with symptoms like impatience, irritability and agitation.

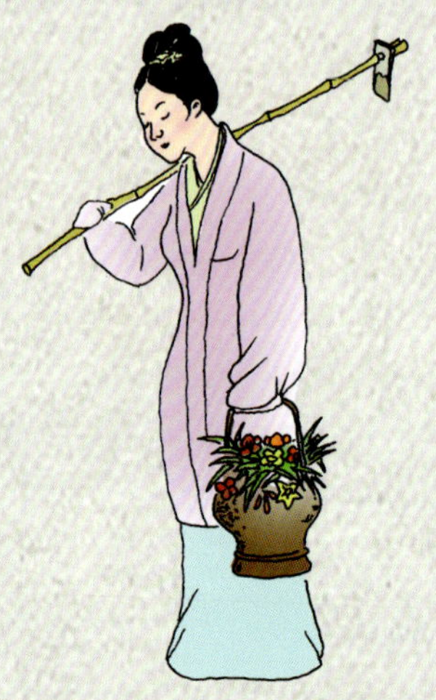

其三是促進消化吸收。若肝失疏泄，則脾氣不升而眩暈、清氣下陷而泄瀉，且使胃氣上逆而噯氣；濁氣不降而脘腹脹滿疼痛、便秘。肝失疏泄，可影響膽汁分泌與排泄，出現脅痛、口苦，甚則黄疸等。

Thirdly, it promotes digestion and absorption. The Liver's failure to govern free coursing can cause the Spleen to fail to raise the clear qi, which will manifest as dizziness and vertigo; and descending the clear qi may even result in diarrhea. Additionally, Stomach qi counter flowing upwards can give rise to hiccup, if the turbid qi fails to descend, it may cause abdominal pain and constipation. The Liver's failure to conduct and dispersing functions influences Gallbladder bile secretion and excretion, and manifests as pain in the rib-side (the area between the armpit and the bottom rib), bitter taste in the mouth, and even jaundice.

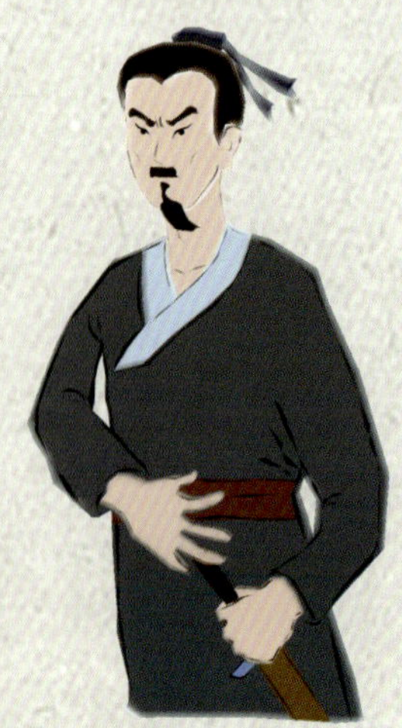

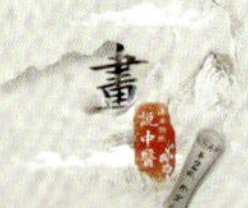

2）肝主藏血

肝能貯藏血液和調節血流量。故稱肝爲“血海”。

（4）肝的生理聯係

1）肝合膽，膽附於肝

經絡相互絡屬，構成表裏關係。肝與膽的疾病可以相互影響。

2）主筋、其華在爪。筋、爪依賴肝血滋養。

2) Storing Blood

The Liver stores the blood and regulates the volume of blood flow. Thus, it is known as "the sea of blood".

(4) The Relationship among the Liver's Physiological Functions

1) The Liver and Gallbladder are connected with each other. Physically, the Gallbladder is attached to the Liver, they are connected by channels and collaterals and form an exterior-interior relationship. Therefore, diseases in the Liver and the Gallbladder can affect each other.

2) The Liver controls the tendons, and manifests in the nails. The tendons and the nails depend on being nourished by Liver's blood.

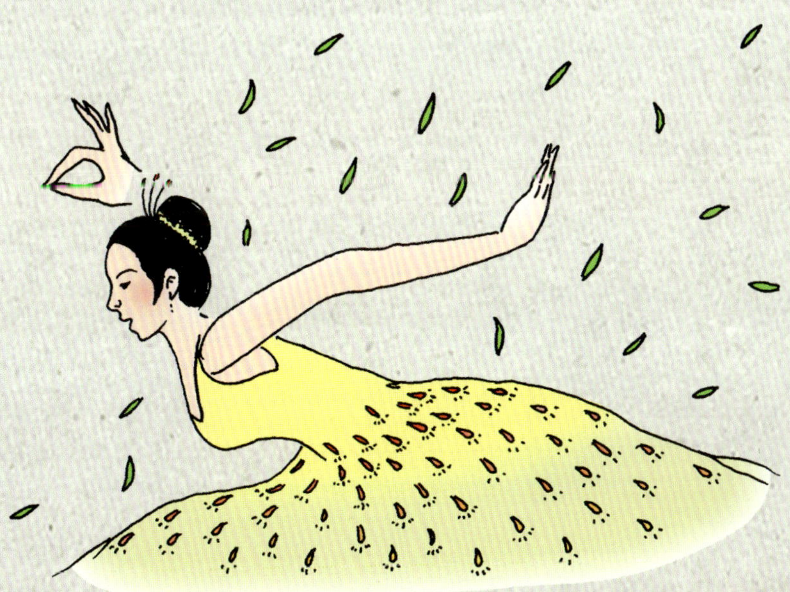

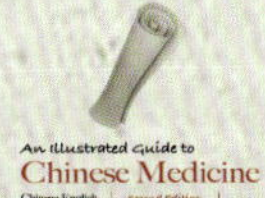

3）肝在誌爲怒

突然大怒，或經常發怒極易傷肝。故有暴怒傷肝之説。

3) In five-phase theory, anger is the emotion of the Liver. Sudden or frequent anger, called excessive anger, can damage the Liver.

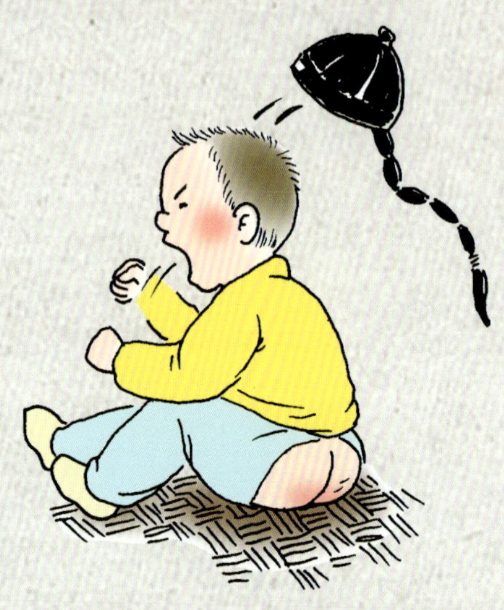

4）肝開竅於目

在液爲淚，目的視力有賴於肝氣之疏泄和肝血之營養。肝血不足可發生兩目幹澀、雀盲，或視物昏花；肝火上炎可見目赤腫痛。

4) The Liver opens into the eyes, and tears are its fluid manifestation. Normal eyesight depends on Liver qi being conducted and dispensed, and the nourishment by Liver blood. Liver blood insufficiency manifests as dry eyes, night blindness or blurred vision. Liver fire flaming upward may cause painful and swollen red eyes.

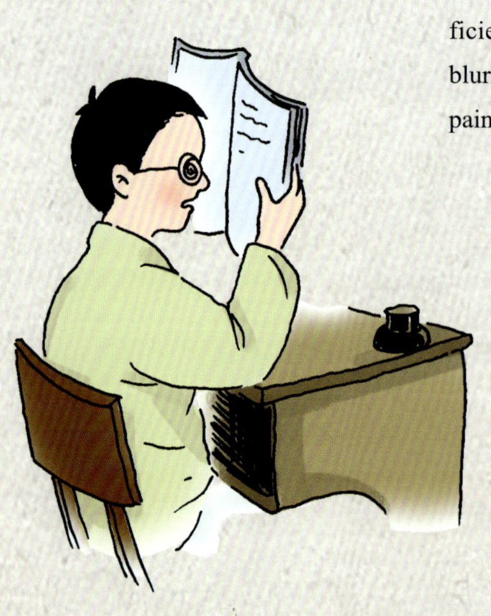

3. 脾

主要生理功能是主運化、主升清、主統血。

（1）脾的位置

脾位於人的橫膈下。

（2）脾的比喻

《内經》稱脾爲倉禀之官。“後天之本”、“氣血生化之源”。藏象學説中的脾作爲解剖學單位包括了現代解剖學中的胰和脾，但其生理功能又遠非脾和胰所囊指。

3. The Spleen

The main physiological functions of the Spleen are to control transportation and transformation, raise the clear qi, and control the blood.

(1) The Location of the Spleen

The Spleen is located underneath the diaphragm muscle.

(2) The Spleen's Metaphor

The Yellow Emperor's Classic of Internal Medicine <Huáng Dì Nèi Jīng> says: "The Spleen is the official of the storage barn." The Spleen is considered to be the "root of the acquired constitution" and the "source of qi and blood".

In Zang-fu manifestation theory, the Spleen is an organ that includes both the pancreas and the spleen, although the physiological functions of the Spleen in Chinese medicine are very different than those of the pancreas and spleen in modern medical theory.

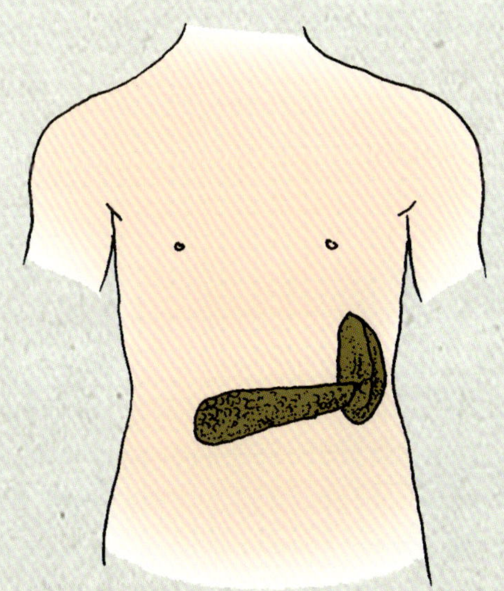

（3）脾的生理功能

1）脾主運化

其一是運化水谷。飲食經胃的受納熟腐之後，由脾進一步消化，並吸收其中的營養物質（水谷精微），再“上輸於肺”，“灌溉四旁”，滋養全身各組織。所以脾的運化功能健全（稱脾氣健運），則生化之源豐富，全身精氣充足。

(3) Physiological Functions of the Spleen

1) The Spleen Controls Transportation and Transformation.

This function has two aspects: firstly, is the transportation and transformation of water and food. After the Stomach decomposes the food and drink, it is further digested by the Spleen, which absorbs the nourishment (the refined essence of food and water) from the diet, and lifts it to the Lung, where it is distributed throughout the body, to nourish and moisten every tissue. Therefore, only when Spleen functions are normal, is the source of transportation and transformation abundant, and the whole body will be full of essential qi.

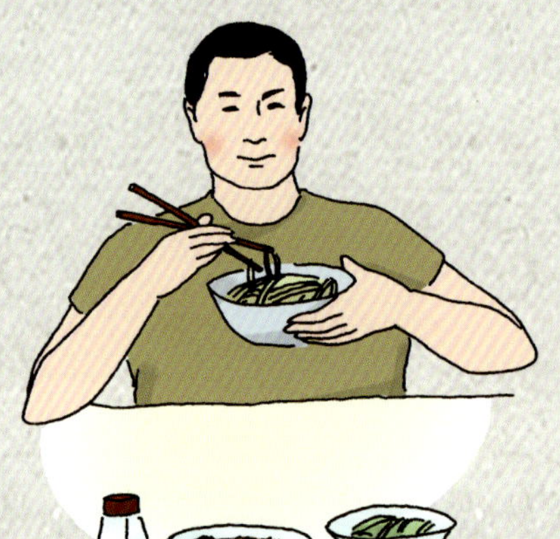

脾主運化

其二是運化水液。人體津液由脾上輸於肺，其清者內而灌養五臟六腑，外而滋潤肌腠皮毛，其濁着，化爲汗液和尿液排出體外。脾失健運，可致痰飲，水腫等癥。

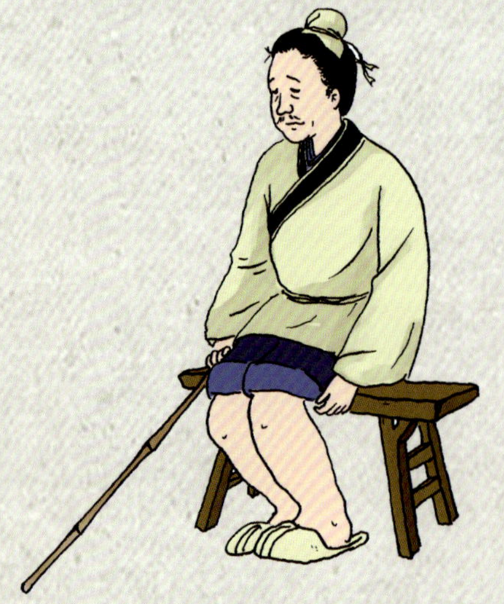

Secondly, is the transportation and transformation of liquids and secretions: The Spleen raises the body fluids to the Lung, where it is divided to clear and turbid. Internally, the clear fluids nourish the five Zang-organs and the six Fu-organs, and externally, they moisten the skin and body hair. The turbid fluids are changed into perspiration and urine, and excreted from the body. Failure of the Spleen in the transportation and transformation of fluids can result in edema, and retention of phlegm and fluids.

2）脾主統血

脾主統血是指脾具有統攝血液在經脈之中流行、防止逸出脈外的功能。其實就是氣對血的固攝作用。脾不統血，則出現各種出血癥。

3）脾主升清

脾氣具有上升爲主的特點，同時，對體内的臟器具有升舉固攝作用。脾氣不升，可出現腹脹、腹瀉等脾失健運癥狀，脾氣下陷，則可見久瀉脱肛，甚至内臟下垂。

2) The Spleen Controls the Blood

The function of the Spleen is to control the circulation of the blood throughout the blood vessels and to hold the blood inside the vessels, thus preventing it from spilling out. In fact, it is the Spleen qi in particular which holds the blood in the vessels. The failure of these functions manifests in various types of hemorrhagic diseases.

3) The Spleen Controls the Rising of Qi in General and Clear Qi in Particular.

The Spleen qi is characterized by its raising function, and at the same time it holds the organs in their proper place. Failure of the Spleen qi to raise the qi may result in abdominal distension and diarrhea. If the Spleen qi descends, it may result in long-term diarrhea, prolapse of the anus or even of internal organs.

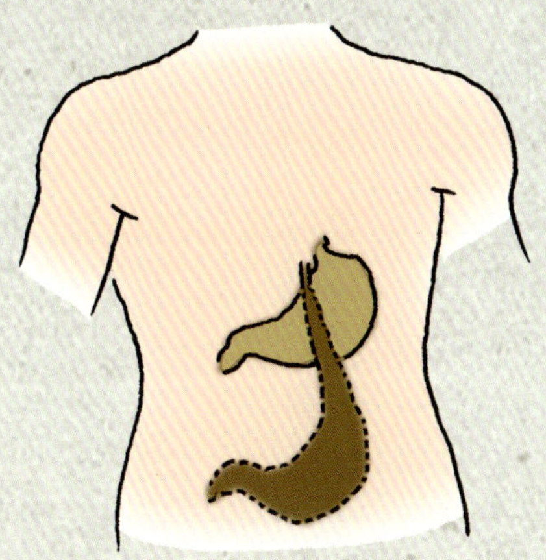

（4）脾的生理聯係

1）脾合胃

脾與胃同屬中焦，以膜相連，經絡相互絡屬，構成表裏關係。脾與胃的疾病可以相互影響。

(4) The Relationship among the Physiological Functions of the Spleen

1) The Spleen and the Stomach connect with each other. The Spleen and Stomach are located in the Middle Jiao and are linked by channels and collaterals, forming an exterior-interior relationship. Therefore, diseases in the Spleen and the Stomach can affect each other.

2）脾開竅於口

其華在唇，脾運化功能旺盛，可將飲食中的營養物質輸送全身，可表現爲肌肉健壯、活動有力、食欲旺盛、口味正常、口唇紅潤有光澤。

3）脾主肌肉與四肢

脾氣健運，精氣四布，則四肢肌肉營養充足，肌肉豐厚，活動輕勁有力。若脾失健運，則四肢營養不足，可見倦怠乏力，甚至萎弱不用。

4）在誌爲思

思即思慮，若思慮太過，或相思不解，就會影響氣的運動而導致氣機的鬱結，易妨礙脾胃的運化功能，導致消化吸收輸布失常，從而出現不思飲食，脘腹脹悶等癥。

5）在液爲涎

涎爲口津，是唾液中較清稀的部分，由脾陰所化生。脾氣不攝，則可導致涎液分泌異常增多，若脾胃陰虛，則可使涎液分泌量減少。

2) The Spleen opens into the mouth, and manifests in the lips. If the Spleen qi is normal in both transportation and transformation actions, then the food and water essence will spread throughout the body, and manifest in strong muscles which can move easily, a good appetite, a normal sense of taste and moist and rosy lips.

3) The Spleen controls the muscles and the four limbs. If the functions of Spleen qi are normal, the four limbs and the muscles will be well nourished and strong. If the Spleen qi functions are weak, the muscles will suffer from lack of nourishment, which manifests as lassitude, weak muscles or even atrophy.

4) In five-phase theory pensiveness is the emotion of the Spleen. Overthinking or inability to explain one's thoughts may affect the movement of the qi, causing qi stagnation and easily obstruct the transportation and transformation function of the Spleen and Stomach, leading to abnormal digestive and absorbing function, manifesting in the loss of appetite, distention and fullness in the upper abdomen.

5) The Spleen's fluid is the saliva, which is thin in nature, and formed by the Spleen yin. Failure in the Spleen's function of holding will manifest in ptyalism (excessive salivation). Spleen and Stomach qi deficiency may result in xerostomia (decreased salivation).

4. 肺

主要功能是主氣、司呼吸、主行水、朝百脈。

（1）肺的位置

肺位於胸腔，五臟六腑中肺位置最高，故稱華蓋。

4. The Lung

The main functions of the Lung are to govern qi and respiration, move the water and control all the channels and blood vessels.

(1) The Location of the Lung

The Lung is located in the thorax. Among the five Zang-organs and the six Fu-organs, the Lung is located at the highest point, and it is known as the Florid Canopy.

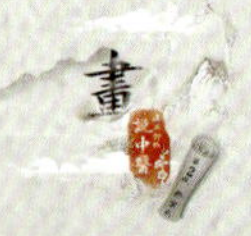

（2）肺的比喻

肺與心同居膈上，位高近君，猶如宰相，故《内經》稱其爲“相傅之官”。肺葉嬌嫩、又易受外邪侵襲，故又有“嬌臟”之稱。

(2) The Lung's Metaphor

Both Lung and Heart are located in the thorax. The Lung's location is next to the monarch (Heart), and its role is similar to a prime minister. *The Yellow Emperor's Classic of Internal Medicine <Huáng Dì Nèi Jīng>* says that the Lung is "the premier who is responsible for coordinating functions." Since the Lung is the highest and the most exterior organ, it can easily be attacked by evil qi, therefore the Lung is called a delicate organ.

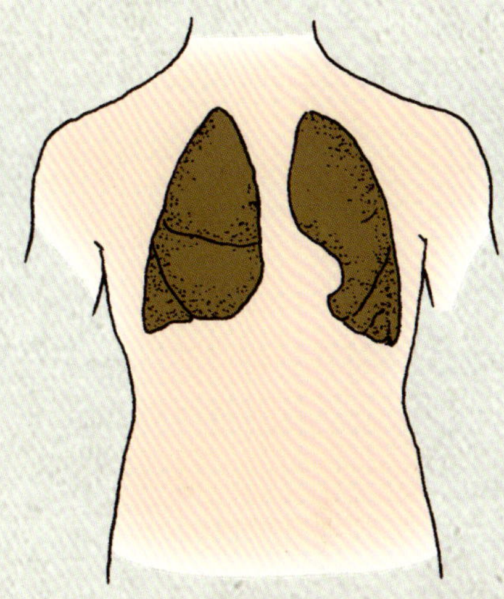

（3）肺的生理功能

1）肺主氣

其一是主呼吸之氣。肺從自然界吸入氧氣，呼出體内二氧化碳等濁氣，以保證人體新陳代謝的正常運行。人體氣的生成、氣血運行、津液輸布等，均要依賴於肺呼吸運動，否則會出現多種病理變化。

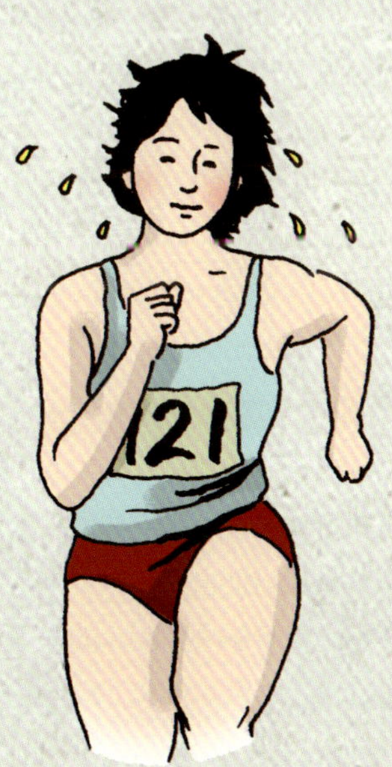

(3) Physiological Functions of the Lung

1) The Lung governs qi. This function has two aspects: firstly, controlling the qi of respiration. The Lung inhales oxygen from Nature and exhales carbon dioxide (turbid air) in order to maintain normal metabolic processes in the human body. Qi generation, the movement of qi and blood, and the distribution of the body fluids, are all dependent on the Lung's respiration. If the Lung's respiration is abnormal, various types of diseases will emerge.

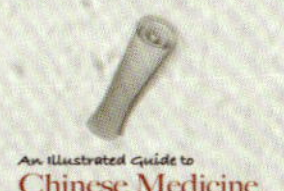

其二，是主一身之氣。肺具有主持調節全身各臟腑經絡的作用。若肺喪失呼吸功能，人的生命活動也就終結。

Secondly, it controls the qi of the whole body, which means that the function of the Lung is to spread the qi to all the Zang-fu organs and channels and collaterals. If the Lung's function of respiration is lost, life will end.

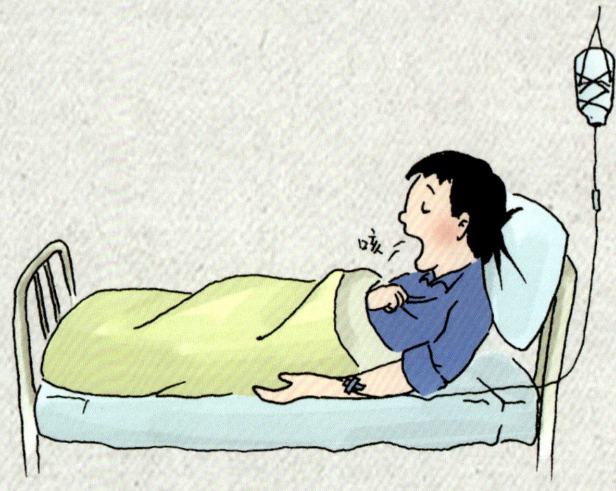

2）肺通調水道

肺對體内水液的運行、排泄有疏通和調節的作用，肺氣宣發使水液布散到肌膚化爲汗；肺的肅降，將水液不斷向下輸送到腎，經腎的氣化作用生成尿液，若肺通調功能減退，水液則停聚引起痰飲、水腫。

2) The Lung regulates the waterways. It has the function of dredging and regulating the circulation and excretion of fluids in the body. The Lung disperses the body fluids throughout the muscles and skin and transforms it into perspiration. Because it has a descending and purifying function, the fluids descend downward to the Kidney, where they are transformed into urine. If the Lung fails in this function, the fluids will accumulate, resulting in phlegm and fluids retention, and edema.

3）肺朝百脈

全身的血液都經過經脈而聚合於肺，通過肺的呼吸進行氣體交換，然後輸布全身。即血液的運行必須依賴於肺氣散布和調節。

3) The Lung controls the circulation in all the vessels. The blood from the all the body's organs and tissues passes through the channels and returns to the lungs for gas exchange, then redistributes as oxygenated blood back to the body through the channels. Blood circulation depends on the function of the Lung qi distribution and regulation.

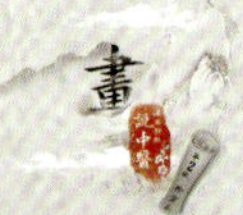

（4）肺的生理聯係

1）肺合大腸

肺與大腸通過經絡的相互絡屬構成表裏關係，兩者的疾病可以相互影響。

2）在體合皮

其華在毛：皮毛，包括皮膚、汗腺、毫毛等組織，爲保衛抵御外邪的屏障。肺合皮毛，是指由肺輸布的衛氣和津液溫養皮毛。若肺氣虛弱，不能宣發衛氣和津液於皮毛，則皮毛憔悴、枯槁，衛氣不固，易感外邪。

(4) The Relationship among the Physiological Functions of the Lung

1) The Lung and the Large Intestine connect with each other, and form an exterior & interior relationship due to the interconnection of their meridians. Therefore, diseases in the Lung and the Large Intestine can affect each other.

2) The Lung joins to the skin and its qi flourishes in the body hair, which includes the sweat glands. So, the Lung serves to screen the body against attacks from external pathogens. The defensive qi and the body fluids, which are transported by the Lung, warm and nourish the skin and the body hair. If Lung qi is deficient, it will not be able to diffuse fluids and secure defensive qi. This can result in withered and dry body hair and skin, and insecure defensive qi. Under these conditions, external evils can easily afflict the body.

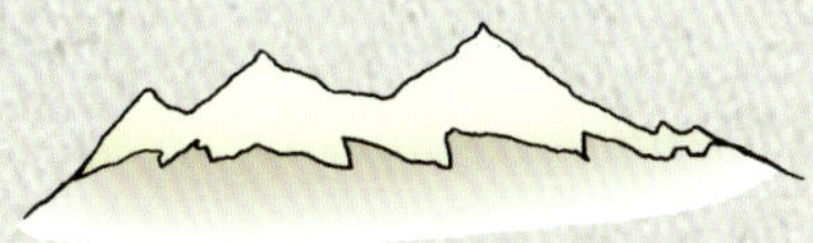

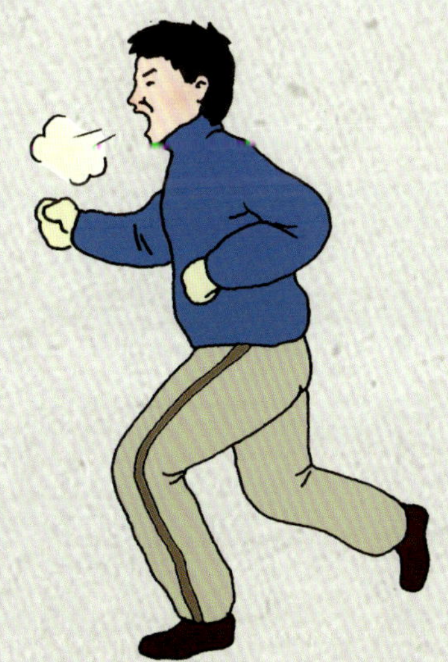

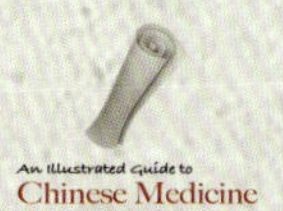

3）開竅於鼻

鼻的通氣和嗅覺功能，都依賴於肺氣的宣發作用。若肺氣宣暢，呼吸平和，則鼻竅通暢，呼吸自如，且嗅覺靈敏，香臭明辨；若肺失宣肅，呼吸不利，則鼻塞不通，氣體交換不利，嗅覺遲鈍。

4）在誌爲憂（悲）

憂、悲均爲人體正常的情緒變化或情感反映，但過度悲哀或過度憂傷，有礙身體健康，最易消耗肺氣。反之，肺虛亦易生悲憂而情緒低落。

5）在液爲涕

涕，即鼻涕，若寒邪襲肺，則鼻流清涕；若肺熱壅盛，則流涕黄濁；若燥邪犯肺，則可見鼻幹而痛。

5. 腎

主要功能是藏精、主水、主納氣。

（1）腎的位置

腎位於腰部，脊柱兩側，形如豇豆，左右各一個。《内經》雲“腰者，腎之府”。

（2）腎的比喻

腎藏先天之精，主生殖，爲生命之本源，故稱爲“先天之本”。腎宅真陰真陽，故又稱“水火之臟”。腎能資助、促進、協調全身各臟腑之陰陽，故稱腎爲“五臟陰陽之本”。

3) The Lung opens into the nose. The nose's olfactory function relies on its ability to diffuse the qi. If Lung qi is properly diffused, the breathing will be calm, the nasal passages will be open, and the sense of smell will be keen. If the Lung fails to diffuse and purify, then a stuffy nose, uneven breathing, and lessened sense of smell can result.

4) In five-phases theory, sorrow is the emotion of the Lung. While sorrow is a normal emotional response, in excess it is harmful and can easily disperse and consume the Lung qi. And also, deficiency of Lung qi gives rise to sorrow and low spirits.

5) The Lung's fluid is nasal mucus. If cold evil attacks the Lung, clear nasal mucus is manifested. If heat congests the Lung, yellow and turbid nasal mucus will be seen. If dryness evil attacks the Lung, it may result in a painful and dry nose.

5. The Kidney

The main functions of the Kidney are to store the essence, govern water and grasp qi.

(1) The Location of the Kidney

The Kidney is located in the limbs, on either sides of the spinal column, and its shape resemble black-eyed peas. *The Yellow Emperor's Classic of Internal Medicine <Huáng Dì Nèi Jīng>* states: "The lumbus is the house of Kidney".

(2) The Kidney's Metaphor

The Kidney stores congenital essence, governs reproduction, and is the source of life. Therefore the Kidney is the root of congenital constitution. It houses the true yin and the true yang, therefore it is called the organ of water and fire. The Kidney can support, promote and harmonize the yin and the yang of every Zang-fu organ, so therefore it is called the root of yin, yang and organs.

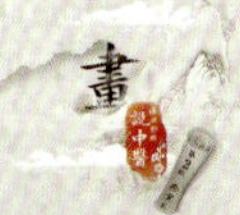

(3) 腎的生理功能

1) 腎藏精

主生長、發育和生殖。腎藏之精包括"先天之精"和"後天之精"。先天之精禀受於父母的生殖之精,後天之精來源於攝入的飲食物。腎中的生殖之精是孕育人體胚胎的原始物質,即精子和卵子。腎藏之精可以化爲腎氣,腎氣通過三焦布散到全身,促進機體及生長發育和生殖,以調節人體的代謝和生理功能。人體的生長壯老死,就是腎中精氣由未盛到逐漸充盛,由充盛到逐漸衰少繼而耗竭的演變過程。

(3) Physiological Functions of the Kidney

1) The Kidney stores essence, governs growth, development and reproduction. The essence stored by the Kidney includes congenital essence and acquired essence. Congenital essence is a reproductive essence inherited from the parents. Acquired essence's origin is the food and drink that enters the body and is absorbed. The Kidney's reproductive essence is an original substance of the embryo, namely from the sperm and the ovum. The Kidney essence can be changed into the Kidney qi which is distributed through the San Jiao to the whole body. It promotes growth, development, and reproduction, and regulates the body's metabolism and physiological functions. Birth, youth, maturity, aging and death are the life processes of the Kidney's essential qi as it gradually changes states from abundance to waning and finally to exhaustion.

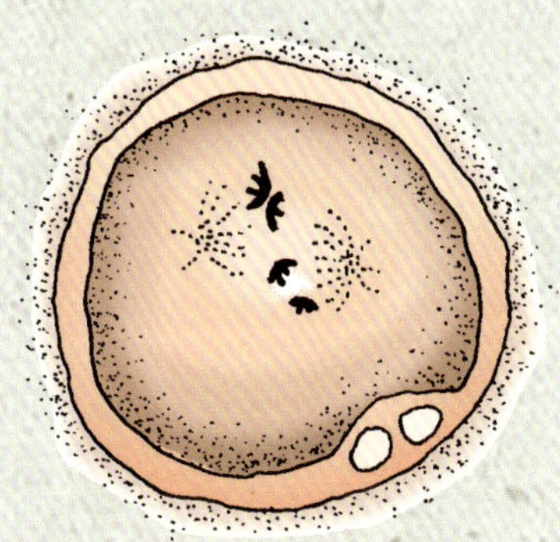

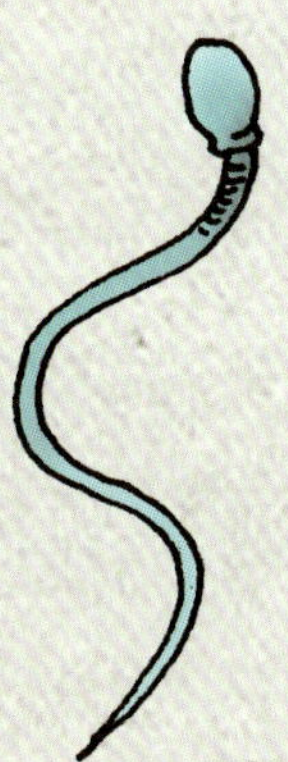

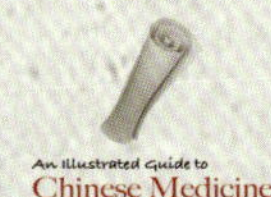

女子一生腎氣的節律

The stage of kidney-qi during a woman's life

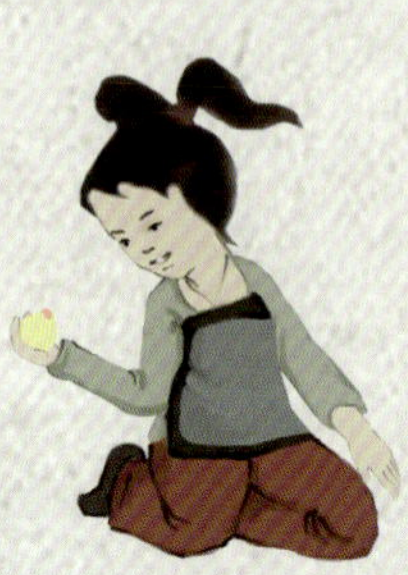

七歲
seven years old
腎氣盛，更换牙齒
The kidney-qi is prosperous and the baby teeth are replaced by permanent teeth.

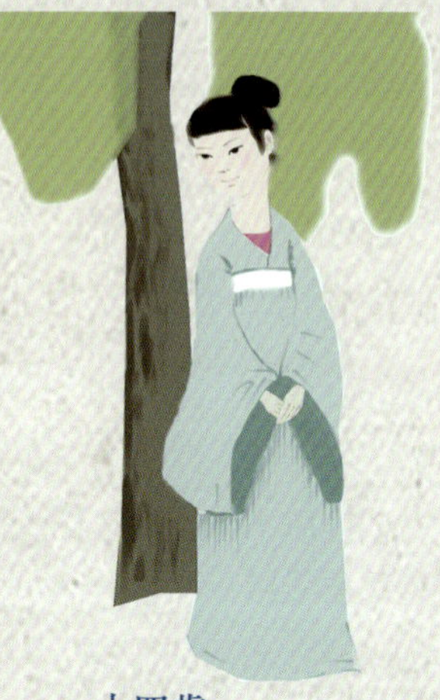

十四歲
foureen years old
天癸至， 月經來潮
Tiangui comes and menstruation beginning.

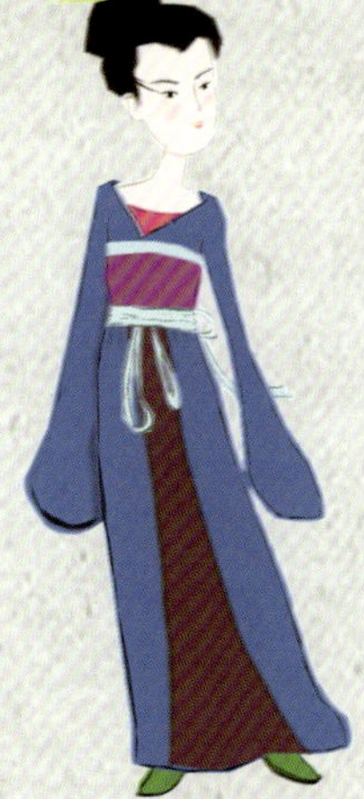

二十一歲
twenty-one years old
腎氣平均， 真牙生而長極
The kidney-qi is average and the teeth are strong.

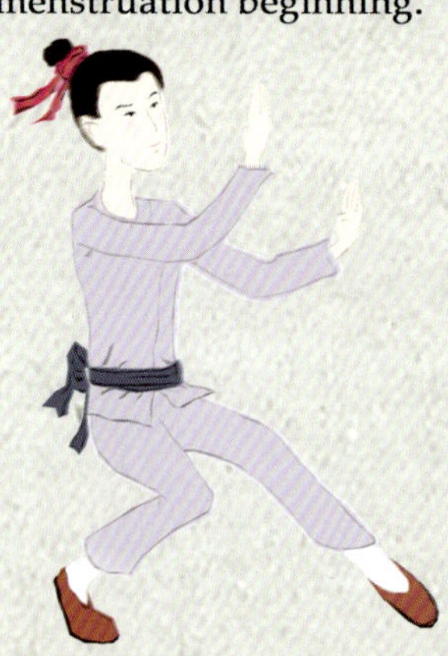

二十八歲
twenty-eight years old
筋骨堅， 發長極， 身體盛壯
The bones are strong, hair is shiny and the human body is healthy.

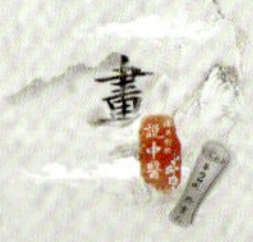

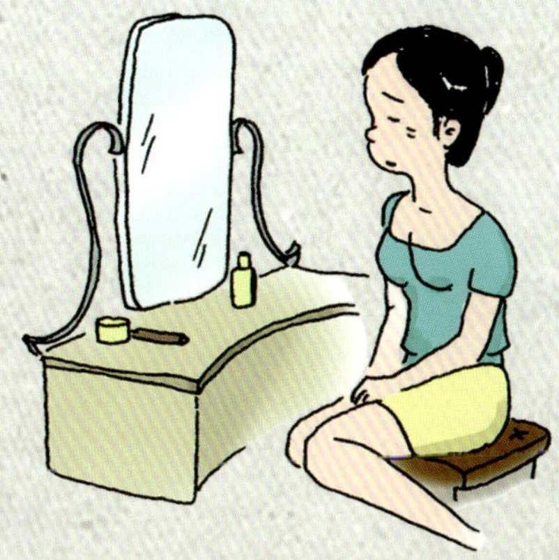

三十五歲
thirty-five years old
陽明脉衰， 面始焦， 發始在墮
Meridian of Yangming decline, the complexion is pale, the hair begins loss.

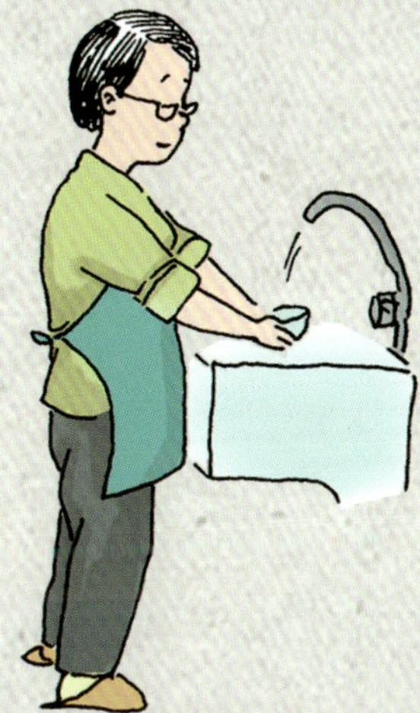

四十二歲
forty-two years old
三陽脉衰于上， 面皆焦， 發始白
Three upper yang veins decline, the complexion is pale and the hair is grey.

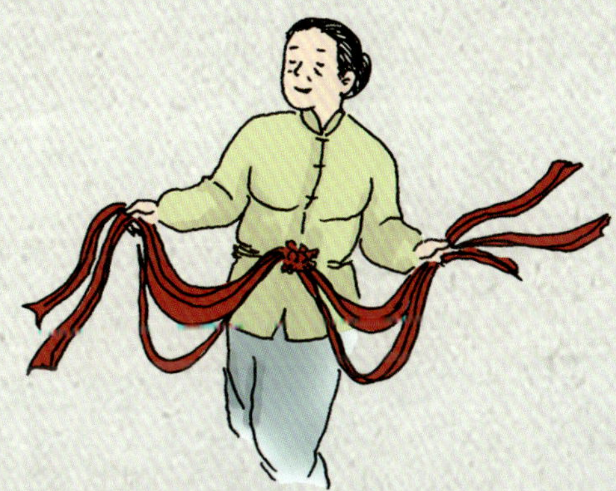

四十九歲
forty-nine years old
天癸竭， 月經斷絶
Tiangui and menstruation exhaust.

男子一生腎氣的節律

The stage of kidney-qi during a man's life

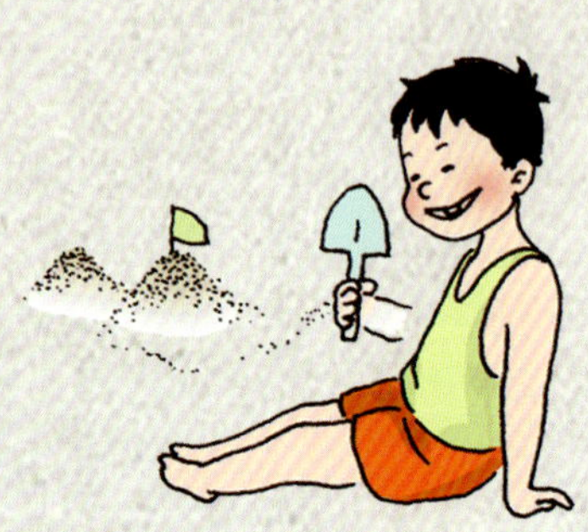

八歲

eight years old

腎氣實， 發長齒更

The kidney-qi is solid, the hair grows longer and faster and the baby teeth are replaced by permanent teeth.

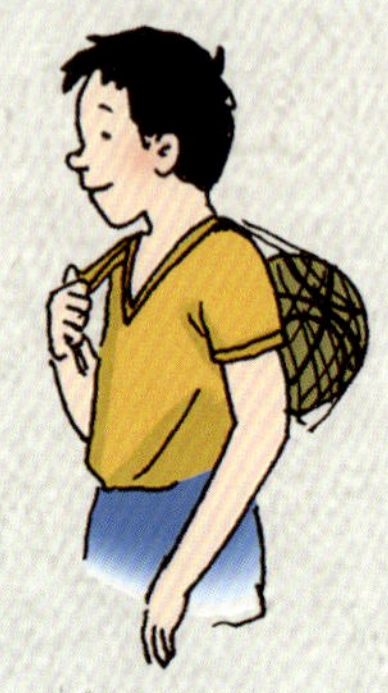

十六歲

sixteen years old

腎氣盛， 天癸至， 精氣溢

The kidney-qi is prosperous, Tiangui comes and the essential qi of the kidney spills.

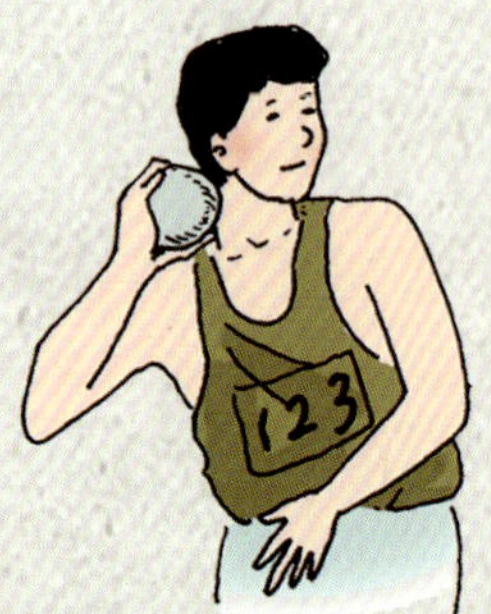

二十四歲

twenty-four years old

腎氣平均， 筋骨勁强

The kidney-qi is average and the bones are strong.

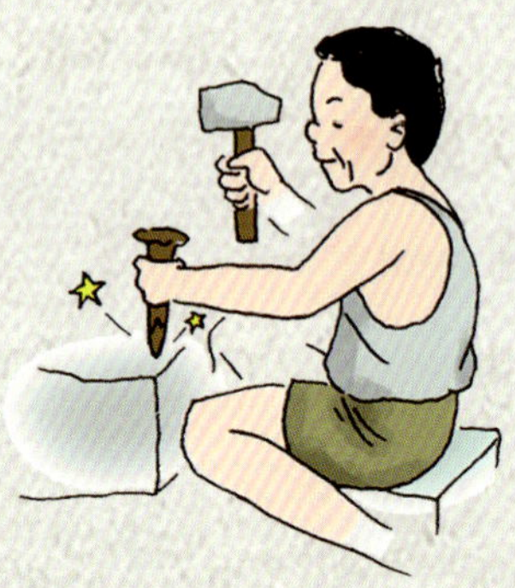

三十二歲

thirty-two years old

筋骨隆盛， 肌肉滿壯

The bones and muscles are extremely strong.

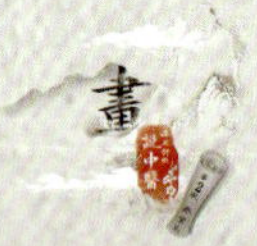

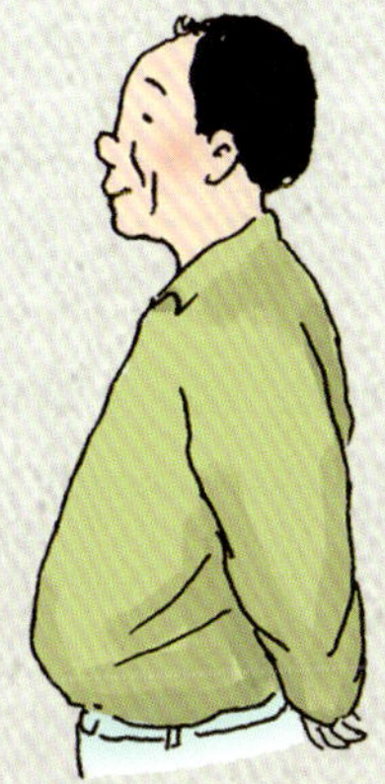

四十歲
forty years old
頭發始脱， 腎氣衰， 發墮齒槁
The hair begins loss, the kidney-qi declines and the teeth loosen.

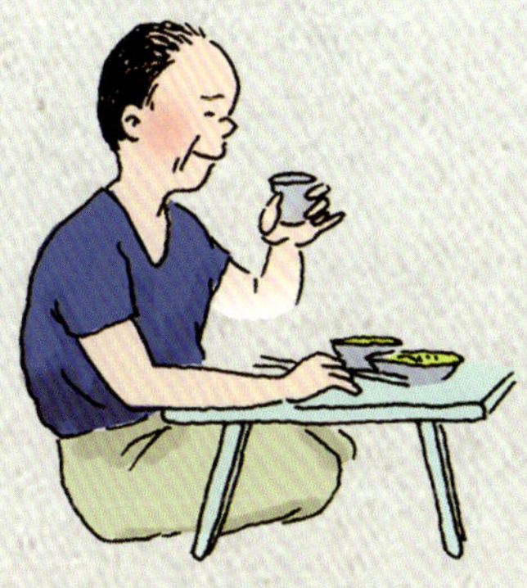

四十八歲
forty-eight years old
陽氣衰竭于上， 面焦， 發鬢斑白
The upper yang-qi declines, the complexion is pale and the hair is grey.

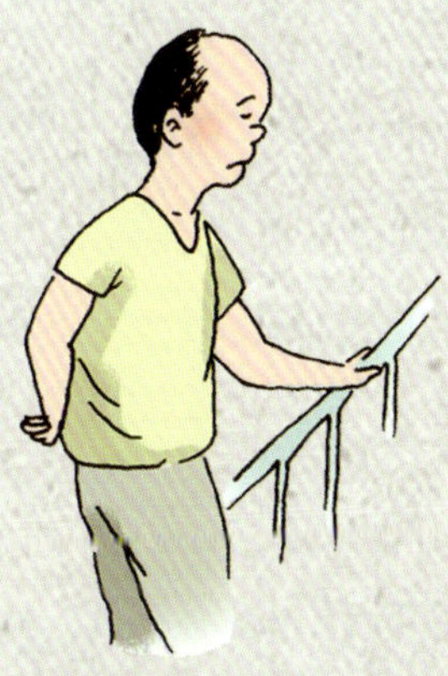

五十六歲
fifty-six years old
肝腎衰， 筋弱精少
The function of the liver and kidney declines.

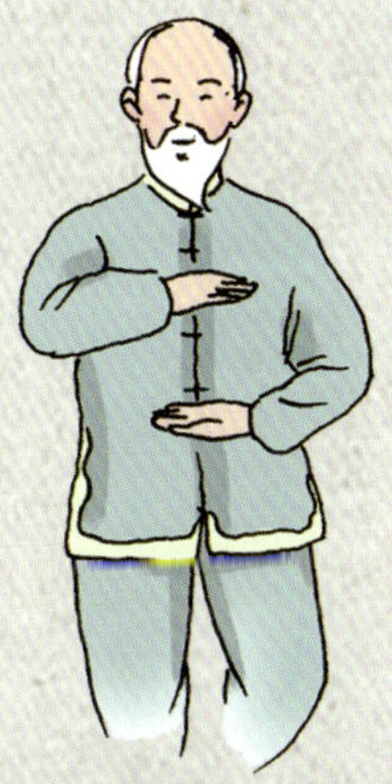

六十四歲
sixty-four years old
腎精衰少， 齒脱發落
The kidney essence declines, the teeth and the hair loosen.

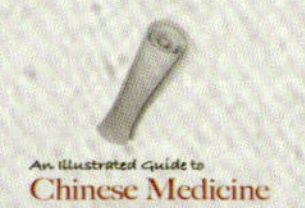

2）腎主水

調節體内水液平衡。它將臟腑組織代謝後的水份及代謝産物化爲尿液、排出體外。

3）腎主納氣

腎有攝納肺吸入之氣而調節呼吸的作用。肺吸入之氣，必須下歸於腎，由腎氣爲之攝納，呼吸才能通暢、調匀。

2) The Kidney governs water and regulates its balance. The Kidney turns water and other metabolic products from the Zang-fu organs into urine, and then discharges it.

3) The Kidney governs grasping qi. This function of the Kidney is to grasp the Lung's inhaled air and to regulate breathing. The Lung's inhaled air must descend to the Kidney to be absorbed and received, thus resulting in smooth and even breathing.

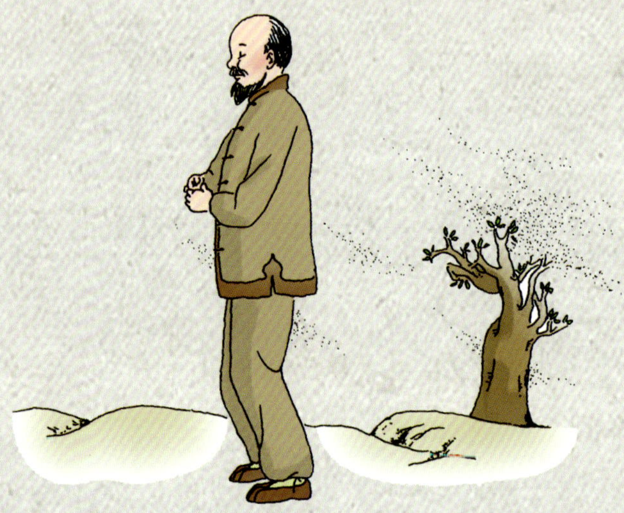

（4）腎的生理聯係

1）腎合膀胱

腎，下通於膀胱，經絡相互絡屬，構成表裏關係。兩者的疾病可以相互影響。

2）腎在誌爲恐

長期或突然的過度恐懼可使腎氣不固，耗精傷腎。

(4) The Relationship among the Physiological Functions of the Kidney

1) The Kidney and the Bladder connect with each other, and form an exterior— interior relationship due to their meridians interconnection. Therefore, diseases in the Kidney and the Bladder affect each other.

2) In five-phase theory, fear is the emotion of the Kidney. Long-term or sudden excessive fear may result in insecure Kidney qi, consumption of essence, and Kidney damage.

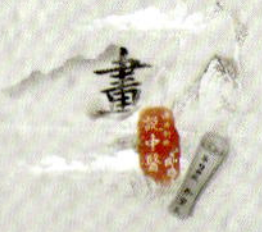

3）腎主骨

腎精能促進骨骼的生長發育和影響骨髓、脊髓、腦髓的充盈和發育。

3) The Kidney governs bones. Kidney essence can promote the skeletal growth and development, and influence the filling and development of the bone marrow, spinal cord and the Brain.

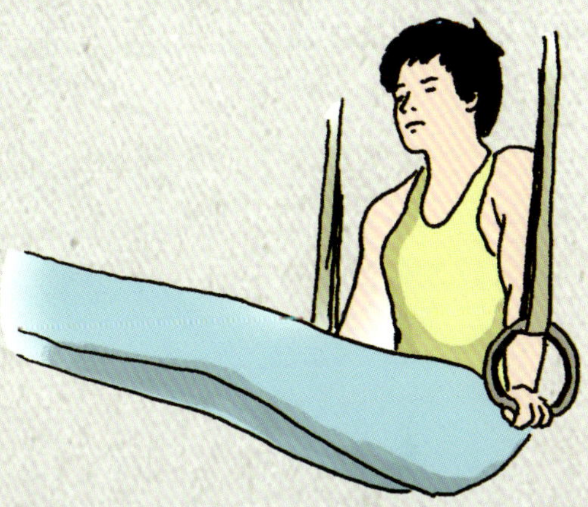

4）腎開竅於耳及前、後陰

腎的精氣不足，就會出現耳鳴、聽力減退。大小便的排泄要依賴腎氣的控製。二陰，即前陰和後陰。前陰是外生殖器和尿道，有排尿和生殖的作用；後陰是指肛門，有排泄糞便作用。

4) Kidney opens into the ears, and to the front and back yin (the two yin are the genitalia and anus orifices). Insufficiency of Kidney essential qi may give rise to tinnitus and diminished hearing. Discharging urine and stools depend on Kidney qi. The two yin include the anterior yin and posterior yin. The anterior yin includes the urethra and genitalia, their function is in discharging urine and reproduction. The posterior yin is the anus, which discharges the stool.

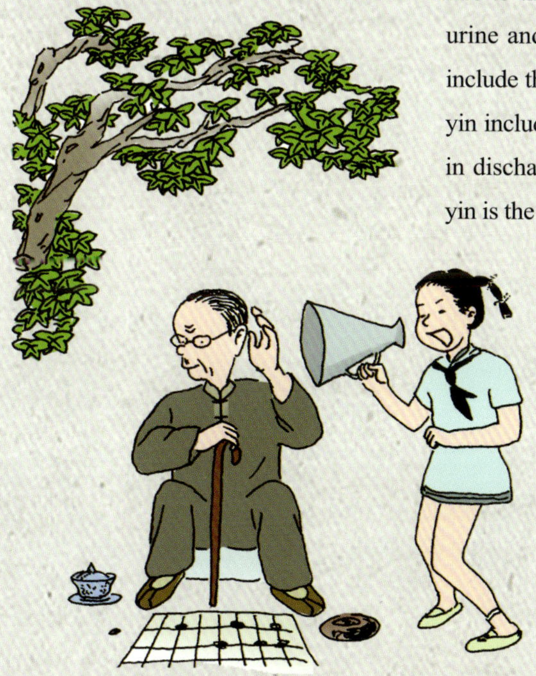

二陰主司二便，而二便的排泄均與腎有關。尿液的貯藏和排泄雖由膀胱所司，但尿液的生成及排泄必須依賴腎的氣化和固攝作用才能完成。若腎之氣化和固攝作用失常，則可見尿少、尿閉、水腫或尿頻、遺尿、尿失禁等小便異常的病證。

大便的排泄，本屬大腸傳化糟粕的功能，但也與腎氣的推動和固攝作用相關，若腎氣不足，推動無力則可致氣虛便秘、固攝無權則可致大便失禁，久瀉滑脫。

前陰是人體的外生殖器，其生殖功能與腎中精氣密切相關。若腎精腎氣不足，則可導致人體性器官的發育不良和生殖能力的減退。從而出現男子陽痿、早泄、少精、滑精，遺精及不育等，女子則見性冷漠，月經異常及不孕等病證。

5）其華在發

發的生長與脱落、潤澤與枯槁是腎中精氣盛衰的反映。發的生長，賴血以養，故有“發爲血之餘”之説。若腎中精氣衰退，則頭發變白、枯槁而易脱落。

6）在液爲唾

唾，是唾液中較稠厚的部分，能潤澤口腔，並能滋養腎精。

The main function of the two yin, related to the Kidney, is in discharging urine and stool. Although the storage and discharge of urine are controlled by the Bladder, urine formation and discharge rely on the function of Kidney qi to transform, secure and contain. If Kidney qi fails in these functions, it may lead to frequent urination, enuresis and urinary incontinence.

Although the function of discharging stool is governed by the Large Intestine, it is also relies on the securing and containing function of the Kidney qi. Insufficiency of Kidney qi may cause qi deficiency which may give rise to constipation, or insecurity of Kidney qi may cause long term diarrhea and rectal prolapse.

The anterior yin is the external genitalia. Its reproductive function relies on Kidney qi. Kidney essence and qi deficiency may cause abnormal development of genitalia and decrease the reproductive ability. About men, this may result in impotency, seminal emission, premature ejaculation, and nocturnal emission. About women, low libido, irregular menstrual cycle and infertility.

5) The Kidney Flourishes in the Hair

The waxing and waning of Kidney essential qi is reflected in the growth, loss, glossiness and dryness of the hair on the head. It also relies on blood nourishment, thus it is named the surplus of the blood. If the Kidney essential qi declines, the hair will turn white, dry and fall out.

6) The Kidney fluid is spittle. Spittle is a thick fluid, which can moisten the oral cavity, and enrich and nourish the Kidney essence.

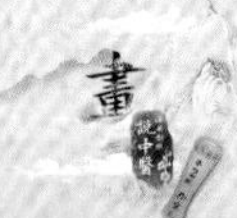

三、六腑

六腑是膽、胃、小腸、大腸、膀胱、三焦的總稱。它們的生理功能是“傳化物”。

1. 膽

是中空的囊狀器官，膽與肝相連，具有貯存和排泄膽汁的功能。

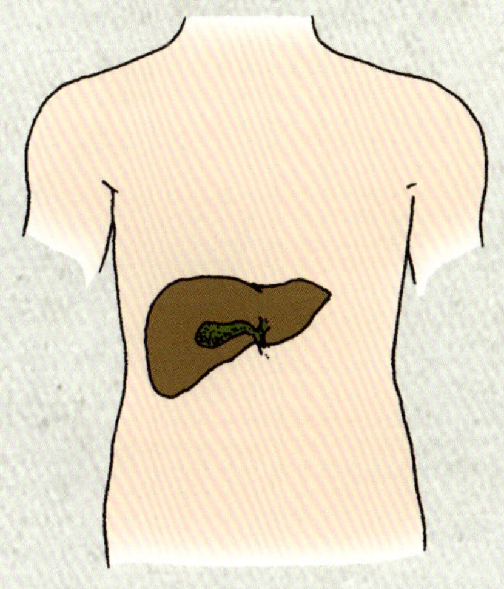

膽汁來源於肝臟，味苦，呈黄綠色，貯存於膽。並通過膽道排泄於小腸。膽汁具有促進飲食物消化的作用。

The Six Fu-organs

The six Fu-organs are the Gallbladder, Stomach, Small Intestine, Large Intestine, Bladder, and San Jiao. Their physiological functions are to pass and transform substances.

1. The Gallbladder

The Gallbladder is a hollow sac organ, located under the right lobe of the Liver. Its functions are to store and excrete bile.

Gallbladder bile forms in the Liver. The bile is bitter in taste, has a yellow-green color and it is stored in the Gallbladder. The bile passes through the Gallbladder passages into the small intestine, where it aids the digestion.

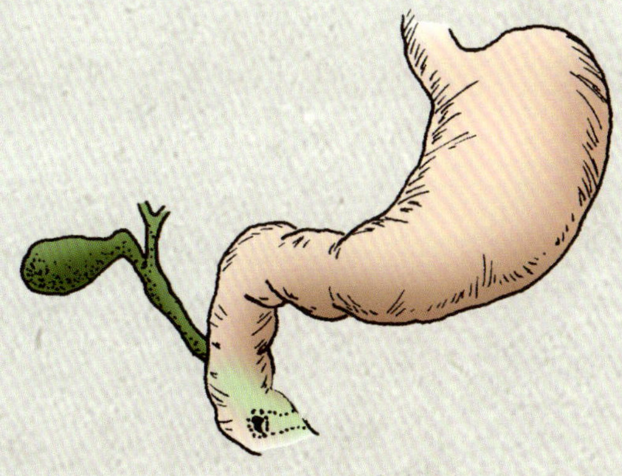

肝失疏泄，膽汁的分泌與排泄受阻，會出現厭食，厭油膩，腹脹，腹瀉等癥。若膽汁上逆，則可見口苦，嘔吐黃綠苦水，若濕熱蘊結肝膽，膽汁外溢發爲黃疸。

If the Liver fails in the function of free coursing, the secretion and excretion of the bile will be obstructed, which may result in loss of appetite, aversion to greasy and oily food, abdominal distention, and diarrhea. Gallbladder bile counterflows upwards, it will cause bitter taste in the mouth and vomiting yellow-green bitter fluids. If damp-heat accumulates in the Liver and Gallbladder, the bile flows out towards the body's exterior, resulting in jaundice.

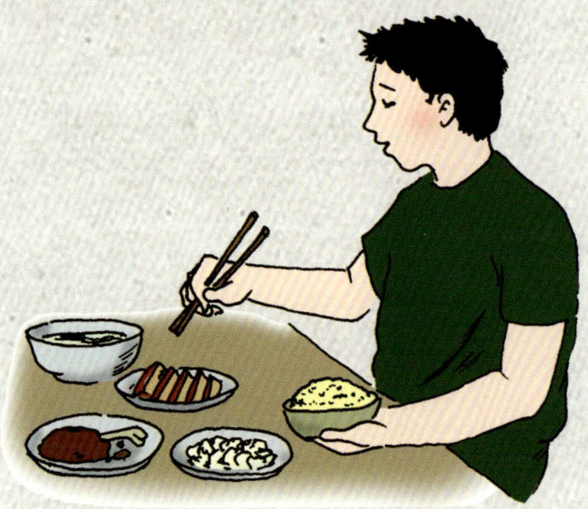

膽爲六腑之一，但它貯藏精汁而不接受水谷或糟粕，所以與其他五腑有所不同，故又稱奇恒之府。

The Gallbladder is one of the six Fu-organs, but it stores refined bile and does not receive water, food, or waste, therefore it differs from the other five Fu-organs, and belongs to the extraordinary organs.

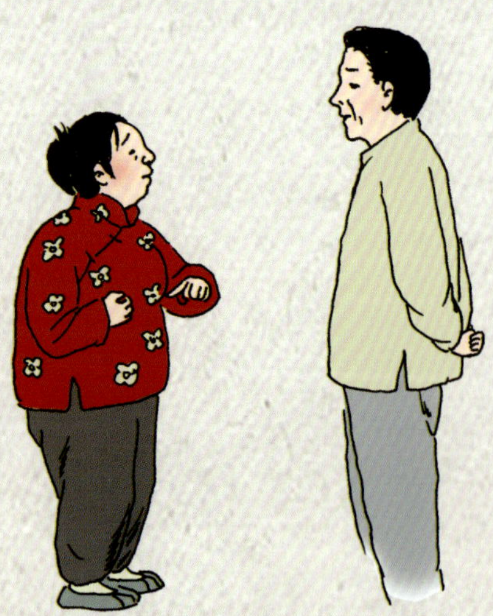

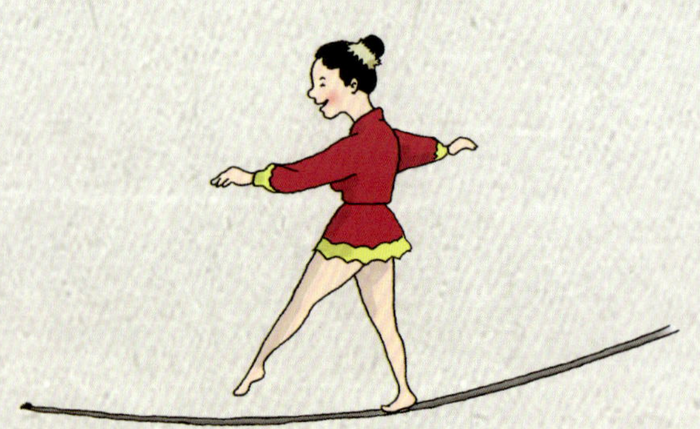

膽主決斷。人的勇怯與膽氣的强弱密切相關。

The Gallbladder governs decision-making. People's bravery and cowardliness are closely related to the strength or weakness of their Gallbladder qi.

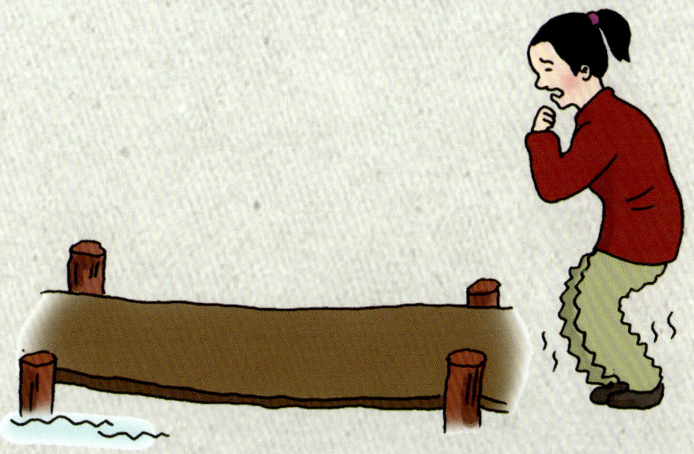

2. 胃

位於膈下，腹腔上部，上接食道，下通小腸。上口爲賁門，下口爲幽門。胃又稱胃脘，主要功能是受納與腐熟水谷。

2. The Stomach

The stomach is located under the diaphragm. Its upper part, the cardia, connects with the esophagus, and its lower part, the pylorus, connects to the small intestine. Another name for the Stomach is epigastrium. The Stomach's main functions are receiving and decomposing food and drink.

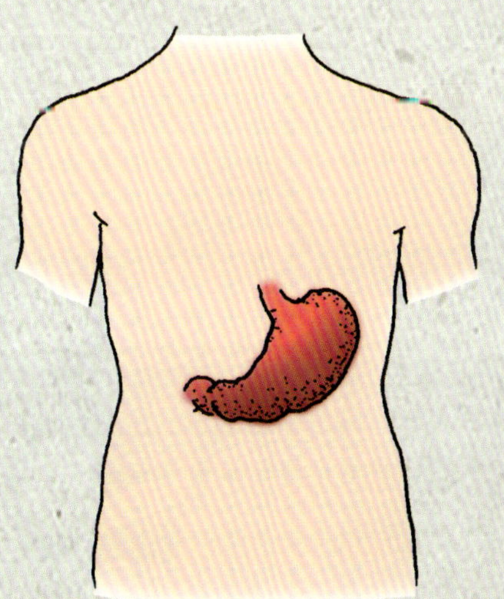

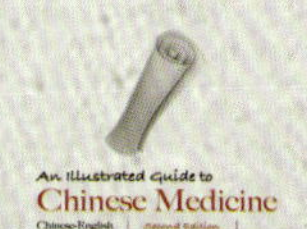

主受納，腐熟水谷。受納，指胃具有接受和容納飲食物的作用。腐熟，是指飲食物經過胃的初步消化，形成食糜的讀思，故胃稱爲“太倉”、“水谷之海”。

The Stomach receives and contains food and drink. Decomposing is an early stage of digestion, forming chyme (thick semi-fluid mass of party digested food that is passed from the stomach to the duodenum). Therefore, the Stomach is named the great granary and sea of grain and water.

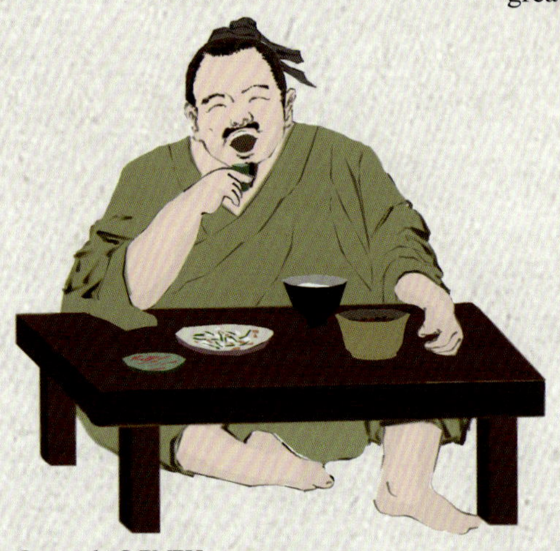

胃主通降，以降爲和。胃之通降是降濁。降濁是受納的前提條件。若胃氣不降，反而上升，則可出現嗳氣酸腐、惡心、嘔吐、呃逆等癥。

The Stomach governs descending, when it is balanced, its qi will descend. Stomach descending turbid matter is a precondition for receiving food. If Stomach qi fails to descend, it will give rise to counterflow ascent as seen in putrid belching, acid regurgitation, nausea, vomiting and hiccups.

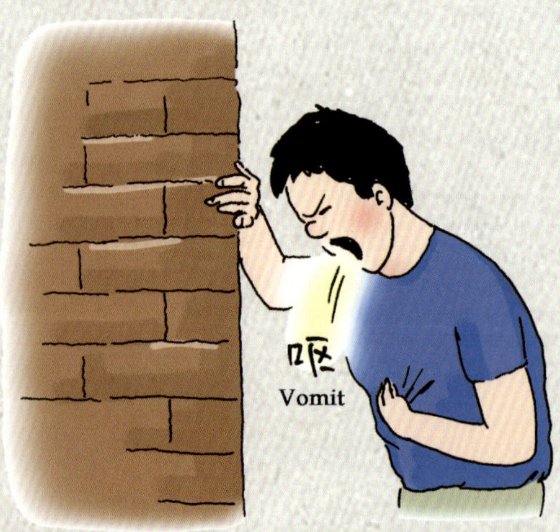

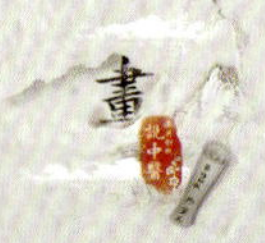

3. 小腸

上接胃，下接大腸。其生理功能是泌別清濁。即將胃傳下來的食糜，作進一步的消化，並將清者吸收，濁者下注大腸，小腸有病則清濁不分，而出現大便稀溏，小便短少等。

4. 大腸

位於腹中，上接闌門，與小腸相通，下端緊接肛門。

3. The Small Intestine

The Small Intestine's upper part meets the Stomach while the lower part meets the Large Intestine. The physiological function of the Small Intestine is to separate clear from turbid. Small Intestine further digests chyme that was already descended by the Stomach by absorbing the clear (qi) and descending the turbid (qi) to the Large Intestine. If the Small Intestine fails to separate clear from turbid, it may result in loose stools and scanty urine.

4. The Large Intestine

The Large Intestine is located in the abdomen, its upper end meets the ileocecal valve and connects to the Small Intestine, and its lower end is the anus.

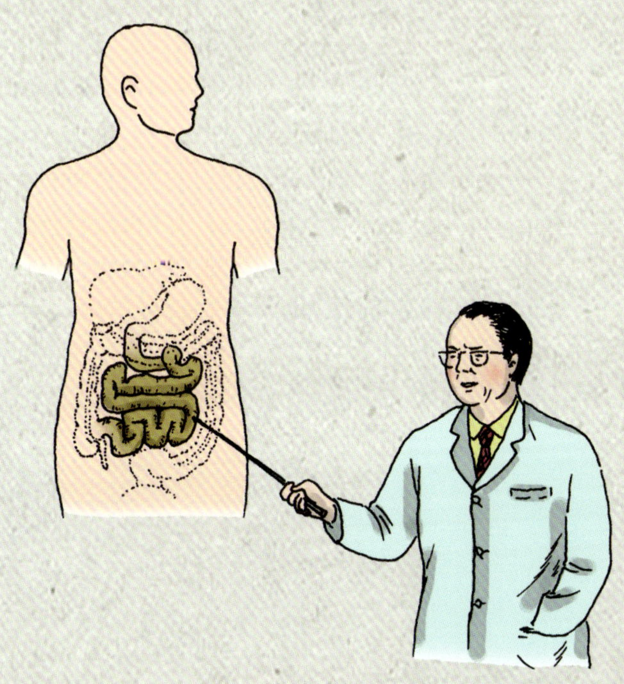

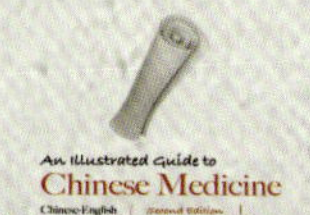

大腸的生理功能是傳化糟粕，吸收水分。飲食物的殘渣由小腸下注大腸，經大腸吸收其中的部分水分，使之成爲成形的糞便，然後傳導下行，經肛門排出體外，如果大腸的吸收傳導功能失常則出現腸鳴、腹瀉或大便秘結等癥。

The physiological functions of the Large Intestine are to transform waste and absorb fluids. The Large Intestine receives the waste of food and drink from the Small Intestine. It absorbs fluids and forms feces, which later descend and exit through the anus. If the Large Intestine fails in these functions, it can lead to borborygmus, diarrhea and constipation.

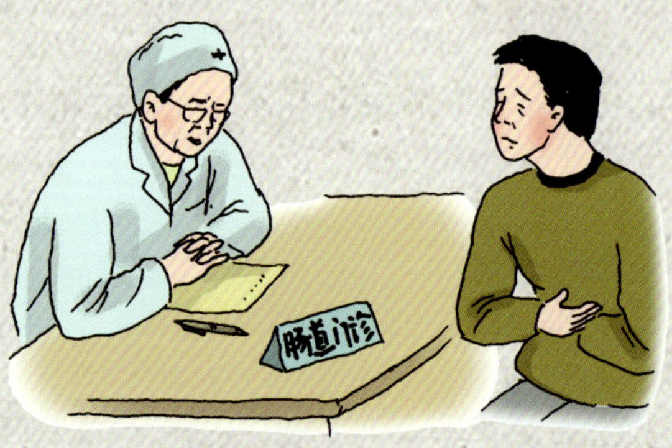

5. 膀胱

位於小腹中央，其上有輸尿管與腎臟相通，其下有尿道，開口於前陰。

膀胱生理功能是貯尿和排尿。在人體水液代謝過程中，多餘的水液在腎的氣化作用下形成尿液，下輸膀胱，並可及時自主地排出體外。

5. The Urinary Bladder

The urinary Bladder is located in the lower abdomen. Its upper end connects to the kidney by the Ureter; its lower end connects to the urethra, which opens to the genitalia.

The physiological functions of the Bladder are to store and discharge urine. During the process of water metabolism the Kidney qi transforms waste fluids into urine, which descend to the Bladder for discharge.

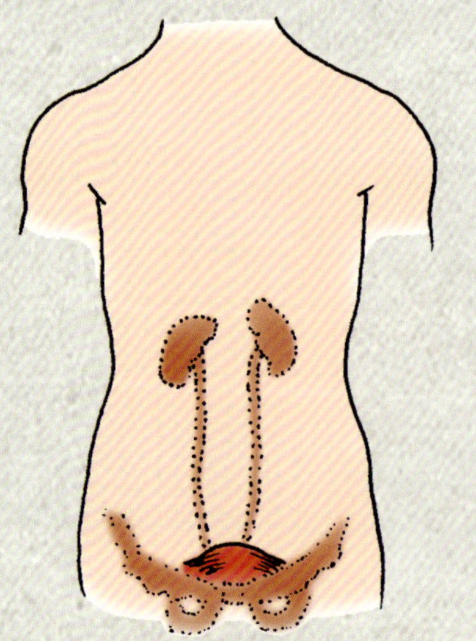

膀胱的貯尿和排尿功能，全賴於腎的氣化功能。如果膀胱氣化不利就可出現尿少或癃閉，若膀胱不能約束，就會出現尿頻，小便失禁等癥。

The Bladder's functions of storing and discharging urine rely on the Kidney qi transformation function. If this function fails it can result in scanty urine and urinary difficulty. Failure of the Bladder to retain urine can result in frequent urination and incontinence of urine.

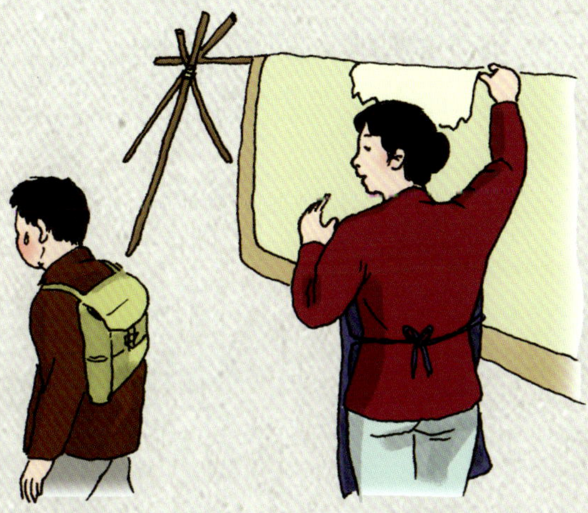

6. 三焦

爲中醫六腑之一，也是中醫學一個特殊概念。横膈以上的胸部爲上焦，膈下臍上的上腹部爲中焦，臍以下的下腹部爲下焦。

6. The San Jiao

The San Jiao is one of the six Fu-organs, and it is an exceptional concept. The Upper Jiao is located above the diaphragm; the Middle Jiao is between the diaphragm and the umbilicus; and the Lower Jiao is below the umbilicus.

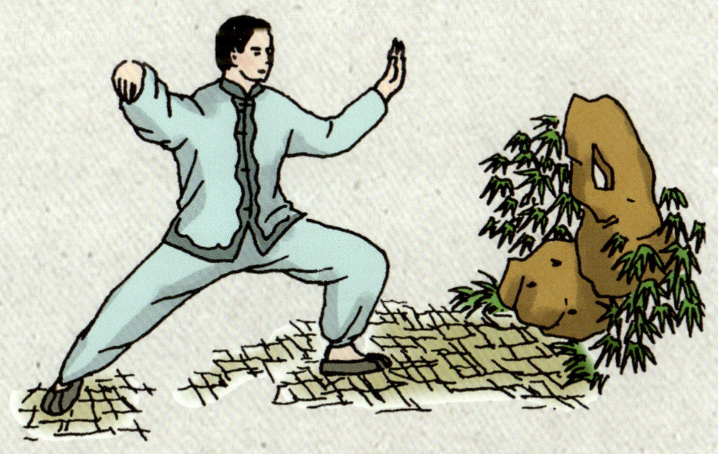

三焦的生理功能：一是通行元氣。元氣根於腎，通過三焦而輸布到五臟六腑，充沛於全身，以激發、推動各個臟腑組織的功能活動。

三焦的生理功能之二是爲水谷、水液運行之道路。人體的飲食水谷，特别是水液的運化吸收，輸布與排泄，都是通過三焦的通道來完成的。

上焦如霧　通過心臟的搏動，肺部的氣體交換，將飲食物的精微和肺部的清氣布散全身。以溫養臟腑、經絡、形體、官竅，故又稱“上焦主宣”。

One of the San Jiao's physiological functions is to distribute original qi. Original qi is rooted in the Kidney, and transported by the San Jiao to the five Zang-organs and the six Fu-organs. This stimulates the activities of organs and tissues.

The second physiological function of the San Jiao is as the passageway for food and fluids. The absorption and distribution, transport and transformation, and excretion of food, and especially of fluids, are all accomplished through the San Jiao passageway.

The Upper Jiao is as a mist. The refined essence and the Lung's clear qi are spread to the whole body by the Heart's beating and the Lung's qi exchange, in order to warm and nourish the Zang-fu organs, channels and collaterals. This explains the saying that the Upper Jiao governs diffusion.

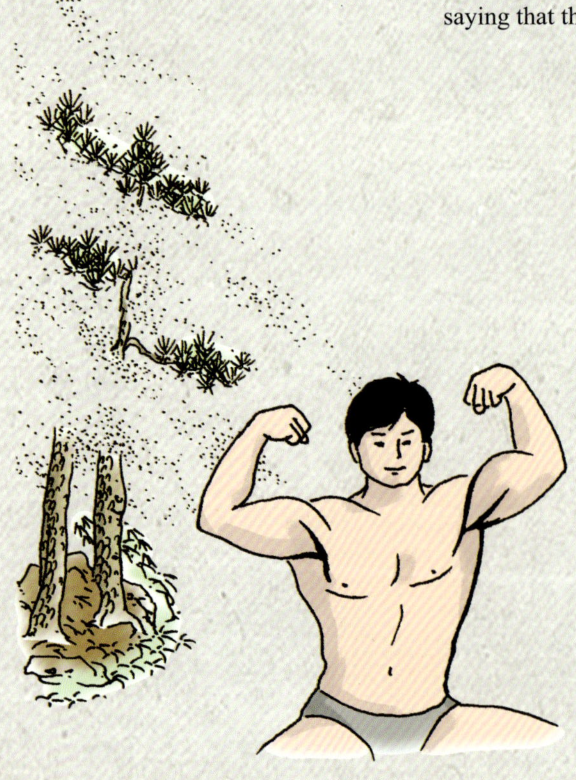

中焦如漚　即腐熟水谷，運化精微，以化生氣血，與脾胃功能有關，故又稱“中焦主化”。

下焦如瀆　水谷分别清濁之後的糟粕，經大小便排出體外，與腎、膀胱、大腸功能有關。故又稱“下焦主出”。

The Middle Jiao is as a maceration chamber. The functions of the Spleen and Stomach are related to the actions of receiving and decomposing food and drink, transforming and transporting the refined essence, and transforming qi into blood. Thus, it is said that the Middle Jiao governs transformation.

The Lower Jiao is as a drain. The waste separated from food and water exit the body as feces, and is related to the functions of Kidney, Bladder and Large Intestine. Thus, it is said that the Lower Jiao governs excretion.

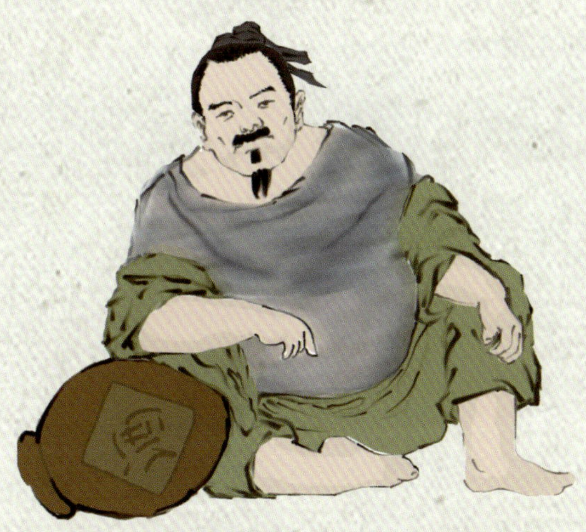

四、奇恒之府

Extraordinary Organs

腦、髓、骨、脈、膽、女子胞，總稱爲奇恒之府。它們的形態結構多爲中空，與臟相似，但其功能多主藏精氣，與腑有别而類於臟，故稱之爲奇恒之臟。

The extraordinary organs include the brain, marrow, bone, blood vessels, Gallbladder, and Uterus. Their structure is hollow, similar to the Fu-organs. However, their main function is to store the essential qi, which differs from the Fu-organs and is similar to the Zang-organs.

1. 腦

爲奇恒之腑之一，位於顱内，由髓匯集而成，故稱“腦爲髓之海”。中國古人很早就十分重視腦的功能，稱腦爲“元神之府”“精明之府”。由於中醫藏象學説是以五臟爲中心，所以把大腦的功能分屬於五臟，即“心藏神、肺藏魄，肝藏魂，脾藏意，腎藏志”。

腦的生理功能，一是主精神思維，二是主感覺的接受，三是主運動的支配。

1. The Brain

The brain is one of the extraordinary organs. It is located inside the skull and produced from the marrow, thus it is said that the brain is the sea of marrow. The ancient Chinese people value the brain's functions, they called it the house of the original mind and of intelligence. Since the five Zang-organs is the core of the Zang-fu manifestation theory, the functions of the brain correspond respectively within the five Zang-organs. The Heart stores the mind; the Lung stores the corporeal soul; the Liver stores the ethereal soul; the Spleen stores the thought, and the Kidney stores the will.

The physiological functions of the brain are to govern thinking, receive sensory perceptions and control movement.

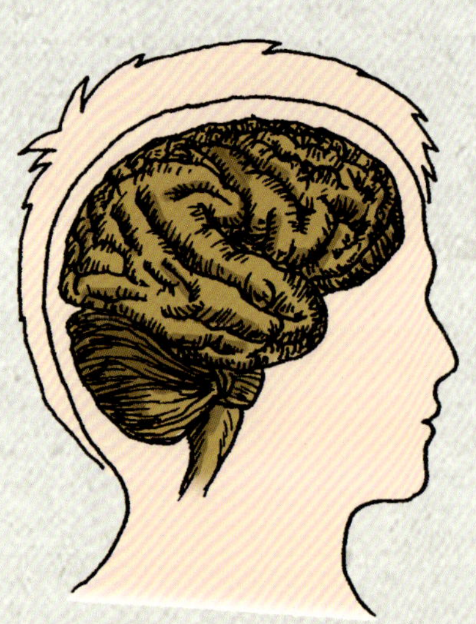

2. 髓

是一種膏狀物質，有骨髓、脊髓和腦髓之分。

髓的生理功能：充養腦髓、滋養骨骼、化生血液。

2. The Marrow

The marrow is a fatty substance, which includes the bone marrow, spinal cord and brain.

The physiological functions of the marrow are to nourish the brain and bones, and to generate blood.

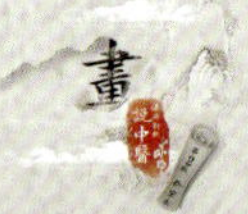

骨髓、脊髓和腦髓三者均爲腎中精氣所生，因此，腎中精氣直接影響着髓的化生。

The bone marrow, spinal cord and the brain are engendered by the Kidney's essential qi. Therefore, the Kidney's essential qi directly affects the generation of marrow.

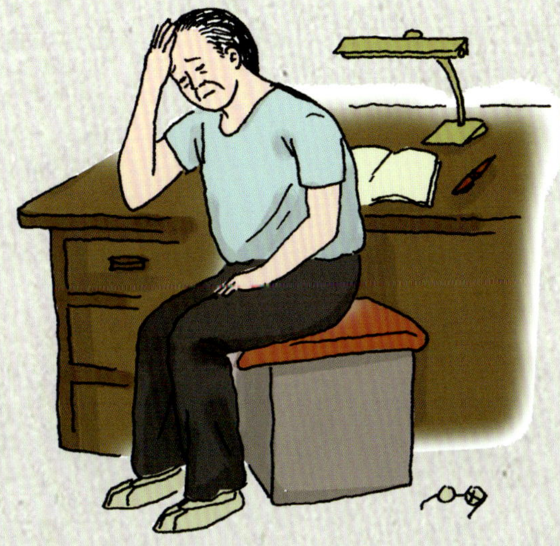

3. 骨

是構成人體的支架。其具有支撑人體、保護内臟貯藏骨髓和進行運動的功能。

4. 女子胞

又稱胞宫、子宫，位於小腹，有主月經和孕育胎兒的作用。與肝、腎、衝任二脈關係最爲密切。

5. 脈

爲血之府。脈是血氣運行的信道。脈和心臟構成一個相對獨立的密閉的血氣運行管道。人體氣血和臟腑功能活動正常與否均可顯現於脈，故脈象可以反應五臟的生理狀態及病理變化。

3. The Bone

The bone's structure supports the body, protects the internal organs, stores bone marrow and conducts movement.

4. The Uterus

The uterus is located in the lower abdomen. Its main functions are to govern menstruation and pregnancy. The Uterus is closely related to the Liver, Kidney and the penetrating vessel and conception vessel.

5. The Vessels

The vessels are the house of blood. The vessels and the Heart form an independent, self-contained passageway inside which blood and qi circulate. Vessels reflect the status of the functions of qi, blood, and Zang-fu organs. Therefore the pulse is a mirror of the physiological conditions and the pathological changes of the five Zang-organs.

第三章 精氣血津液
Chapter 3 Essence, Qi, Blood and Body Fluids

精、氣、血、津液，是構成人體和維持人體生命活動的基本物質。

Essence, qi, blood and body fluids are the basic components of the body and maintain its life activities.

一、精

Essence

精是體内的精微物質，是構成人體和維持人體生命活動的基本物質之一，精有廣義和狹義之分，廣義之精泛指體内一切精微的物質，包括氣、血、津液以及從飲食物中吸收的水谷精微等，統稱爲“精氣”。狹義之精，指腎中所藏之精，又稱“腎精”，分爲先天之精和後天之精。先天之精又稱“生殖之極”，是禀受於父母，與生俱來，爲生命的基礎，後天之精又稱“臟腑之精”是機體從飲食物中攝取的營養精華和臟腑代謝化生的精微物質。

Essence is a refined substance in the body, and it is one of the basic components that maintain the human body's life activities. The broad meaning of essence refers to all the refined substances in the body, which include qi, blood, body fluids and substances absorbed from dietary intake, all of these are called essence qi. The more narrow meaning is essence stored in the Kidney, called the Kidney essence which is divided into two parts: congenital constitution and acquired constitution. Congenital constitution is inherited from the parents and it is essence used for reproduction, therefore it is the fundamental substance of life. Acquired constitutional essence is also called the Zang-fu essence, it comes from the essential nutritional substances absorbed from the diet as well as those produced by the normal metabolism of the Zang-fu organs.

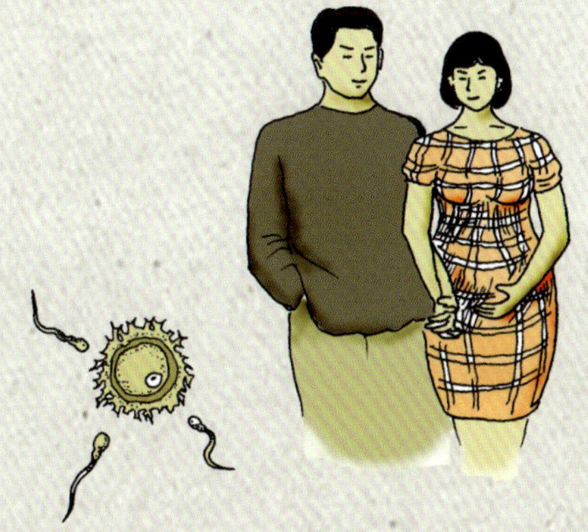

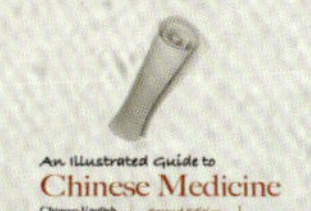

精的生理功能是繁衍生命，促進生長發育，濡養臟腑、生髓化血。

The physiological functions of essence are to generate life, promote growth and development, nourish the viscera, produce marrow and generate blood.

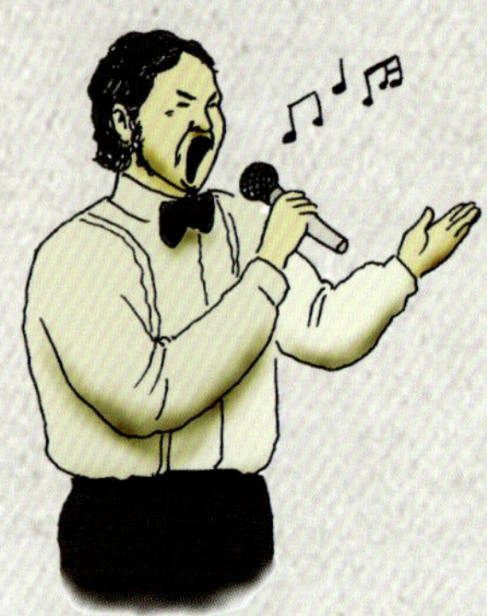

二、氣

Qi

氣是構成人體、維持人體生命活動的基本物質。

Qi is a basic substance which maintains the human body's life activities.

1. 氣的概念

構成人體的氣有兩種狀態，一是聚而成形的，如人身的血、精、津液等；另一種是彌散狀態，難以直接察知其態，如人體内宗氣、元氣、衛氣等。

1. The Concept of Qi

In the human body, there are two different states of qi, one refers to an accumulated state, which has taken forms, such as blood, essence and body fluids. The other refers to a spreading state, which is effused and hard to see, such as gathering qi, original qi and defensive qi.

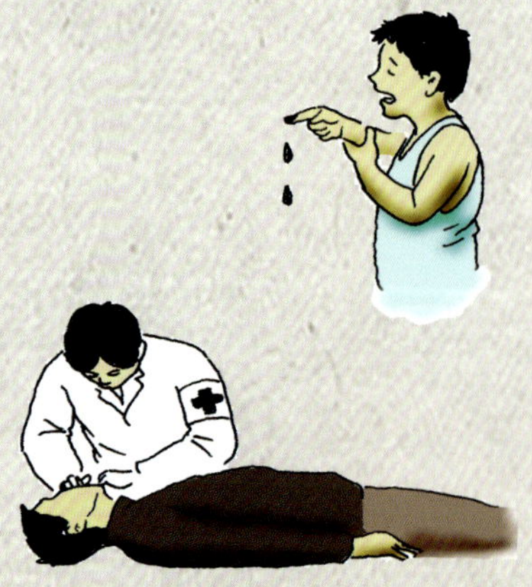

2. 氣的生成

氣的生成來源爲藏於腎的精氣，化生於飲食物的水谷之氣和來自於自然界的清氣。腎中的精氣禀受於父母，是先天之氣。水谷之氣由脾胃功能所化生，存在於自然界的清氣經肺吸入體内，兩者都是後天之氣。

2. The Formation of Qi

The qi of the human body comes from three sources: the essential qi stored in the Kidney, the essential qi from drinks and food, and the clear qi (air) which comes from nature. Congenital qi essence is inherited from one's parents and stored in the Kidney. Acquired constitutional essence is the food essence absorbed from the diet and generated in the Spleen and Stomach, and the clear qi is inhaled from nature into the Lung.

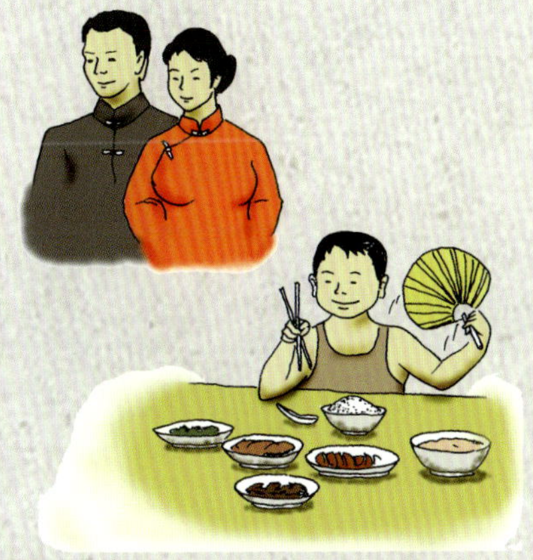

3. 氣的生理功能

（1）推動作用：人的生長發育，各臟腑、經絡的生理活動，血的生成和運行、津液生成、輸布和排泄，都要依靠氣的推動作用。

3. The Physiological Functions of Qi

(1) Promoting Function: one function of qi is to promote the normal activities in the body, such as its development and growth, the physiological function of every organ and meridians, the circulation and generation of blood, and the generation, supply, distribution and drainage of body fluids.

幾年不見，長成大姑娘了！
You have grown into a young lady since I saw you several years ago

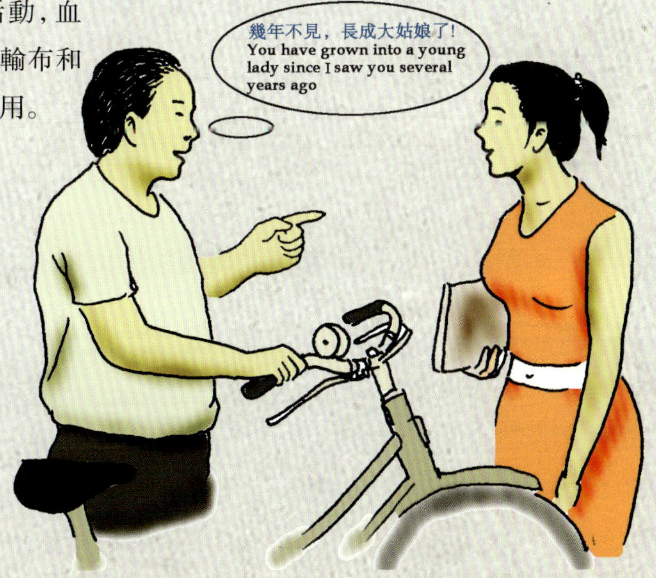

（2）溫煦作用：氣對機體各臟腑、經絡、皮膚和血、津液具有溫煦的作用。人體依靠氣的溫養，以維持正常體溫。

(2) Warming function: qi warms the viscera, meridians, skin, blood and body fluids. The human body relies on the warm function of qi to maintain normal temperature.

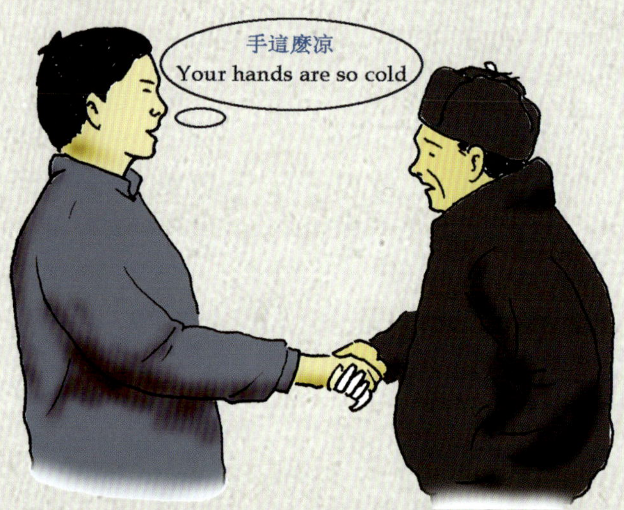

（3）防御作用：氣能護衛肌表防御外邪的入侵。正氣存内，邪不可幹。

(3) Defending function: qi guards the body surface from the invasion of an exterior evil. When the right qi is inside the body, the evil qi will not be able to attack.

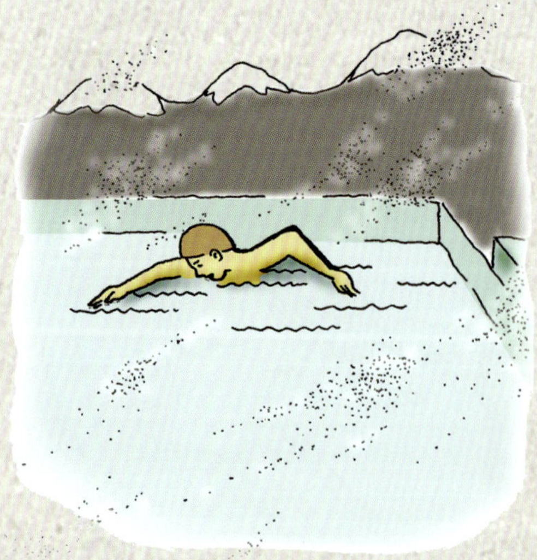

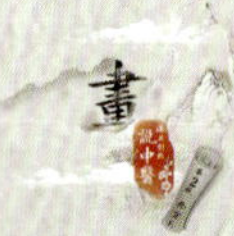

（4）固攝作用控製血液，防止其逸出脈外，控製汗液與尿液，使其有節製的排出，以及固攝精液等。

(4) Securing and containing function: qi's securing and containing function holds the blood inside the vessels and prevents it from overflowing, it also controls the excretion of sweat, urine and sperm.

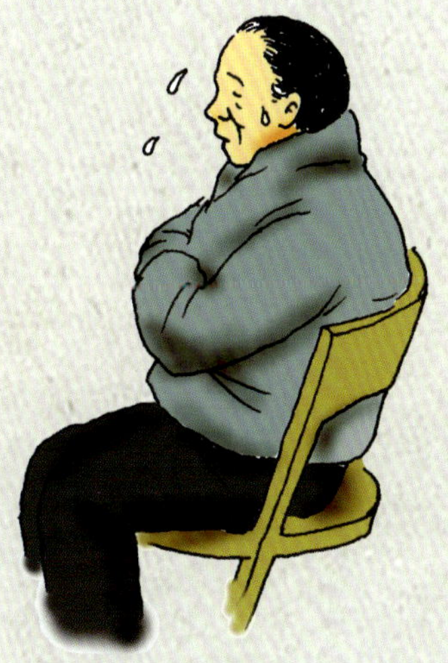

（5）氣化作用通過氣的運動而產生的各種變化。具體説是指精、氣、血、津液各自的新陳代謝及其相互轉化。氣化功能是通過氣的作用而產生的。

(5) Transforming function: qi movement causes various changes in the body in turn, like the metabolism of essence, qi, blood, and body fluids and their mutual transformation.

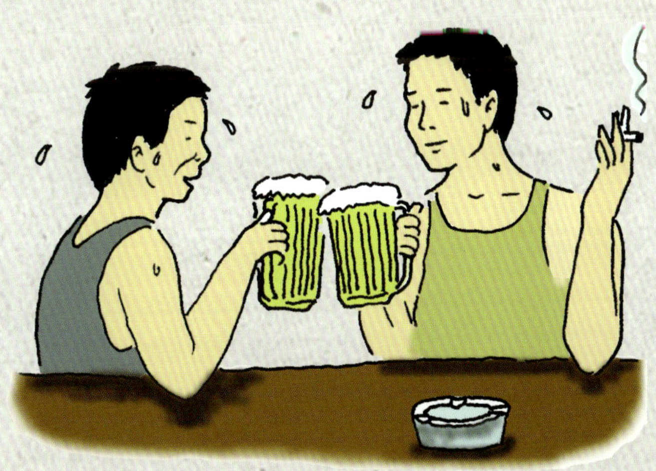

4. 氣的運動

氣的運動稱爲“氣機”。氣的基本運動形式可歸納爲升、降、出、入四種。升是氣由下向上運動；降是氣由上向下運動；出是氣由内向外的運動；入是氣由外向内的運動。

4. Qi Movement Direction

The movement of qi is called qi mechanism, and can be divided into four basic patterns: ascending, descending, exiting and entering. Ascending refers to a movement from below, descending, from above, exiting, from the interior, and entering from the exterior.

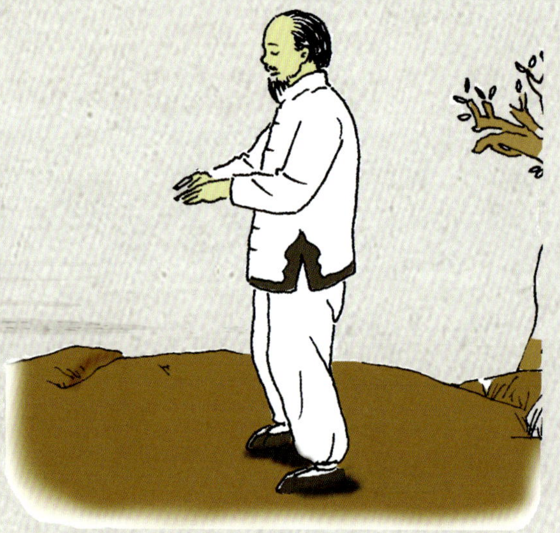

氣的運行正常稱爲“氣機調暢”。若氣機阻滯不通稱“氣滯”，氣的上升太過或不降而反升稱爲“氣逆”，氣的上升不及或應升而反降稱“氣陷”；氣不内守，大量外逸稱“氣脱”等。

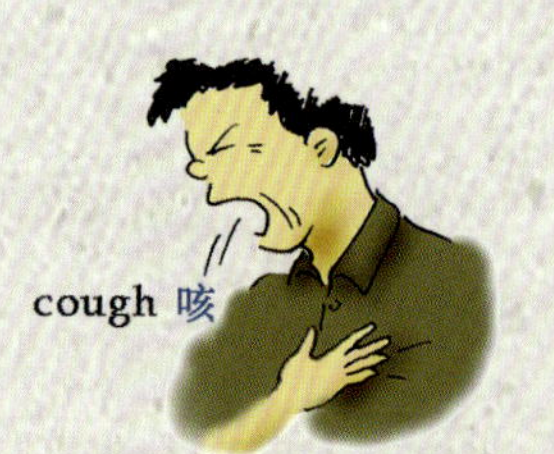

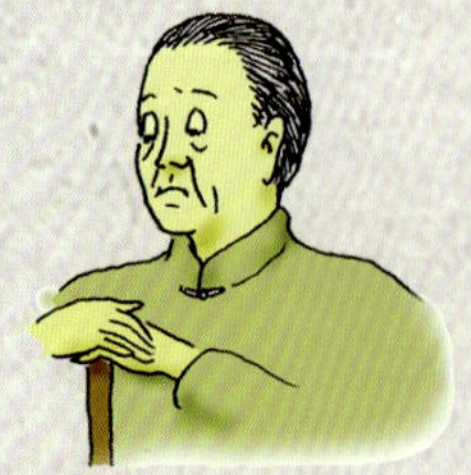

Stagnation of qi is obstruction of the qi movement, qi counterflow is abnormal qi descending and ascending, qi sinking describes an insufficient motion of qi ascending or when the qi is descending instead of ascending, qi desertion is inability of the qi to conserve the body's interior so that a large amount of qi is leaking out from the body.

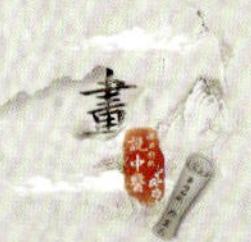

5. 氣的分類

（1）元氣

元氣是人體的本原之氣，是人體生命活動原動力，它禀受於父母的先天之精氣，並靠後天水谷之氣所滋養。是人體的本原之氣，是人體生命活動原動力，它禀受於父母的先天之精氣，並靠後天水谷之氣所滋養。元氣充沛則活力强盛而體健少病。元氣充沛則活力强盛而體健少病。

（2）宗氣

宗氣是聚於胸中之氣，是由肺吸入的清氣與脾運化而來的水谷之氣結合而成，宗氣的主要生理功能爲：走息道以行呼吸，貫心脈而行氣血。

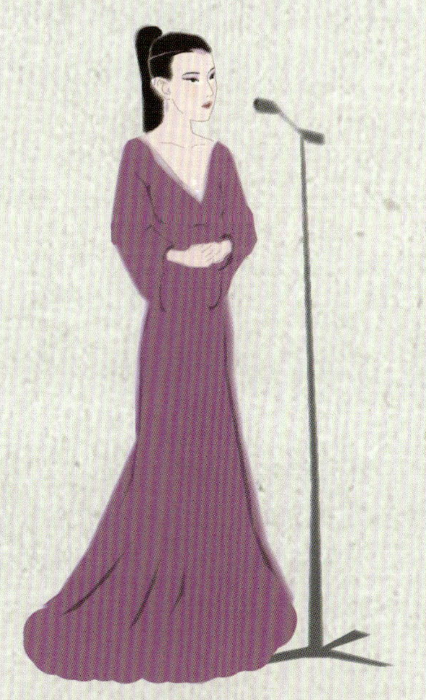

5. The Classification of Qi

(1) Original Qi

Original qi is the body's most fundamental and important qi, and the basic motivating force for life activities. It is inherited from the parents' congenital constitutions and also relies on the acquired constitution, which is nourished by the essence of drinks and food. If original qi is sufficient, then life activities will be normal, and so the body is healthy and rarely sick.

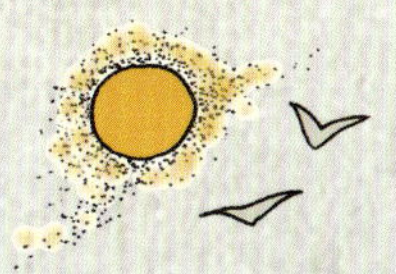

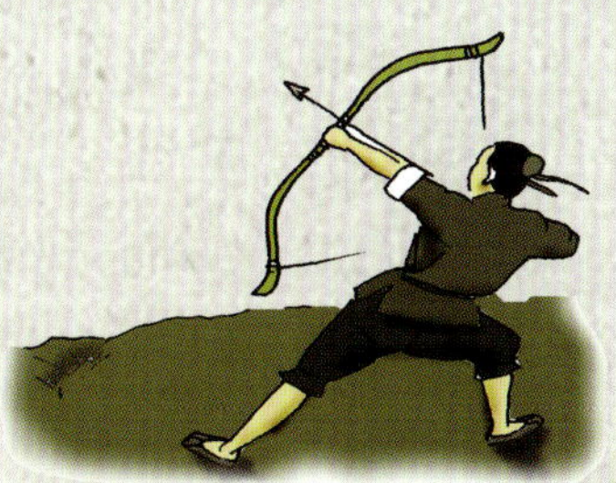

(2) Gathering Qi

Gathering qi is assembled in the chest, by combining the clear qi inhaled by the Lung and the essential qi transformed by the Stomach and Spleen from the essence of food and drink. The main physiological functions of gathering qi are to promote the Lung's respiratory function by passing through the respiratory tract, the Heart and the blood vessels in order to move qi and blood.

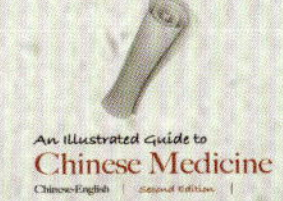

（3）營氣

營氣是水谷之氣中較爲輕柔富有營養的部分。營氣行於脈中，營養全身，營氣與血的關係密切，故常“營血”並稱。

（4）衛氣

衛氣是水谷之氣中較爲慓悍滑利的部分。衛氣行於脈外，具有護衛機體，不使外邪侵犯作用。主要生理是：

1）護衛肌表以抗御外邪；

2）溫養臟腑、肌肉皮毛；

3）調節控製腠理汗孔的開合。

(3) Nutritive Qi

Nutritive qi is a gentle and nourishing component of the essence of food and drink. It flows together with the blood in the vessels and nourishes the entire body, therefore blood and nutritive qi are closely related and are called nutrient-blood.

(4) Defensive Qi

Defensive qi is a relatively quick-moving and smooth component of the essence from food and drink. It flows on the exterior of the vessels and its function is to guard the human body from attacks of evil qi. Its main physiological functions are:

1) to defend the body surface and prevent exterior evil attacks.

2) to warm and nourish the Zang-fu organs, muscles, skin and hair.

3) to control the opening and closing of the interstitial spaces in order to prevent leaking of sweat.

三、血

Blood

1. 血的概念

血是行於脈中的紅色液體，是構成人體和維持人體生命活動的基本物質之一，具有營養滋潤作用。

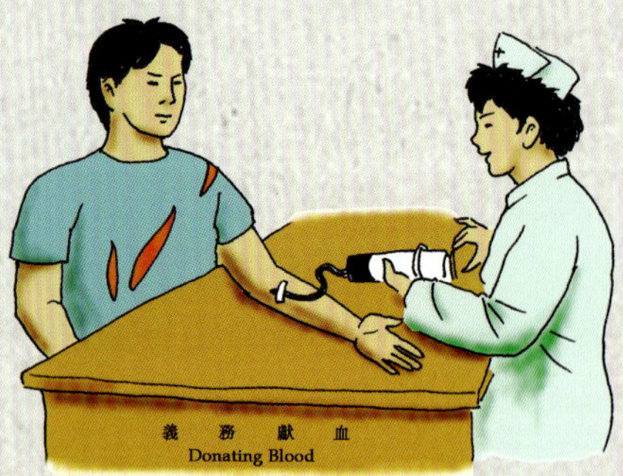

1. The Concept of Blood

Blood is a red fluid containing rich nutrients which flows in the vessels, it has nourishing and moistening functions, and is a basic material for maintaining life activities.

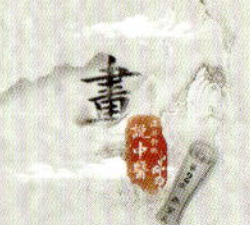

2. 血的生理功能

（1）對全身組織器官起着營養和滋潤作用。

如果血液不足，就可能出現面色萎黄，肌肉瘦削，皮膚幹燥，毛發枯槁，臟腑脆弱。機體的活動都需要血液的濡養。血液充盈則運動與感覺正常。血虚則常見頭暈眼花、四肢麻木、視物不清、運動無力或筋骨拘攣。

2. The Physiological Functions of Blood

(1) Blood nourishes and moistens the tissues and organs in the body.

If blood is insufficient, it can cause yellow complexion, emaciated muscles, dry hair and skin, and weak functions of Zang-fu organs. All human physical activities need enough blood nourishment. Blood deficiency may cause dizziness, blurred vision, numbness of the limbs and muscle and joint spasms.

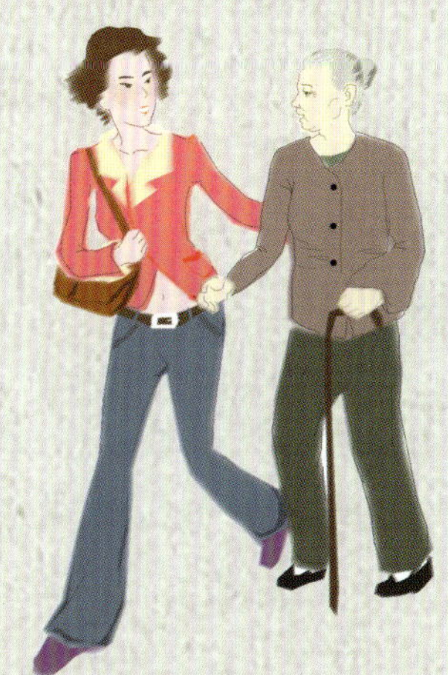

（2）神誌活動的物質基礎。氣血充盈，才能神誌清晰，精神旺盛。心肝血虚，常有驚悸，失眠，多夢等神誌不安的表現。

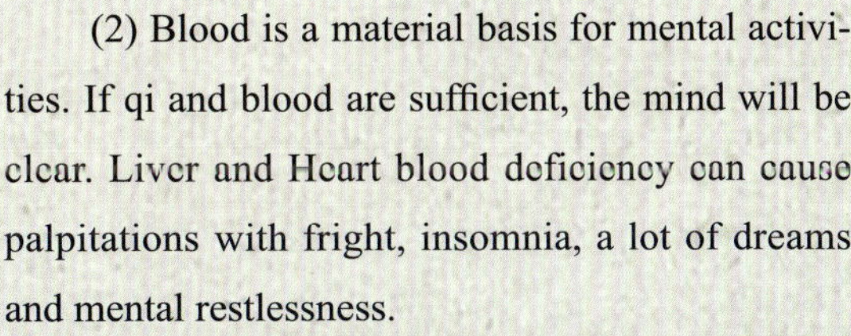

(2) Blood is a material basis for mental activities. If qi and blood are sufficient, the mind will be clear. Liver and Heart blood deficiency can cause palpitations with fright, insomnia, a lot of dreams and mental restlessness.

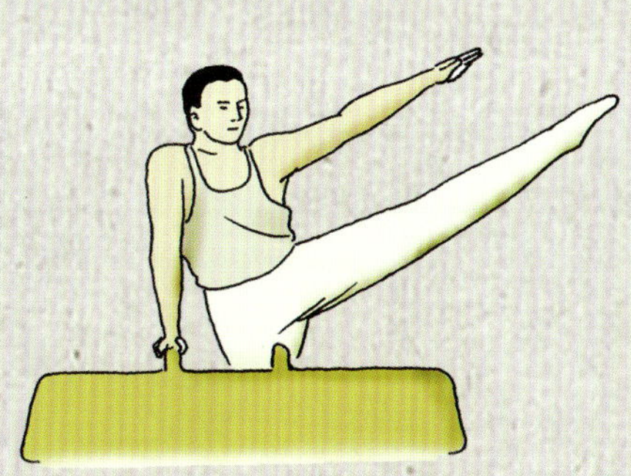

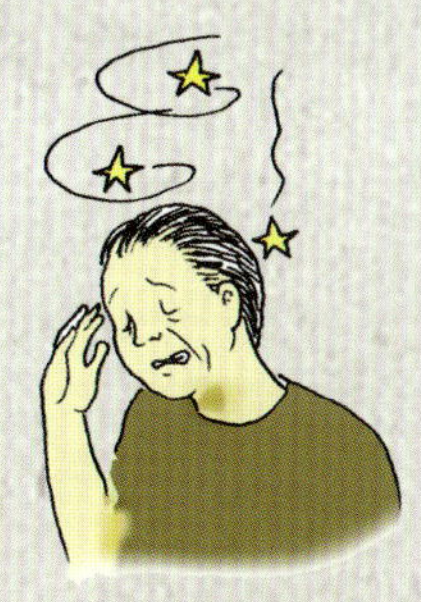

四、津液

1. 津液的概念

津液是機體内一切正常水液的總稱。包括各臟腑組織器官的内在體液及其正常的分泌物，如胃液、腸液和涕淚等。津液是構成人體和維持人體生命活動的基本物質。

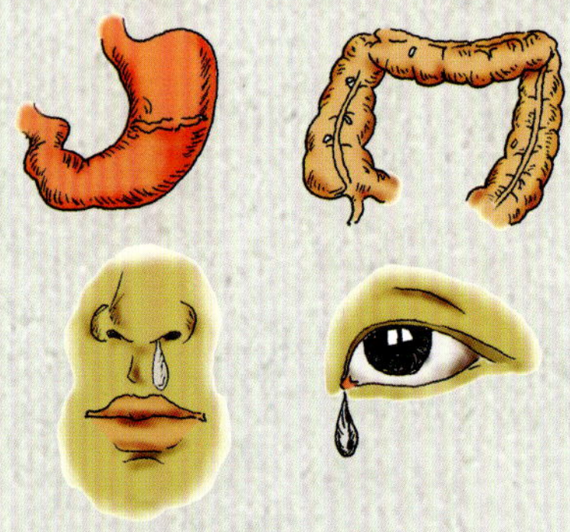

2. 津液的來源

津液來源於飲食，經過脾胃的吸收運化而生成。津液的輸布和排泄，主要與脾的轉輸，肺的宣降，腎的蒸騰氣化以及三焦氣化有關。

Body Fluids

1. The Concept of Body Fluids

Body fluids is a general term for all kinds of normal liquids and secretions in the organs and tissues of the body, such as gastric acid, digestive fluids, snivel, tears and et cetera. Like qi and blood, body fluids are also a basic substance for maintaining the normal life activities of the human body.

2. The Formation of Body Fluids

The body fluids originate from food and drink, and are formed through the functions of transportation and transformation by the Spleen and the Stomach. The distribution and excretion of body fluids is accomplished mainly by the Spleen's functions of transportation and transformation, the Lung's dispersing function, the Kidney's vaporizing function and the San Jiao's transformation function.

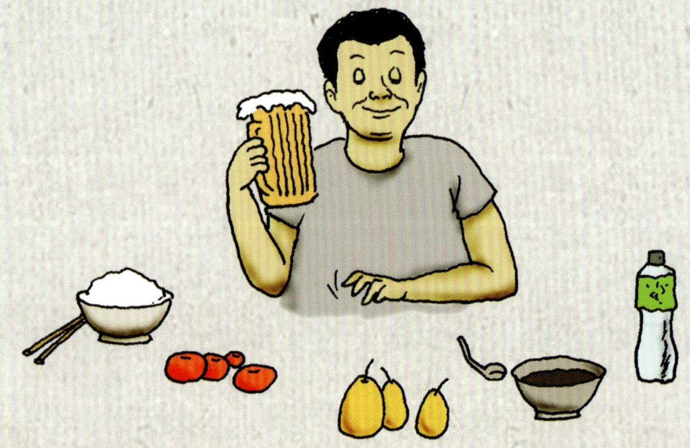

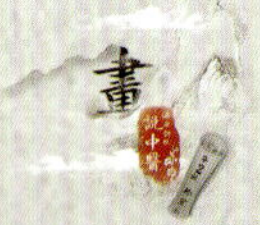

3. 津液的代謝

肺具有通調水道的作用。肺將從脾轉輸的津液，通過宣發、外達皮毛和鼻中，另一方面下向內輸布到腎、膀胱。通過肅降，把津液向腎爲水臟。腎臟氣化作用，將代謝後的津液化生成尿液，下注膀胱而排出體外。

4. 津液的作用

津液的作用主要是滋潤和營養。能滋潤皮毛肌膚，滑利關節，充養骨髓腦髓，滋潤臟腑，孔竅等。津液滲入血脈之内就成爲血液的組成部分。

3. The Excretion of Body Fluids

One of the Lung's functions is to regulate the water passages. By diffusion, the Lung distributes the fluids, transported by the Spleen, to all the parts of body, such as skin, hair and nose. The Lung also directs the fluids downward to the Kidney and the Bladder. These metabolized fluids are changed into urine. The Kidney's function of qi transformation is responsible for the discharge of urine from the body.

4. The Functions of Body Fluids

The main functions of the body fluids are to moisten and nourish the body. They moisten the skin, hair and muscles, and nourish the bone marrow, spinal core, brain, organs and the orifices. When the body fluids go into the vessels, they become a part of the blood.

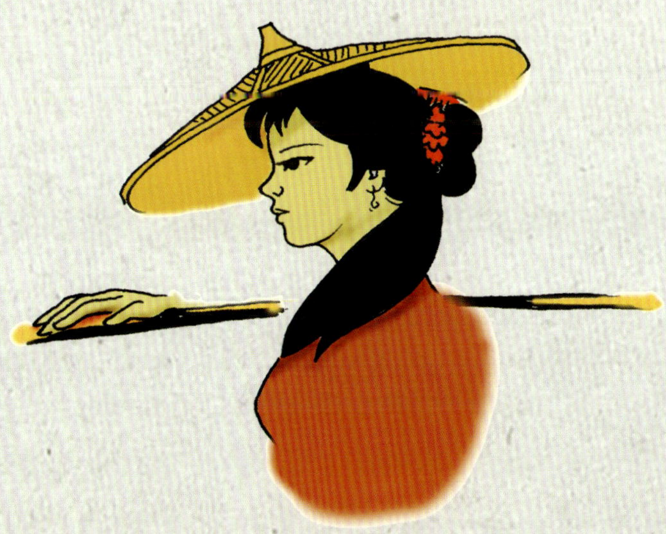

精、氣、血、津液的關係表

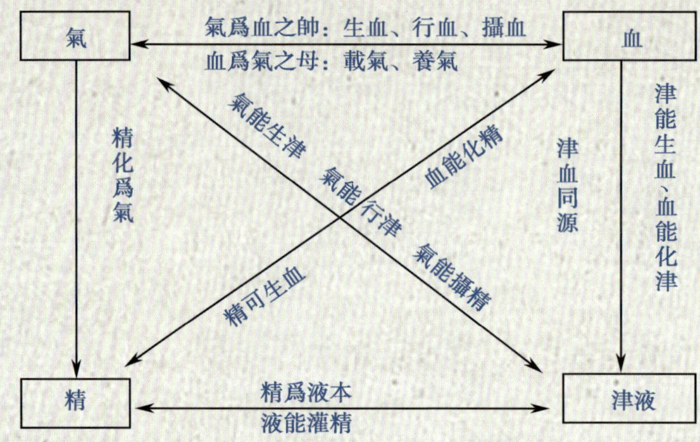

The Relationships between Qi, Blood and Body Fluids

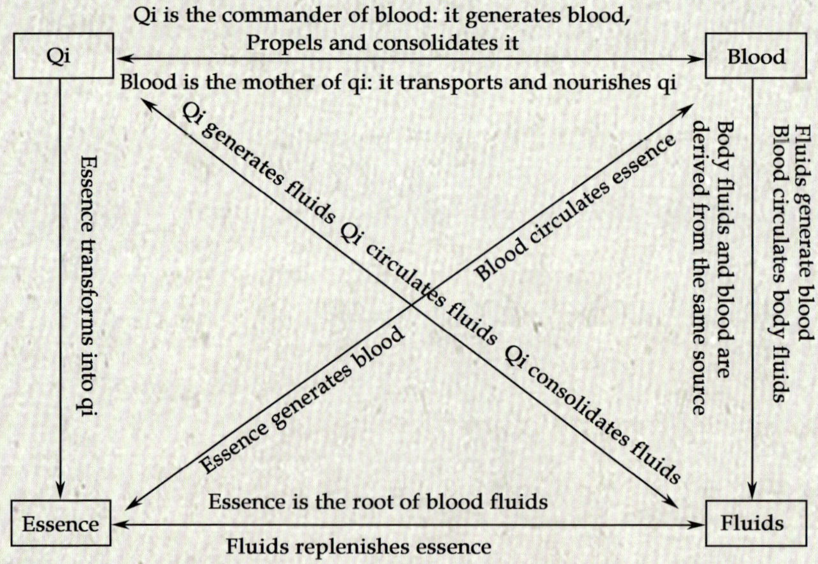

第四章 經絡 Chapter 4 Channels & Collaterals

經絡學説，是研究人體經絡係統的生理功能、病理變化及其與臟腑形體官竅、氣、血、津液等相互關係的學説，是中醫理論體係的重要組成部分。

經絡學説是古人在長期的醫療實踐中，從針灸、推拿、氣功等方面積累的經驗，並結合當時的解剖知識，逐步上升爲理論的基礎上形成的。它不僅是針灸、推拿、氣功等學科的理論基礎，而且對指導中醫臨床各科，均有十分重要的諠義。

The theory of the channels and collaterals is concerned with the physiology and pathology of the channels and collaterals and with their relationships with the Zang-fu organs, orifices, qi, blood, and body fluids. It is an essential part of the theory of Chinese medicine.

The theory of channels and collaterals was formed over a long time of medical practice. It is based on the gradual accumulation of experience in acupuncture & moxibustion, tui na and qi gong, combined with contemporary anatomical knowledge. The theory of channels and collaterals is not only the basic theory underpinning these arts, but also is the great significance in guiding every field of Chinese medicine.

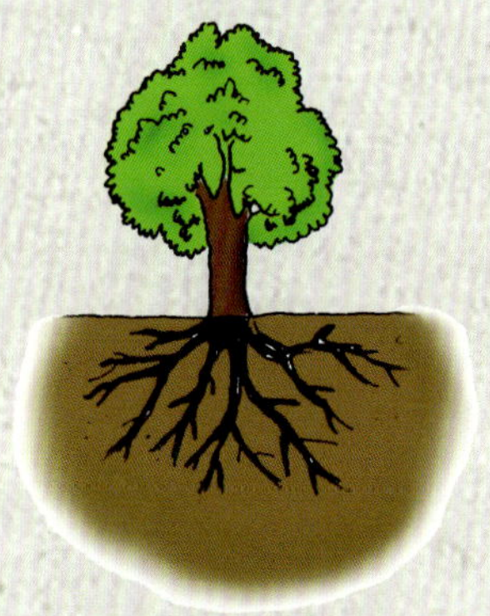

一、經絡的概念和經絡係統的組成

The Concept and Contents of the System of Channels and Collaterals

1. 經絡的概念

經絡是運行全身氣血，聯絡臟腑肢節，溝通上下内外的通路。

1. The Concept of the Channels and Collaterals

The channels and their collaterals are the pathways through which qi and blood circulate in the body and by which the Zang-fu organs and limbs are connected. They allow communication to occur between the upper & lower and interior & exterior parts of the body.

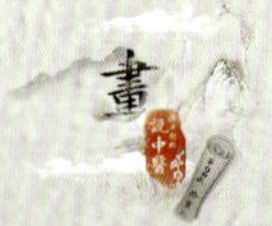

經絡，是經脈和絡脈的總稱。經，有路徑的意思，經脈是經絡係統中縱行的主幹綫，大多循行於深部，有固定的循行路綫；絡，有網絡的意思，是經脈的分支，縱橫交錯，網絡全身。經脈和絡脈，相互溝通聯係，將人體所有的臟腑、形體、孔竅等部分緊密地聯結成一個統一的有機整體。

The term "channel" indicates a pathway, it is the main trunk path which runs lengthwise in the system of the channels and collaterals. Most channels run through the deeper parts of the body along fixed courses. The term "collateral" means net, and they are the branches of the channels. Collaterals travel in crisscross directions in the body, forming a network which links the Zang-fu organs, physical body, and orifices into one organic whole.

乾隆銅人
(上海中醫藥大學)

2. 經絡係統的組成

經絡係統由經脈、絡脈及連屬部分組成。經脈和絡脈是主體，在内連屬於臟腑，在外連屬於筋肉皮膚。

2. The Composition of the System of Channels and Collaterals

The system of the channels and collaterals consists of the channels, collaterals, and their subsidiary parts. The channels and collaterals connect internally to the Zang-fu organs, and externally to the tendons, muscles and skin.

（1）經脈

分正經和奇經兩大類，爲經絡係統的主要部分。此外，還有十二經别。

(1) Channels

The channels can be divided into two types: the primary and extraordinary. These are the core of the system of channels. Also, there are twelve divergent channels.

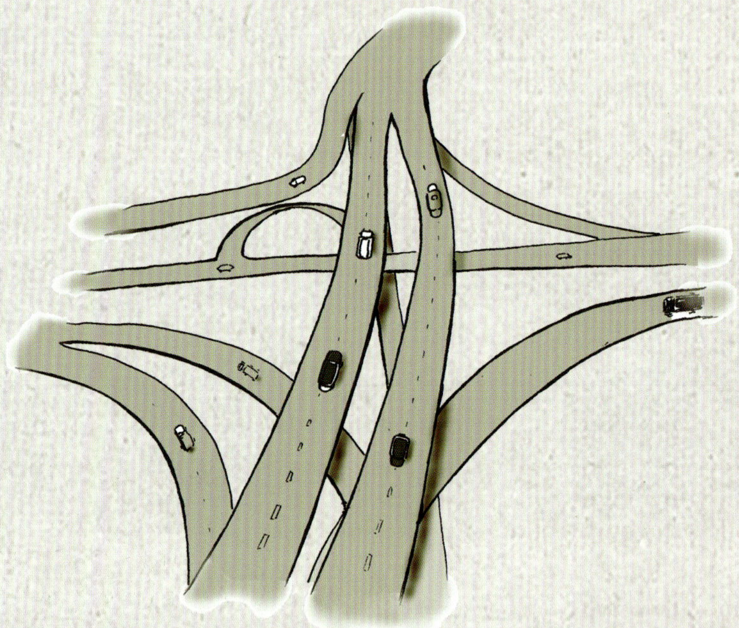

1）十二正經

即手足三陰經（太陰、少陰、厥陰）和手足三陽經（太陽、陽明、少陽），又稱"十二經脈"。十二經脈有一定的起止、一定的循行部位和交接順序，在肢體的分布和走向有一定的規律，與臟腑有直接的絡屬關係，是人體氣血運行的主要通道。

1) The Twelve Primary Channels

The twelve primary channels are the three yin channels of the hand and foot (taiyin, shaoyin & jueyin) and the three yang channels of the hand and foot (taiyang, yangming & shaoyang). They originate and terminate at specific locations, and circulate in distinct courses and sequences. They are regularly distributed over the trunk and limbs, and also pertain to and directly connect with the Zang-fu organs in the interior of the body. They are the main pathways through which qi and blood circulate.

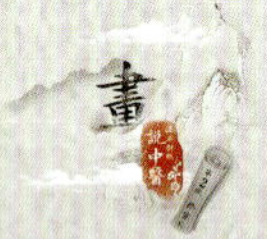

2）奇經八脈

即督、任、衝、帶、陰蹺、陽蹺、陰維、陽維等脈的合稱。有統率、聯絡和調節十二經脈的作用。奇經八脈的分布不像十二經脈那樣規則，且無臟腑絡屬關係，與正經有別，故名奇經。

3）十二經別

是從十二經脈別出的經脈。它們分別起於四肢，循行於體腔臟腑深部，上出於頸項淺部。十二經別的作用，主要是加强十二經脈中相爲表裏的兩經之間的聯係，還由於它能通達某些正經未循行到的器官與形體部位，因而能補正經之不足。

（2）絡脈

有別絡、浮絡、孫絡之分。

1）別絡

是較大的和主要的絡脈。十二經脈與督、任脈各有一支別絡，再加上脾之大絡，合爲“十五別絡”。別絡的主要功能是加强表裏兩經之間在體表的聯係。

2) The Eight Extraordinary Vessels

The Governing vessel, Conception vessel, Penetrating vessel, Girdling vessel, Yin heel vessel, Yang heel vessel, Yin link vessel, and Yang link vessel are commonly referred to as the Eight Extraordinary Vessels. They function in governing, communicating between and regulating the twelve channels. They are called the "Extraordinary Channels" because their pathways do not resemble those of the Twelve Channels, and because they have no direct relationships with any of the internal organs.

3) The Twelve Divergent Channels

The twelve divergent channels spread from the primary channels, starting from the four limbs and transfusing into the deep portion of the Zang-fu organs, and then emerging at the superficial levels of the neck and nape. Their main functions are to strengthen interconnection between the two interior-exterior primary channels and to replenish the primary channels, as the divergent channels can reach the organs and body areas where some primary channels cannot traverse.

(2) Collaterals

The collaterals can be classified as the divergent collaterals, superficial collaterals and minute collaterals.

1) The Divergent Collaterals

These are the larger, main collaterals. All the Twelve Channels, the Governing vessel and the Conception vessel each has one divergent channel. These divergent channels with the great divergent channel of the spleen total fifteen. Their main functions are to strengthen the relations of interiorly-exteriorly related channels.

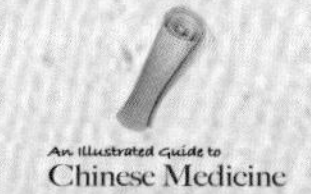

2）浮絡

是循行於人體淺表部位而常浮現的絡脈。

3）孫絡

是最細小的絡脈。

3. 連屬部分

（1）十二經筋

是十二經脈與筋肉的連屬部分。人體的經筋是十二經脈之氣"結、聚、散、絡"於筋肉、關節的體係，即是十二經脈循行部位上分布於筋肉係統的總稱。它有聯綴四肢百骸，主司關節運動的作用。

2) The Superficial Collaterals

The superficial collaterals are the ones those travel at the surface layer of the human body where they often make their appearances.

3) The Minute Collaterals

The minute collaterals are the smallest collaterals.

3. The Subsidiary Parts

(1) The Twelve Sinew Channels

The twelve sinew channels refer to the connection part of the twelve channels with their conjunctive tissues, including tendons, muscles and joints. The sinew channels form a system where the channel qi accumulates, gathers, disperses, and connects with the tendons, muscles, and joints. They are affiliated with the primary channels and together are called the twelve channels sinew regions. Their functions are to connect the limbs and tissues, as well as to control joint movements.

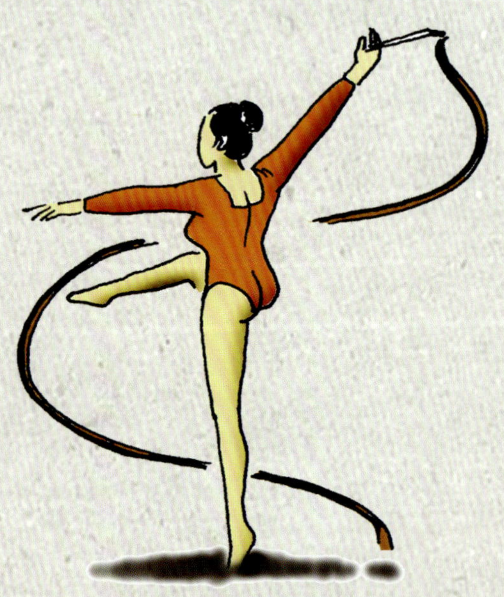

（2）十二皮部

是十二經脈在體表的連屬部分，即是十二經脈在體表一定部位的反應區。全身的皮膚，是十二經脈的功能活動反映於體表的部位，也是經絡之氣的散布所在，所以把全身皮膚分爲十二部分，分屬於十二經脈，故名“十二皮部”。

(2) The Twelve Cutaneous Regions

The twelve cutaneous regions refer to the area on the body surface which is linked to the twelve channels. These areas reflect the twelve channels at certain parts of the body surface. The skin of the body is where the functional activities of the twelve primary channels are reflected and where channel qi is distributed. The skin of the body can be divided into twelve parts, which correspond to the twelve channels, and termed "the twelve cutaneous regions".

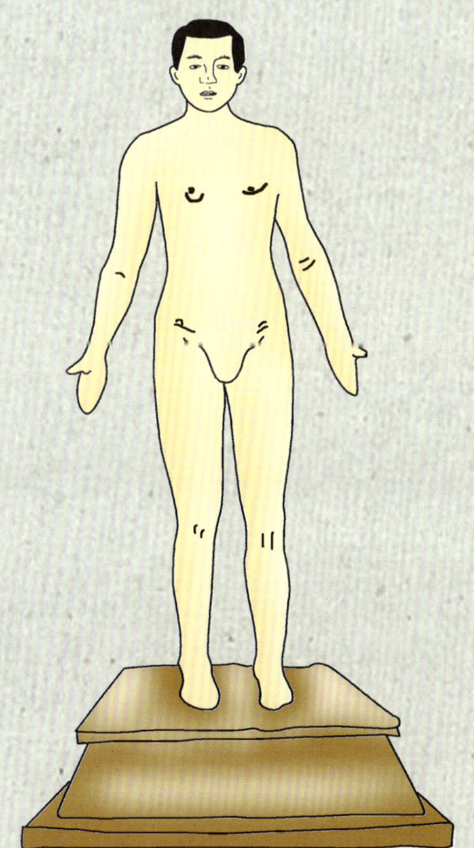

表 4-1　經絡係統簡表

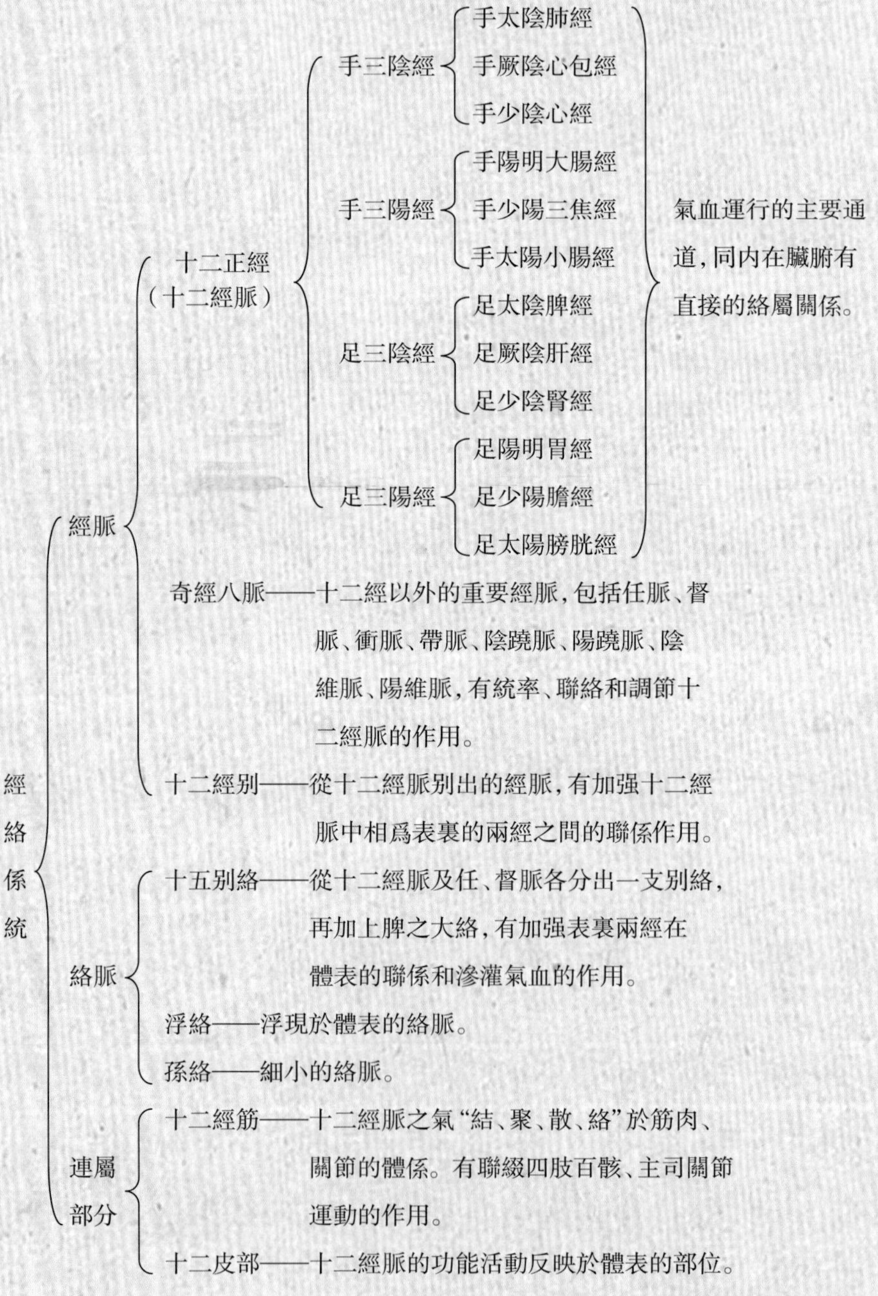

- 經絡係統
  - 經脈
    - 十二正經（十二經脈）——氣血運行的主要通道，同内在臟腑有直接的絡屬關係。
      - 手三陰經
        - 手太陰肺經
        - 手厥陰心包經
        - 手少陰心經
      - 手三陽經
        - 手陽明大腸經
        - 手少陽三焦經
        - 手太陽小腸經
      - 足三陰經
        - 足太陰脾經
        - 足厥陰肝經
        - 足少陰腎經
      - 足三陽經
        - 足陽明胃經
        - 足少陽膽經
        - 足太陽膀胱經
    - 奇經八脈——十二經以外的重要經脈，包括任脈、督脈、衝脈、帶脈、陰蹺脈、陽蹺脈、陰維脈、陽維脈，有統率、聯絡和調節十二經脈的作用。
    - 十二經别——從十二經脈别出的經脈，有加强十二經脈中相爲表裏的兩經之間的聯係作用。
  - 絡脈
    - 十五别絡——從十二經脈及任、督脈各分出一支别絡，再加上脾之大絡，有加强表裏兩經在體表的聯係和滲灌氣血的作用。
    - 浮絡——浮現於體表的絡脈。
    - 孫絡——細小的絡脈。
  - 連屬部分
    - 十二經筋——十二經脈之氣“結、聚、散、絡”於筋肉、關節的體係。有聯綴四肢百骸、主司關節運動的作用。
    - 十二皮部——十二經脈的功能活動反映於體表的部位。

Table 4-1 Classification of the Channels and Collaterals System

1. Channels		
Twelve primary channels (The main pathways in which qi and blood circulate. They pertain to and connect with the Zang-fu organs directly in the interior of the body.)	The three yin channels of hand	Lung channel of hand taiyin Pericardium channel of hand jueyin Heart channel of hand shaoyin
	The three yang channels of hand	Large Intestine channel of hand yangming San Jiao channel of hand shaoyang Small Intestine channel of hand taiyang
	The three yin channels of foot	Spleen channel of foot taiyin Liver channel of foot jueyin Kidney channel of foot shaoyin
	The three yang channels of foot	Stomach channel of foot yangming Gallbladder channel of foot shaoyang Bladder channel of foot taiyang
Eight extra channels	Other important channels in addition to the twelve channels, are the Governing vessel, Conception vessel, Penetrating vessel, Girdling vessel, yin heel vessels, yang heel vessels, yin link vessels, and yang link vessels. The function is to govern, regulate and communicate with the twelve channels.	
The twelve divergent channels	They are the main branches of twelve channels. They strengthen the relationship between the interior and the exterior related channels.	
2. Collaterals		
The fifteen divergent collaterals	The branches derived from twelve channels, the Conception vessel and Governing vessel are together with the large collateral of the Spleen. The function is to strengthen the relationship between the interior and the exterior related channels and to transport qi and blood	
The minute collaterals	All the small collaterals	
The superficial collaterals	The collaterals distributed on the body surface.	
3. Subsidiary Parts		
The twelve sinew channels	The system where the channel qi accumulates, knots, gathers, scatters, and connects with the tendons, muscles, and joints. They connect the limbs and tissues, as well as control joint movement.	
The twelve cutaneous regions	The twelve regions where the reactions caused by the twelve regular channels manifest at the body surface.	

二、十二正經

1. 命名

十二經脈對稱地分布於人的兩側，分別循行於四肢的内（陰）外（陽）側，每一條經脈分别屬於一個臟或一個腑。因此，十二經脈的名稱是依據陰陽、手足、臟腑三個方面而命名的。其命名有以下一些規律：

（1）臟為陰，腑為陽

凡是隸屬於臟的經脈叫陰經；隸屬於腑的經脈叫陽經。

（2）上為手，下為足

循行在上肢的爲手經；循行在下肢的爲足經。

The Twelve Primary Channels

1. Nomenclature

The twelve primary channels distribute symmetrically and bilaterally in the body and pass through the medial and lateral aspects of the upper or lower limbs. Each channel connects with a Zang-organ or a Fu-organ, thus, the name of each channel of the twelve primary channels has three parts: hand or foot, yin or yang, and the Zang-fu organ. These are the rules of nomenclature:

(1) The Zang Pertains to Yin, the Fu Pertains to Yang

Yin channels pertain to the Zang-organs, while the yang channels, pertain to the Fu-organs.

(2) Upper Limbs Refer to the Hand, Lower Limbs Refer to the Feet

The channels flowing along the upper limbs are the hand channels, and also the channels which flow along the lower limbs are the foot channels.

表 4-2　十二經脈名稱分類表

	陰經（屬臟）	陽經（屬腑）	循行部位 （陰經行於內側，陽經行於外側）	
手	手太陰肺經	手陽明大腸經	上肢	前緣
	手厥陰心包經	手少陽三焦經		中綫
	手少陰心經	手太陽小腸經		後緣
足	足太陰脾經 ※	足陽明胃經	下肢	前緣
	足厥陰肝經 ※	足少陽膽經		中綫
	足少陰腎經	足太陽膀胱經		後緣

※ 在小腿下半部和足背部，肝經在前緣，脾經在中綫。至内踝上八寸處交叉之後，脾經在前緣，肝經在中綫。

Table 4-2　Classification of Nomenclature of the Twelve Primary Channels

	Yin channels (Pertaining to Zang-organs)	**Yang channels** (Pertaining to Fu-organs)	**Course** (Yin channels run along the medial aspect, yang channels run along the lateral aspect.)	
Hand	The Lung channel of hand taiyin	The Large Intestine channel of hand yangming	Upper limbs	Anterior border
	The Pericardium channel of hand jueyin	The San Jiao channel of hand shaoyang		Midline
	The Heart channel of hand shaoyin	The Small Intestine channel of hand taiyang		Posterior border
Foot	The Spleen channel of foot taiyin※	The Stomach channel of foot yangming	Lower limbs	Anterior border
	The Liver channel of foot jueyin※	The Gallbladder channel of foot shaoyang		Midline
	The Kidney channel foot shaoyin	The Bladder channel of foot taiyang		Posterior border

※At the lower leg and dorsal foot, the Liver channel lies in the anterior border, and the Spleen channel is in the midline. After they cross at the point 8 cun above the medial malleolus, the Spleen channel is at the anterior border and the Liver channel in the middle.

（3）内為陰，外為陽

循環在肢體内側面的經脈爲陰經；循環在肢體外側面的經脈爲陽經。内側面有前、中、後之分，分别爲太陰、厥陰、少陰；外側面也有前、中、後之分，分别爲陽明、少陽、太陽。

2. 走向與交接規律

十二經脈的走向與交接是有一定規律的。手三陰經，從胸腔走向手指末端，交手三陽經；手三陽經從手指末端走向頭面部，交足三陽經；足三陽經從頭面走向足趾末端，交足三陰經。足三陰經從足趾走向腹腔、胸腔，交手三陰經。

(3) The Medial Side Pertains to Yin, while the Lateral Side Pertains to Yang

The yin channels run along the medial side of the four limbs, while the yang channels run along their lateral side. The rules of distribution of the yin border are: the taiyin channels are distributed at the anterior border, the shaoyin channels are distributed over the posterior border, and the jueyin channels are distributed along the midline. The distributing rules of the yang channels are: the yangming channels are distributed over the anterior border, the taiyang channels are distributed over the posterior border, and the shaoyang channels are distributed along the midline.

2. The Rules of Courses and Connections

There is a specific rule for the courses and connections of the twelve primary channels. The three yin channels of the hand travel from the chest to the tip of the fingers, then connect with the three yang channels of the hand. The three yang channels of the hand travel from the tip of the fingers to head and face, then connect with the three yang channels of the foot. The three yang channels of the foot descend from the face and head down to the tip of the toes, then connect with three yin channels of the foot. The three yin channels of the foot start from the toes and ascend to the abdomen and chest to connect with three yin channels of the hand.

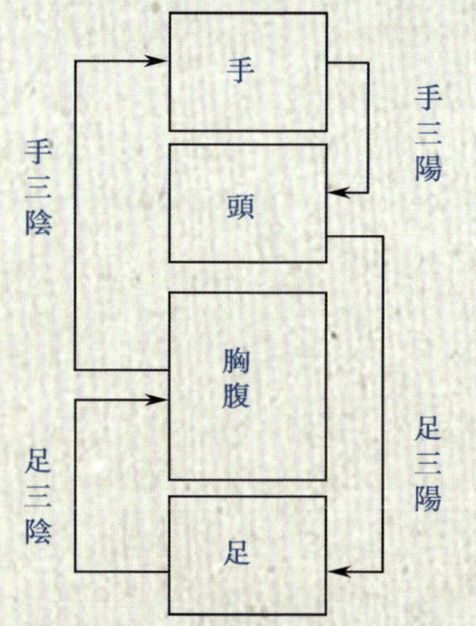

手足陰陽經脈走向交接規律示譩圖

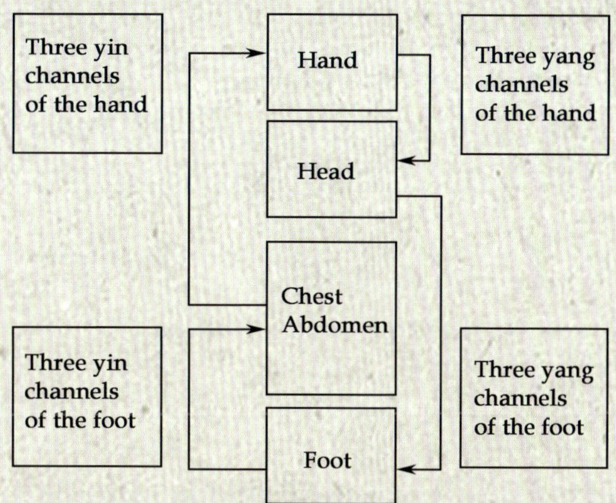

Diagram of the Connections of the Hand-Foot Channels

3. 分布規律

十二經脈在體表的分布，有一定的規律。

（1）頭部

手足陽明經行於面部、額部；手足少陽經行於頭側部；手足太陽經行於面頰、頭頂和頭後部。手足三陽經皆會聚於頭面。

（2）軀幹部

手三陽經行於肩胛部；足三陽經則陽明經行於前（胸、腹面），太陽經行於後陰足陽（背面），少陽經行於側面。手三陰經均從腋下走出。足三陰經均行於腹面。

3. The Rules of Distribution

The distributions of the twelve primary channels on the body surface are fixed.

(1) On the face and head

The yangming channels are distributed on the face and forehead. The shaoyang channels travel along the lateral aspect of the head. The taiyang channels pass through the cheek, vertex and back of the neck. The three yang channels of hand and foot gather on the face and head.

(2) On the body trunk

The three Yang channels of the hand run through the scapular regions. Among the three Yang channels of the foot, the yangming channel runs anteriorly (from chest to abdomen), the taiyang channel travels posteriorly (along the back), and the shaoyang channel laterally. The three yin channels of the hand all emerge from the area below the axilla, and the three yin channels of the foot run through the abdominal regions.

（3）四肢部

陰經行於內側面，陽經行於外側面。內側三陰經，太陰在前緣，厥陰在中綫，少陰在後緣。但下肢內側陰經分布：內踝八寸以下，厥陰在前，太陰在中綫，少陰在後。下肢外側陽經分布：陽明在前，少陽在中，太陽在後。

4. 表裏配合

手足三陰三陽經，通過各自的經別和別絡互相溝通，組成六對“表裏相合”關係。

(3) The four limbs

The yin channels run along the medial side of the four limbs, while the yang channels run along the lateral side of the four limbs. The distributing order of the three yin channels has: the taiyin channels at the anterior border, the shaoyin channels at the posterior border and the jueyin channels along the midline. The two channels of foot taiyin and jueyin cross about eight cun above the tip of the internal malleolus, then the taiyin channel moves to the anterior border and the jueyin channel moves to the midline. The distributing order of the yang channels has: the yangming channels at the anterior border, the taiyang channels at the posterior border, and the shaoyang channels along the midline.

4. Interior-Exterior Relationships

The three yin channels of the hand and foot and the three yang channels of the hand and foot are linked with each other through the divergent channels and collaterals, which constitute six pairs of exterior-interior relationship.

表 4-3　十二經脈表裏關係表

表	手陽明 大腸經	手少陽 三焦經	手太陽 小腸經	足陽明 胃經	足少陽 膽經	足太陽 膀胱經
裏	手太陰 肺經	手厥陰 心包經	手少陰 心經	足太陰 脾經	足厥陰 肝經	足少陰 腎經

Table 4-3　The External and Internal Relationships among the Twelve Channels

External	The Large Intestine channel of hand yangming	The San Jiao channel of hand shaoyang	The Small Intestine channel of hand taiyang	The Stomach channel of foot yangming	The Gallbladder channel of foot shaoyang	The Bladder channel of foot taiyang
Internal	The Lung channel of hand taiyin	The Pericardium channel of hand jueyin	The Heart channel of hand shaoyin	The Spleen channel of foot taiyin	The Liver channel of foot jueyin	The Kidney channel of foot shaoyin

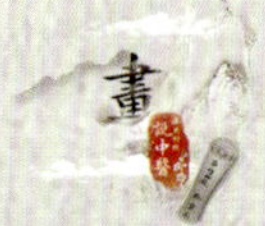

相爲表裏的兩條經脈，分別循行於四肢内外側的相對位置，並於四肢末端交接，其各自絡屬於相爲表裏的臟或腑，即陰經屬臟絡腑；陽經屬腑絡臟。這樣，既加强了表裏兩經的聯係，又促進了表裏的臟與腑在生理功能上的相互協調與配合，表裏兩經在病理上也可相互影響。在治療時，相爲表裏的兩經的俞穴可交叉使用，如肺經的穴位可用以治療大腸或大腸經的疾病。

The two external and internal channels connect at the ends of the four limbs, which run respectively along the medial and lateral aspects of the limbs. The channels which have external & internal relationships pertain to Zang-fu organs which are also related to each other externally and internally. In this way the channels and the Zang-fu organs of external and internal relationships associate with each other. The yin channel pertains to the Zang-organ and connects to the Fu-organs by its collaterals, while the yang channel pertains to the Fu organ and connects to the Zang-organs by its collaterals. The interior-exterior relationship of the twelve primary channels, not only strengthen communication by the connection of the two interior-exterior channels, but also connect with and pertains to the same Zang-fu organs.

This enables the Zang-organs and Fu-organs which have interior-exterior relationships to be mutually coordinated in their physiological functions, and influence each other pathologically. In treatment, the points belonging to the two interior-exterior channels can be mutually selected. For example, the points of the Lung channel can be selected to treat diseases of the Large Intestine Fu organs or also illness of the channel.

5. 流注次序

十二經脈是氣血運行的主要通道。十二經脈分布在人體各部，經脈中氣血的運行是依次循環貫注的，即經脈在中焦受氣後，上注於肺，自手太陰肺經開始，依次傳至足厥陰肝經，再複注於手太陰肺經，首尾相貫，如環無端，構成十二經循環。其流注次序見下表：

5. The Flow and Sequence of the Twelve Channels

The twelve primary channels are the main pathways of qi and blood, distributed all over the body; and the qi and blood circulate constantly in the channels. The qi passes from the middle burner to the Lung, starts from the Lung channel of hand taiyin, and is transported to the Liver channel of foot jueyin in proper order, this process then starts again at the Lung channel of hand taiyin. The interconnection of the beginning and ending points forms a cycle. It is called the cyclical flow of qi in the twelve primary channels. This flow and sequence is demonstrated in the following figure.

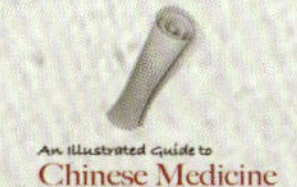

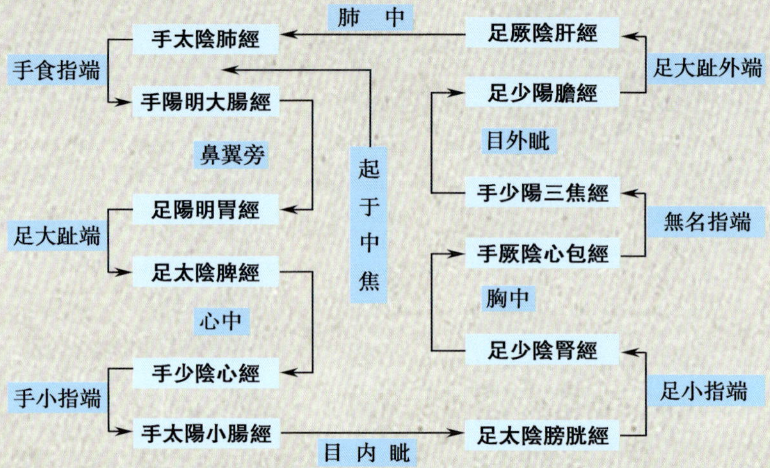

The Flow and Sequence of the Twelve Primary Channels

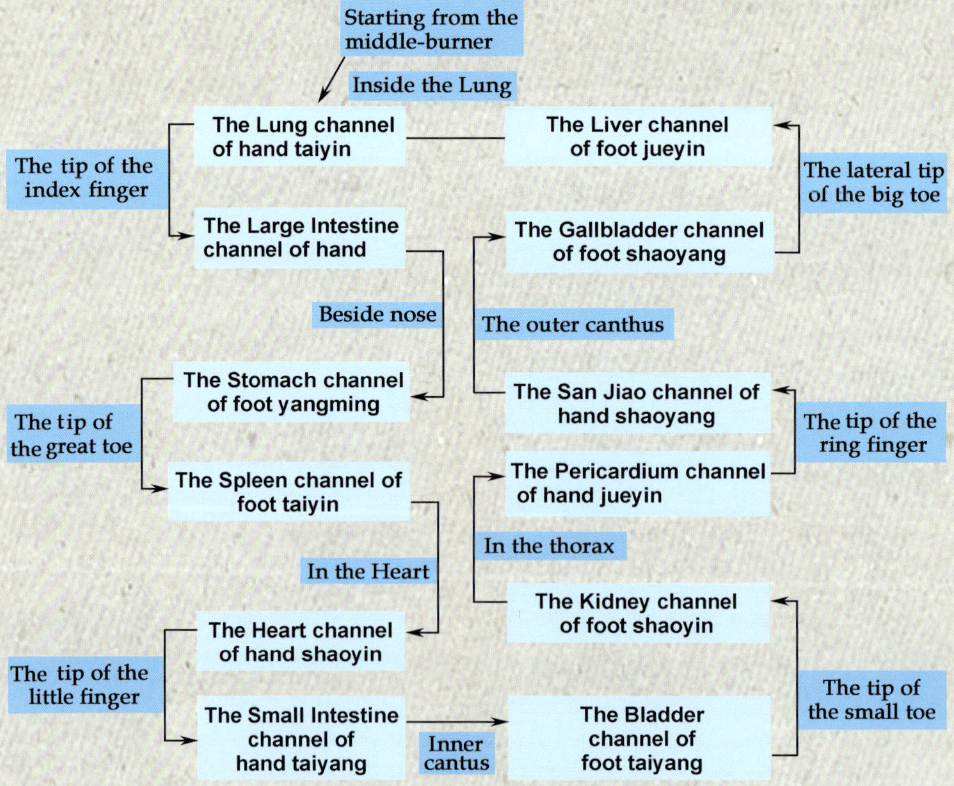

6. 循行路綫

（1）手太陰肺經

中焦→大腸→胃上口→橫膈→肺→肺係→上臂內側→肘窩→前臂內側前緣→寸口→魚際→拇指橈側端。

支脈：腕後方（列缺穴處）→食指橈側端→與手陽明大腸經相接。

6. The Course of the Twelve Primary Channels

(1) The Lung channel of hand taiyin

Middle burner →Large Intestine →upper orifice of the Stomach →diaphragm →Lung →Lung system →medial aspect of the upper arm →armpit →the anterior border of the radial side of the forearm →cun pulse on the wrist →LU 10 (*yú jì*) →the medial side of the thumb tip.

The branch channel: posterior wrist at LU 7 (*liè quē*) →the radial side of the index fingertip →connects to the Large Intestine channel of hand yangming.

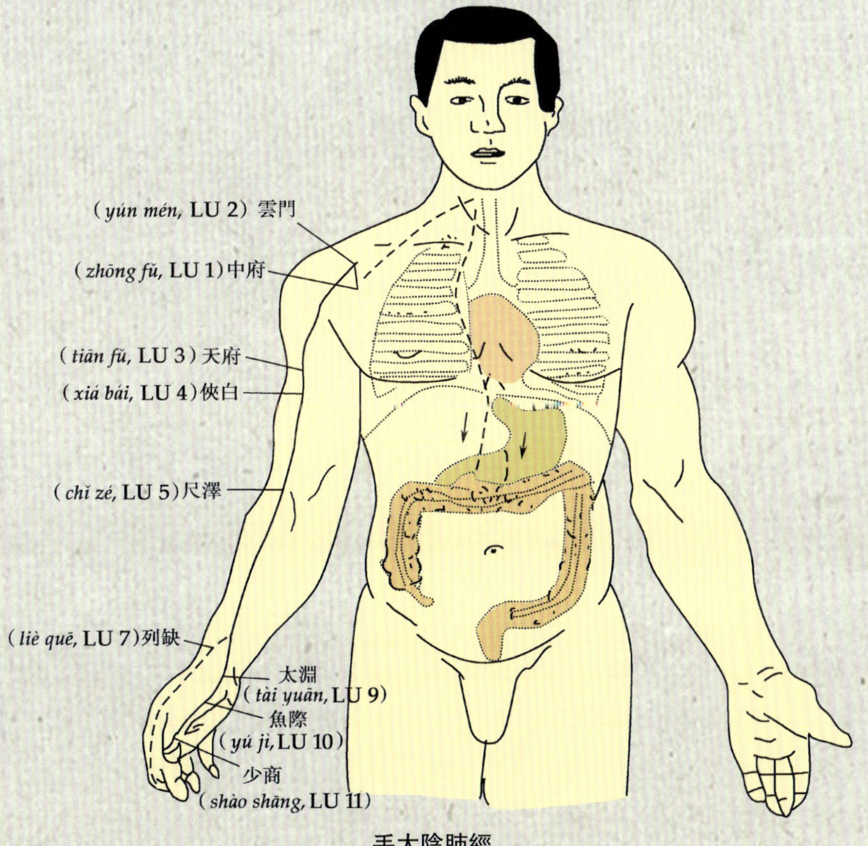

手太陰肺經

The Lung channel of hand taiyin

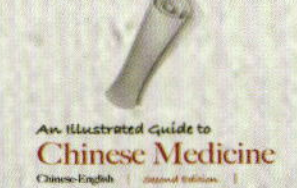

（2）手陽明大腸經

食指橈側端→一、二掌骨間→向上進入兩筋（拇長伸肌腱與拇短伸肌腱）之間→前臂前方→肘外側→上臂外側前緣→肩端→肩峰前緣→大椎→缺盆→肺→橫膈→大腸。

支脈：缺盆→頸→面頰→下齒齦→上唇→人中→（左脈向右，右脈向左）→鼻孔兩側，與足陽明胃經相接。

(2) The Large Intestine channel of hand yangming

The radial side of the index finger →the space between the first and second metacarpal bones → the depression between the tendons of extensor pollicis longus and brevis→the anterior aspect of the forearm →the lateral side of the elbow →the lateral anterior aspect of the upper arm →the highest point of the shoulder →the anterior border of the acromion →DU 14 (*dà zhuī*) →ST 12 (*quē pén*) → the Lung →the diaphragm →the Large Intestine.

The branch channel: ST 12 (*quē pén*) →neck → cheek →the lower gums →the upper lip →LI 17 (*tiān dǐng*), the left channel crosses to the right and the right channel to the left →the contralateral sides of the nose → and links with the Stomach channel of foot yangming.

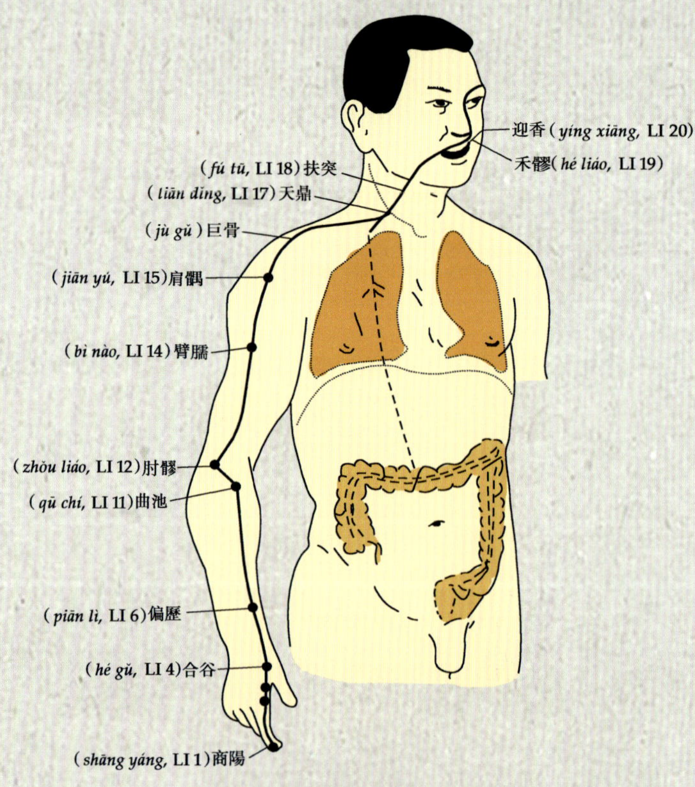

手陽明大腸經

The Large Intestine channel of hand yangming

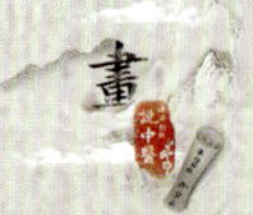

（3）足陽明胃經

鼻翼旁→鼻根部→鼻外側→上齒齦→繞唇→唇溝→口腮後下方→下頜大迎穴處→下頜角頰車→耳前→前額。

面部支脈：大迎→人迎→缺盆→横膈→胃→脾。

缺盆部直行的脈：缺盆→乳頭→臍旁→氣衝。

胃下口部支脈：胃下口→沿腹裏下行→氣衝→髀關→伏兔→膝蓋→脛骨外前緣→足背→第二趾外側端。

脛部支脈：膝下 3 寸處→足中趾外側。

足跗部支脈：足背跗上→足大趾内側端，與足太陰脾經相接。

(3) The Stomach channel of foot yangming

The lateral side of the nose →the bridge of the nose →lateral to the nostrils →the upper gum →round the lips →posterior and lateral to the mouth →the lower portion of the cheek at ST 5 (*dà yíng*) →below the zygomatic bone →in front of the ear →forehead.

The facial branch channel: ST 5 (*dà yíng*) →ST 9 (*rén yíng*) →ST 12 (*quē pén*) →diaphram →Stomach →Spleen.

The direct pathway of the channel arising from the superclavicular fossa: ST 12 (*quē pén*) →nipple →umbilicus →ST 30 (*qì chōng*).

The branch from the lower orifice of the stomach: from inside the abdomen →descends to ST 30 (*qì chōng*) →ST 31 (*bì guān*) →ST 32 (*fú tù*) →the knee →the anterior border of the lateral tibia →the dorsum of the foot →the lateral side of the tip of second toe.

The tibial branch channel: 3 cun below the knee →the lateral side of the middle toe.

The branch from the dorsum of the foot: the dorsum of the foot →ends at the medial side of the tip of the big toe →and links with the Spleen channel of foot taiyin.

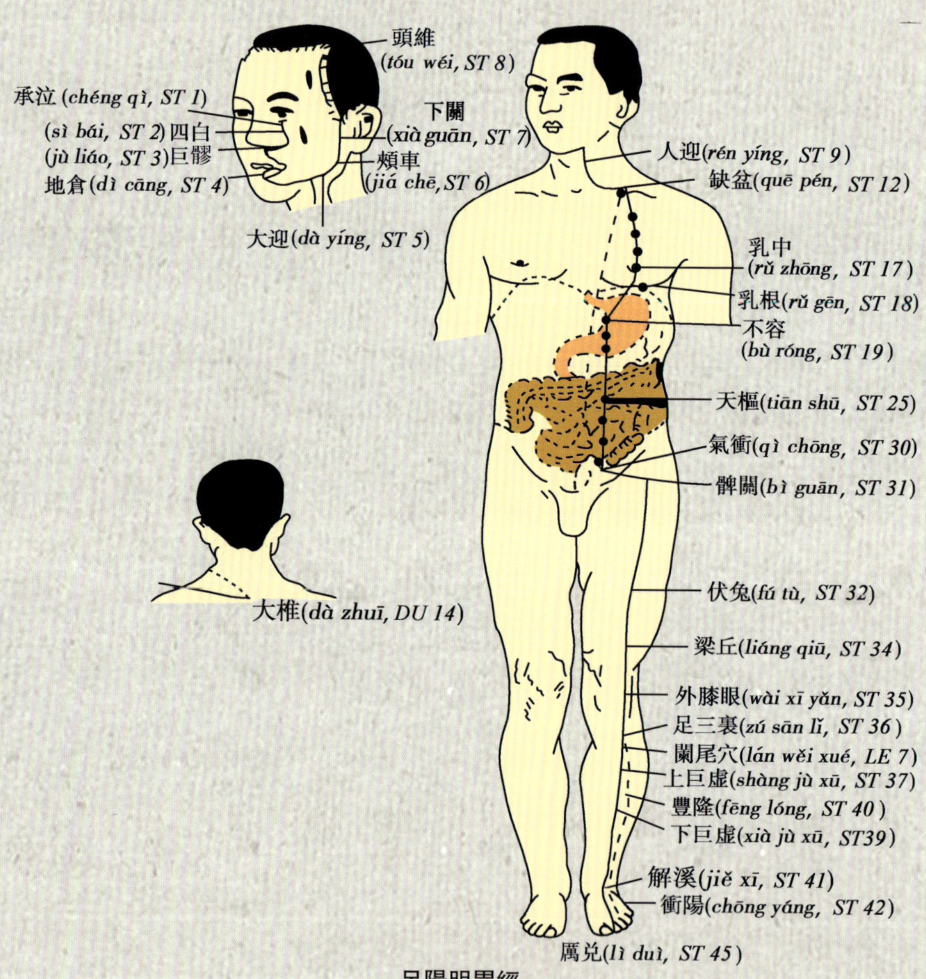

足陽明胃經

The Stomach channel of foot yangming

（4）足太陰脾經

足大趾端内側→第一趾關節後面→内踝前→腿肚→交出足厥陰肝經前面→膝、股部内側前緣→腹部→脾→胃→横膈→咽→舌根→舌下。

胃部支脈：胃→横膈→心中，與手少陰心經相接。

(4) The Spleen channel of foot taiyin

The medial side of the tip of the big toe →the posterior aspect of the toe joint →the anterior medial malleolus →the calf →after connecting, medial to the Liver channel of foot jueyin →the anterior medial aspect of the knee and thigh →abdomen →Spleen → Stomach →diaphragm →esophagus →the root of the tongue →beneath the tongue.

The Stomach branch channel: Stomach → diaphragm →heart →and links with the Heart channel of hand shaoyin.

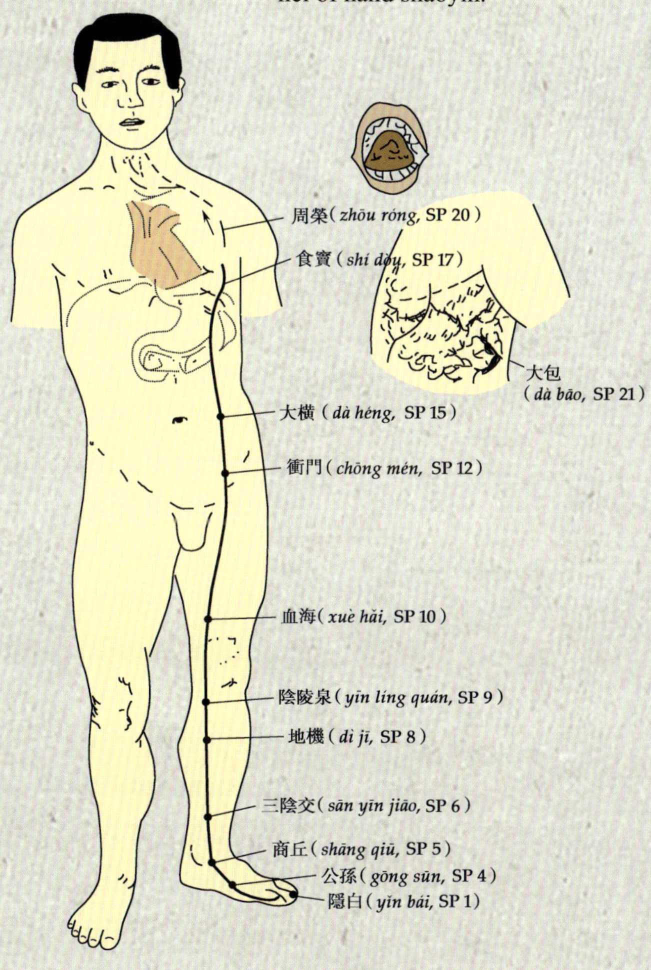

足太陰脾經

The Spleen channel of foot taiyin

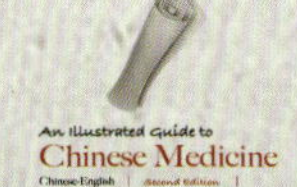

（5）手少陰心經

心中→心係→横膈→小腸。

從心向上的脈：心係→咽喉→目係。

從心係直行的脈：心係→肺→腋窩→上臂内側後緣→前臂内側後緣→掌後豆骨部→掌内→小指内側至末端，與手太陽小腸經相接。

(5) The Heart channel of hand shaoyin

Heart →heart system →diaphragm →Small Intestine.

The ascending branch of the "heart system" channel: heart system →throat →eye system.

The direct pathway of the channel of the "heart system": heart system →Lung →axilla →the posterior border of the medial upper arm →the posterior border of the medial forearm →the pisiform region proximal to the palm →the palm →the medial aspect of the little finger to the tip →and links with the Small Intestine channel of hand taiyang.

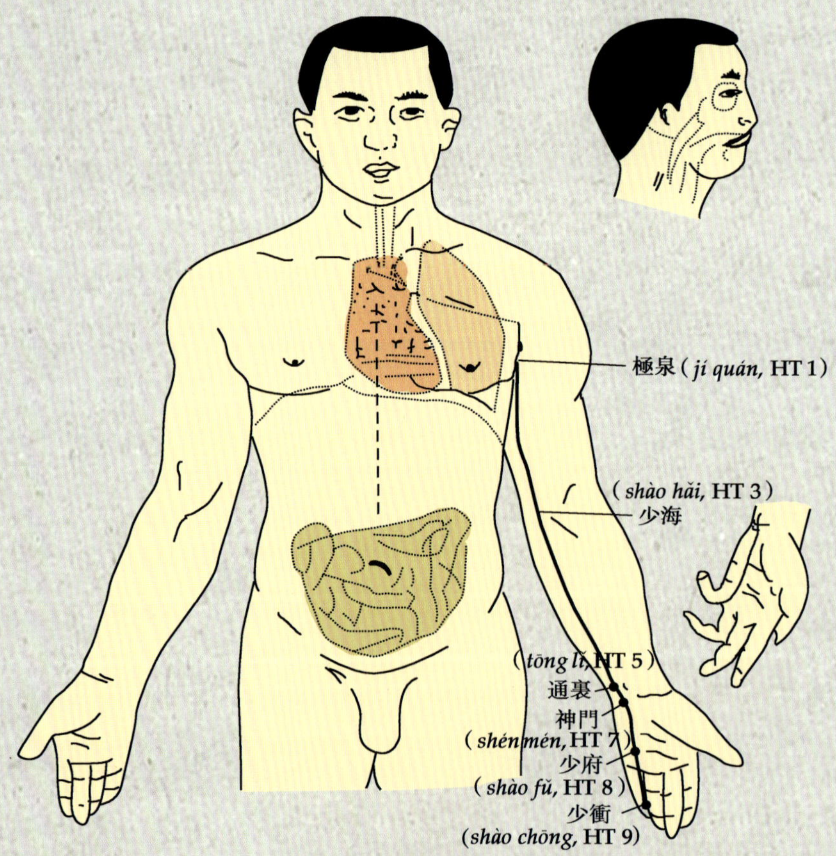

手少陰心經

The Heart channel of hand shaoyin

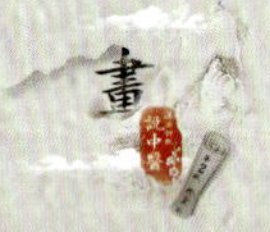

（6）手太陽小腸經

小指外側端→手背外側→腕部→尺骨莖突→前臂外側後緣→尺骨鷹嘴與肱骨内上髁之間上臂外側後緣→肩關節→肩胛部→大椎→缺盆→心→横膈→胃→小腸。

缺盆部支脈：缺盆→頸→面頰→目外眦→耳中。

頰部支脈：頰→目眶下→鼻旁→目内眦，與足太陽膀胱經相接。

(6) The Small Intestine Channel of hand taiyang

The lateral tip of the little finger →the lateral side of the dorsum of the hand →wrist →the styloid process of the ulna →the lateral posterior aspect of the forearm → superior to the olecranon of the ulna and the medial epicondyle of the humerus →the posterior border of the lateral aspect of the upper arm →shoulder joint → scapular region →DU 14 (*dà zhuī*) →ST 12 (*quē pén*) → Heart →diaphragm →Stomach →Small Intestine.

The branch channel of the supraclavicular fossa: ST 12 (*quē pén*) →neck →cheek →the outer canthus →ear.

The branch channel of cheek: cheek → infraorbital region → lateral to the nose → the inner canthus → and links with the Bladder Channel of foot taiyang.

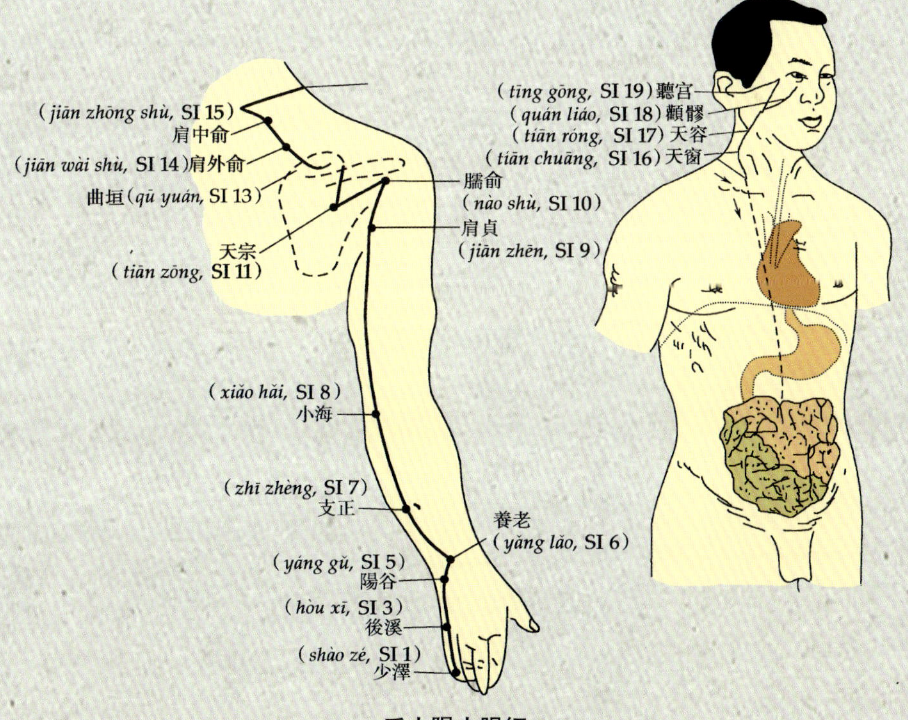

手太陽小腸經

The Small Intestine channel of hand taiyang

（7）足太陽膀胱經

目内眦→額→巔頂。

巔頂部支脈：巔頂→顳顬部。

巔頂部直行的脈：頭頂（入裏）→腦→肩胛内側→腰（從脊旁進入腹腔）→腎→膀胱。

腰部的支脈：腰→臀→膕窩。

後項的支脈：項後→肩胛内緣→臀→大腿後外側→膕窩（與腰部支脈會合）→腓腸肌→外踝後→第五跖骨粗隆→小趾外側端，與足少陰腎經相接。

(7) The Bladder Channel of foot taiyang

The inner canthus → forehead → the vertex.

The branch channel of vertex: the vertex → temple.

The direct pathway of the channel: vertex of the brain → inside of the brain → the medial aspect of the scapular region → the lumbar region (from where it enters the body cavity via the paravertebral muscles) → Kidney → the Bladder.

The branch channel of the lumbar region: the lumbar region → the gluteal region → the popliteal fossa.

The branch channel of the posterior aspect of the neck: the posterior neck → the medial border of the scapula → the gluteal region → the lateral posterior aspect of the thigh → the popliteal fossa (where it meets the branch descending from the lumbar region) → the gastrocnemius muscle → the posterior aspect of the external malleolus → the tuberosity of the fifth metatarsal bone → where it links with the Kidney channel of foot shaoyin.

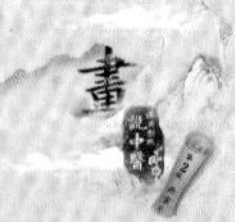

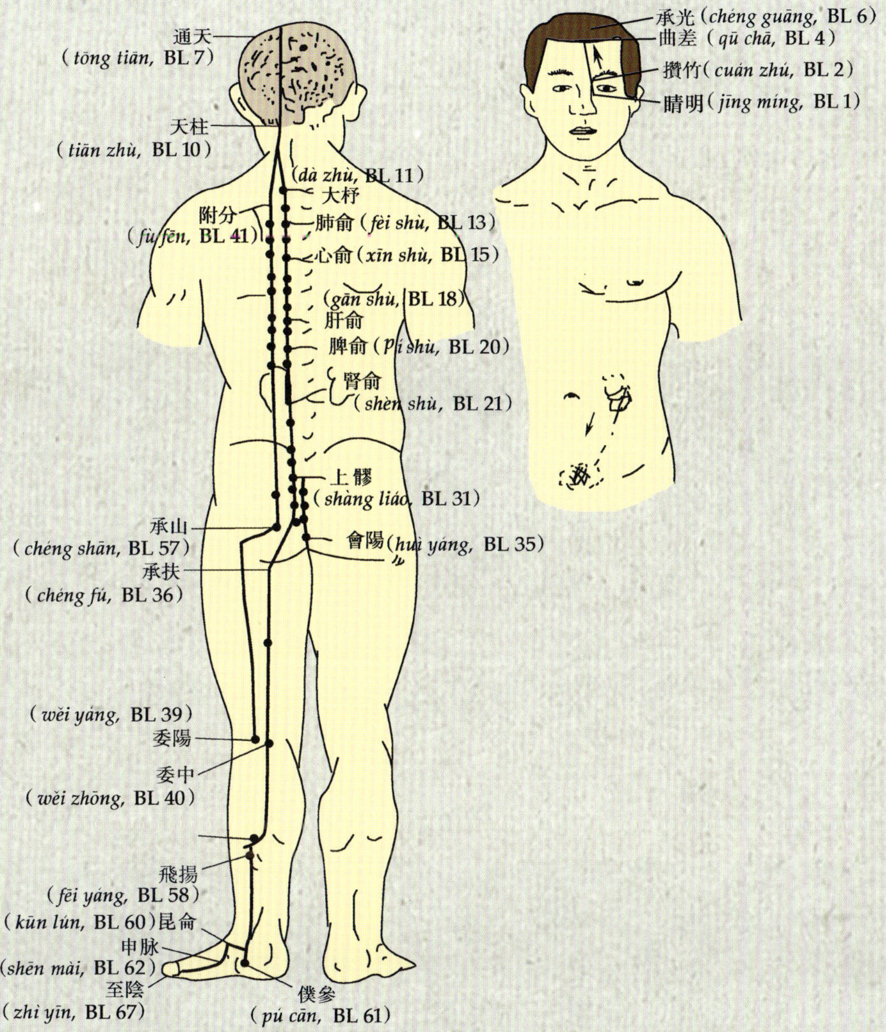

足太陽膀胱經

The Bladder channel of foot taiyang

（8）足少陰腎經

小趾下→足心→舟骨粗隆下→内踝後→足跟→腿内側→股部内後緣→脊柱→腎→膀胱

腎臟部直行的脈：腎→肝→横膈→肺→喉嚨→舌根。

肺部支脈：肺→心→胸中，與手厥陰心包經相接。

(8) The Kidney channel of foot shaoyin

The inferior aspect of the small toe → the sole → the tuberosity of the navicular bone → the medial malleolus → the heel → the medial side of the leg → the medial side of the popliteal fossa → the posterior medial aspect of the thigh → the vertebral column → Kidney → Bladder.

The direct pathway of the channel: the Kidney → Liver → diaphragm → Lung → throat → root of the tongue.

The branch that springs from the Lung: Lung → Heart → chest → and links with the Pericardium channel of hand jueyin.

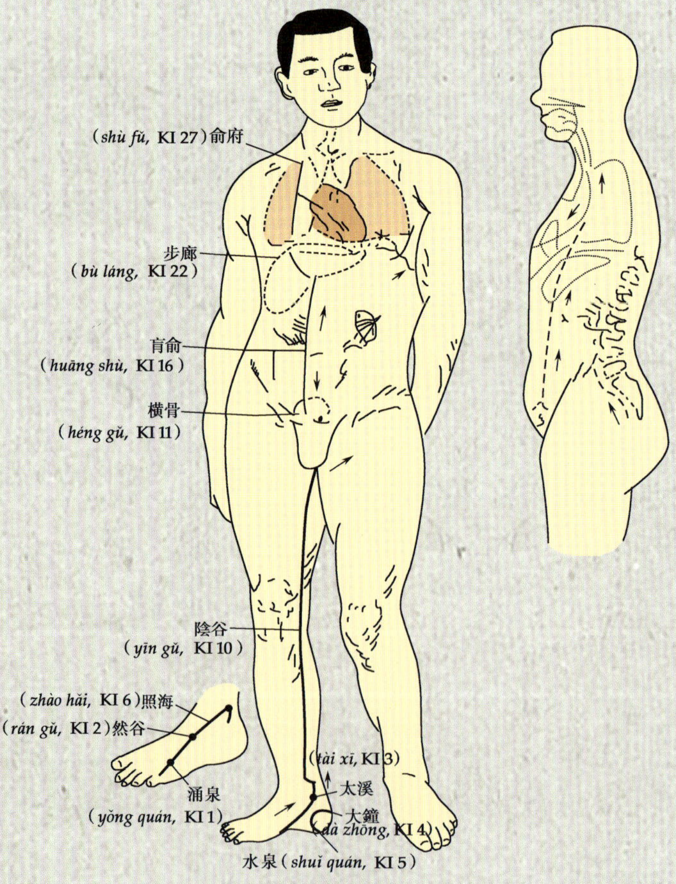

足少陰腎經

The Kidney channel of foot shaoyin

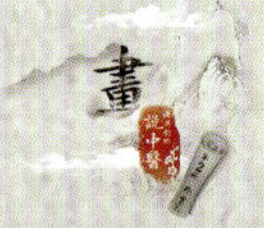

（9）手厥陰心包經

胸中→心包絡→橫膈（從胸至腹聯絡上、中、下三焦）。

胸部支脈：胸中→脅→腋下3寸處→腋窩→上臂內側肘窩中→前臂兩筋之間→掌中→中指端。

掌中支脈：勞宮穴→無名指端→與手少陽三焦經相接。

(9) The Pericardium channel of hand jueyin

Chest → Pericardium → diaphragm (to connect with the upper, middle, and lower burners successively in the chest and the abdomen).

The branch channel of the chest: chest → the costal region → the point 3 cun below the axilla → axilla → the cubital fossa of the medial upper arm → the forearm between the tendons of palmaris longus and flexor carpi → palm → the tip of the middle finger.

The branch channel of the palm: PC 8 (*láo gōng*) → the tip of the ring finger → links with the San Jiao channel of hand shaoyang.

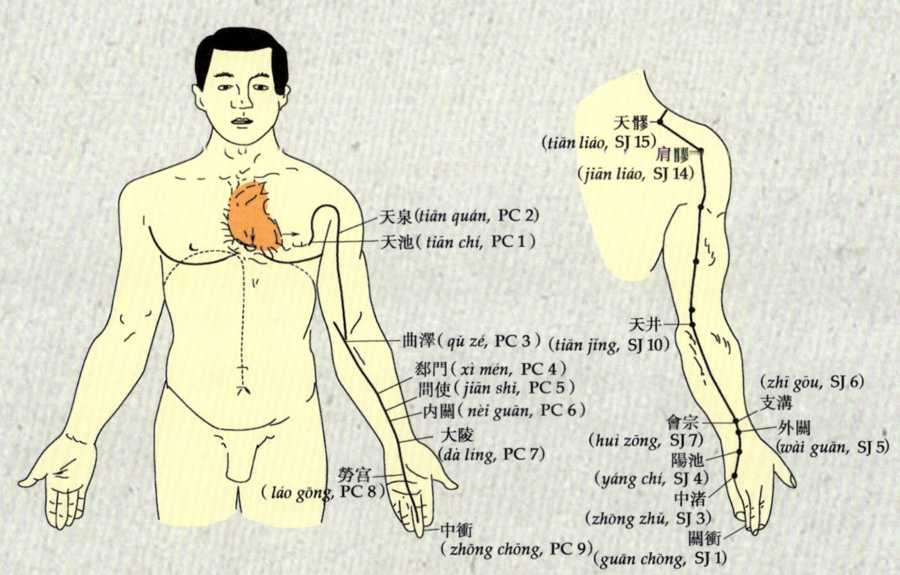

手厥陰心包經

The Pericardium channel of hand jueyin

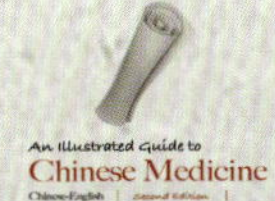

（10）手少陽三焦經

無名指末端→四、五掌骨間→腕背→前臂外側橈、尺骨之間→肘尖→上臂外側→肩部→缺盆→胸中→心包→橫膈，從胸至腹，屬於上、中、下三焦。

胸中的支脈：胸→缺盆→項部→耳後→耳上部→額角→面頰→眶下部。

耳部的支脈：耳後→耳中→耳前→面頰→目外眦，與足少陽膽經相接。

(10) The San Jiao channel of hand shaoyang

The tip of the ring finger → between the 4th and 5th metacarpal bones → the dorsal aspect of the wrist → the lateral forearm between the radius and ulna → the olecranon → the lateral upper arm → the shoulder region → the supraclavicular fossa → chest → pericardium → diaphragm, from where it descends through the abdomen, and joins its pertaining organ, the upper, middle and lower Burners.

A branch channel of the chest: chest → the supraclavicular fossa → neck → posterior border of the ear → above the ear → anterior hairline → cheek → infraorbital region.

The auricular branch channel: from the retro-auricular region → inside the ear → in front of the ear → cheek→ outer canthus, where it links with the Gallbladder Channel of foot shaoyang.

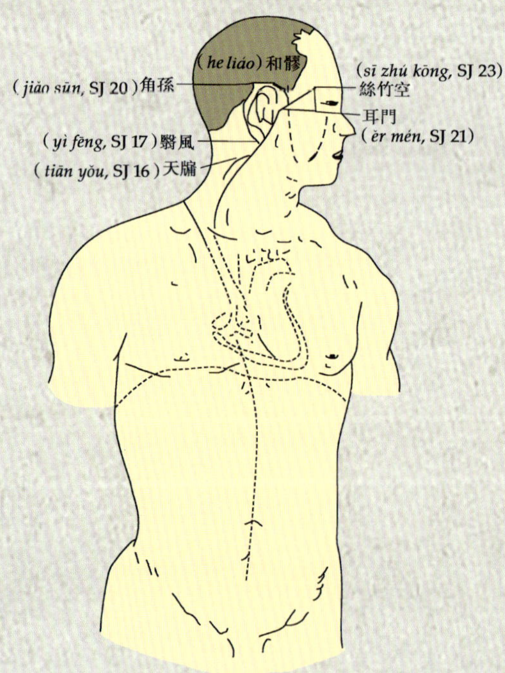

手少陽三焦經

The San Jiao channel of hand shaoyang

（11）足少陽膽經

目外眦→耳前→額角→耳後→乳突後下方→前額→頸→肩→缺盆。

耳部的支脈：耳後→耳中→耳前→目外眦後方。

目外眦的支脈：目外眦→大迎→目眶下→頰車→頸→缺盆→胸中→横膈→肝→膽→脅→腹股溝→外陰部毛際→髖關節。

缺盆部直行的脈：缺盆→腋部→胸側→季脅→髖關節部→大腿外側→膝部外側→腓骨前面→腓骨下段→外踝前→足背→第四趾外側端。

足背部支脈：足臨泣→一、二跖骨之間→大趾端→趾甲後毫毛部，與足厥陰肝經相接。

(11) The Gallbladder Channel of foot shaoyang

The outer canthus → in front of the ear → the corner of the forehead → the retro-auricular region → behind the mastoid → the forehead → the neck → the shoulder → ST 12 (*quē pén*).

The retro-auricular branch: the retro-auricular region → inside the ear→ the pre-auricular region → the posterior outer canthus.

The outer canthus branch channel: The outer canthus → ST 5 (*dà yíng*) point → the infraorbital region → ST 6 (*jiá chē*) point → the neck → ST 12 (*quē pén*) → chest → diaphragm → Liver→ Gallbladder → the hypochondriac region → inguinal groove → the pubic margin → the hip joint.

The direct pathway of the supraclavicular fossa branch channel: ST 12 (*quē pén*)→ the axilla → the lateral chest → the floating ribs → the hip region → the lateral aspect of the thigh → the lateral side of the knee → the anterior aspect of the fibula → the inferior fibula → the anterior aspect of the external malleolus → the dorsum of the foot → the lateral side of the tip of the 4th toe.

The branch of the dorsum of the foot: GB 41 (*zú lín qì*) → the first and second metatarsal bones → the distal portion of the big toe → the hairy region of the area posterior to the toenail, where it links with the Liver channel of foot jueyin.

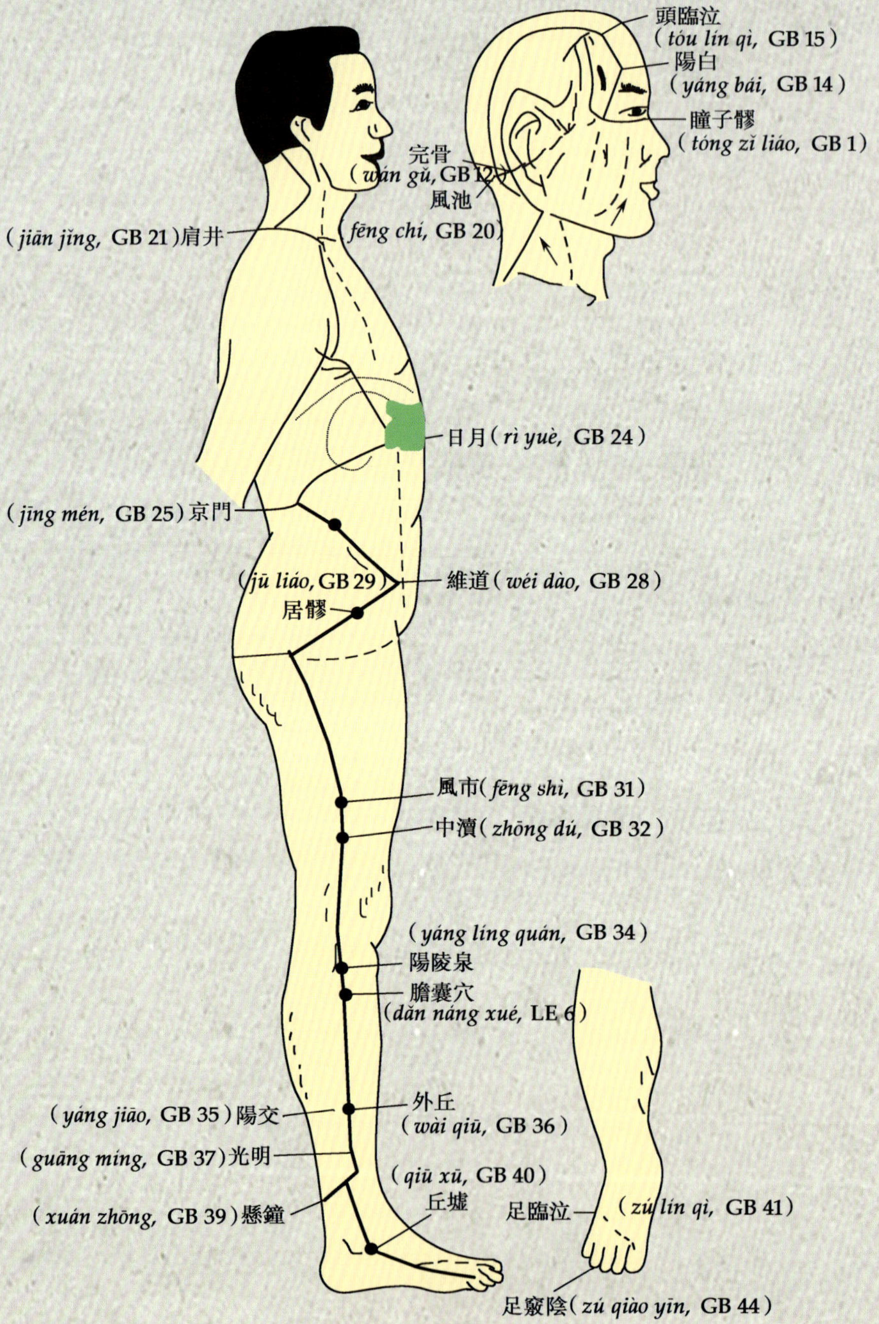

頭臨泣（tóu lín qì, GB 15）
陽白（yáng bái, GB 14）
瞳子髎（tóng zǐ liáo, GB 1）
完骨（wán gǔ, GB 12）
風池（fēng chí, GB 20）
（jiān jǐng, GB 21）肩井
日月（rì yuè, GB 24）
（jīng mén, GB 25）京門
（jū liáo, GB 29）居髎
維道（wéi dào, GB 28）
風市（fēng shì, GB 31）
中瀆（zhōng dú, GB 32）
（yáng líng quán, GB 34）陽陵泉
膽囊穴（dǎn náng xué, LE 6）
（yáng jiāo, GB 35）陽交
外丘（wài qiū, GB 36）
（guāng míng, GB 37）光明
（qiū xū, GB 40）丘墟
（xuán zhōng, GB 39）懸鐘
足臨泣（zú lín qì, GB 41）
足竅陰（zú qiào yīn, GB 44）

足少陽膽經
The Gallbladder channel of foot shaoyang

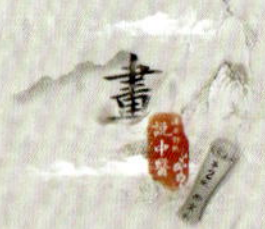

（12）足厥陰肝經

足大趾毫毛部→足背→内踝前→内踝上 8 寸處交出於足太陰脾經之後→膝内側→股内側→陰毛中（繞陰部）→小腹→胃→肝→膽→横膈→脅肋→喉嚨後面→鼻咽部→目係→前額，與督脈會合於巔頂。

目係的支脈：目係→頰裏→唇内（環繞）。

肝部的支脈：肝→横膈→肺，與手太陰肺經相接。

(12) The Liver channel of foot jueyin

The area of hair on the big toe dorsum → the dorsum of the foot → in front of the medial malleolus → an area 8 cun above the medial malleolus, where it intersects with and moves behind the Spleen channel of foot taiyin → the medial side of the knee → the medial side of the thigh → the public hair region (where it curves around the external genitalia) → the lower abdomen → Stomach → Liver → Gallbladder → diaphragm → the costal and hypochondriac regions → the posterior throat → pharynx nasalis → the eye system → forehead, where it meets the Du vessel at the vertex.

The branch channel of the eye system: eye system→ inside the cheek → the inner surface of the lips.

The branch channel of the Liver: Liver→ diaphragm→ Lung, where it links with the Lung channel of hand taiyin.

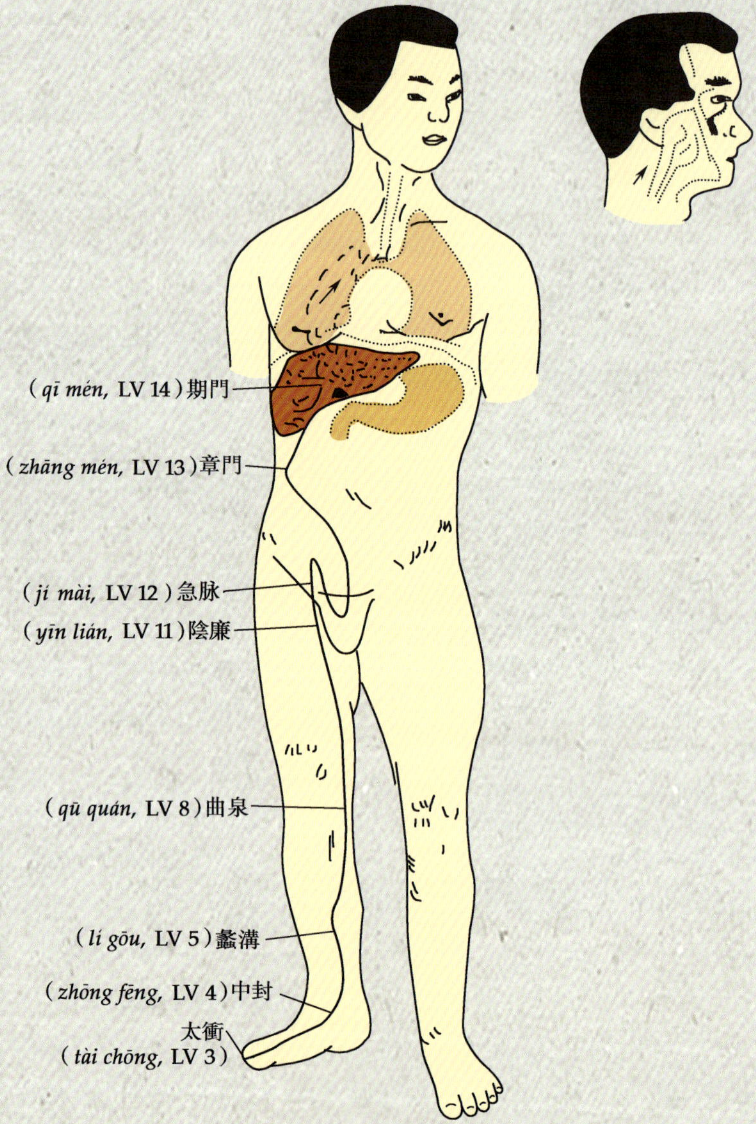

(qī mén, LV 14)期門

(zhāng mén, LV 13)章門

(jí mài, LV 12)急脉

(yīn lián, LV 11)陰廉

(qū quán, LV 8)曲泉

(lí gōu, LV 5)蠡溝

(zhōng fēng, LV 4)中封

太衝
(tài chōng, LV 3)

足厥陰肝經

The Liver channel of foot jueyin

表 4-4　十二經歸納表

經脈名稱	起點	體表主要分布部位			止點	聯係臟腑	聯絡器官
		頭部	軀幹部	四肢部			
手太陰肺經	中焦（胃）		胸部外上方	上肢內側前緣	拇指末端	肺、大腸、胃	氣管、喉嚨
手陽明大腸經	食指末端	面頰、挾口	肩胛部	上肢外側前緣	鼻旁與胃經相接	大腸、肺	下齒、口、鼻
足陽明胃經	鼻旁	鼻根、前額	胸部（乳中綫）、腹部	下肢前外側	二趾（及中趾）	胃、脾、心	上齒、喉嚨、乳、鼻、口
足太陰脾經	大趾		腹部、胸部	下肢內側前緣	舌下	脾、胃、心	咽、舌
手少陰心經	心中		腋下	上肢內側後緣	小指末端與小腸經相接	心、心係、小腸、肺	咽、目係
手太陽小腸經	小指末端	面頰、目眶下緣	肩胛部	上肢外側後緣	目內眦與膀胱經相接	小腸、心、胃	耳、目
足太陽膀胱經	目內眦	額、頂、枕、項	背、腰部	下肢後外側	小趾與腎經相接	膀胱、腎、腦	肛門、目
足少陰腎經	小趾		腹部、胸部	足跟、下肢內側後緣	夾舌本	腎、膀胱、肝、肺、心	喉嚨、舌
手厥陰心包經	胸中		脅部	上肢內側中綫	中指末端	心包、三焦	
手少陽三焦經	無名指末端	耳周圍、頰	肩後側	上肢外側中綫	目眶下	三焦、心包	耳、目
足少陽膽經	目外眦	頭顳側、耳周圍	胸側、腹側	下肢外側中綫	四趾	膽、肝、心	耳、目、咽
足厥陰肝經	大趾	頭頂	少腹、脅肋	下肢內側中綫	頭頂	肝、膽、肺、胃	外生殖器、目係、喉嚨、鼻、目

Table 4-4 The Sum Form of Twelve Channels

The names of channels	Starting point	Distribution			End point	Linking with the Zang-fu organs	Linking with the organs
		Head region	Body region	The trunk			
The hand greater yin Lung channel	Middle burner (Stomach)		The lateral aspect of upper chest	The anterior border of the radial side in the medial aspect of the forearm	The tip of the thumb	Lung, Large Intestine, Stomach	Bronchus, throat
The hand yang brightness Large Intestine channel	The tip of the index finger	Cheek, around the mouth	Scapular region	The lateral anterior aspect of the upper arm	The contra-lateral sides of the nose, links with the Stomach channel of the foot yangming	Lung, Large Intestine	Lower teeth, mouth, nose
The foot yang brightness Stomach channel	The lateral side of the nose	The root of the nose, forehead	The chest region and the abdomen region	The lateral aspect of the lower limbs	The 2nd and middle toe	Stomach, Spleen, Heart	Upper teeth, throat, breast, nose, mouth
The foot greater yin Spleen Channel	The tip of the big toe		Abdomen, chest	The anterior medial aspect of the lower limbs	Under tongue	Spleen, Stomach, Heart	Throat, tongue
The hand lesser yin Heart channel	The heart		The axilla	The posterior border of the medial aspect of upper arms	The tip of the little finger links with Small Intestine channel	Heart, heart system, Small Intestine Lung	Throat, eye system
The hand greater yang Small Intestine channel	The tip of the little finger	Cheek, infraorbital region	Scapular region	The posterior border of the lateral aspect of upper arms	The inner canthus links with the Urinary Bladder channel of foot taiyang	Small Intestine, Heart, Stomach	Ear, eye

(Continued)

The names of channels	Starting point	Distribution			End point	Linking with the Zang-fu organs	Linking with the organs
		Head region	Body region	The trunk			
The foot greater yang Urinary Bladder Channel	The inner canthus	Forehead, the vertex, the posterior aspect of the neck	Back, waist	The lateral aspect of the upper limbs	The little toe links with the Kidney channel	Bladder, Kidney, Brain	The anus, the eye
The foot lesser yin Kidney Channel	The small toe		Abdomen, chest	Hell, the posterior border of medial aspect of lower limbs	The root of the tongue	Kidney, Urinary, Bladder, Liver, Lung, Heart	Throat, tongue
The hand revering yin Pericardi-um channel	The chest		The costal region	The middle line of medial aspect of upper limbs	The tip of middle finger	Pericardium, San Jiao	
The hand lesser yang San Jiao channel	The tip of the ring finger	The region of the ear the cheek	The back side of shoulder region	The middle line of lateral aspect of the upper limbs	The infraorbital region	San Jiao, pericardium	Ear, eye
The foot lesser yang Gallbladder channel	The outer canthus	The region of the ear	The front of the axilla	The middle line of lateral aspect of the lower limbs	The forth toe	Gallbladder Liver Heart	Ear, eye, throat
The foot reverting yin Liver Channel	The big toe	The vertex	The lower abdomen, the costa	The middle line of medial aspect of the lower limbs	The vertex	Liver, Gallbladder, Lung, Stomach	Eye system, throat, nose

三、奇經八脈

1. 概念

奇經八脈是督脈、任脈、衝脈、帶脈、陽蹺脈、陰蹺脈、陰維脈、陽維脈的總稱。由於它們的分布不像十二經脈那樣規則，與臟腑沒有直接的相互絡屬，相互之間也沒有表裏關係，與十二正經不同，故稱奇經。

2. 作用

奇經八脈縱橫交叉於十二經脈之間。

主要作用是：

（1）進一步密切十二經脈之間的聯係，如督脈能＂總督諸陽＂，任脈爲＂諸陰之海＂等。

（2）調節十二經脈的氣血。十二經脈氣血有餘時，則流注於奇經，蓄以備用；十二經脈氣血不足時，可由奇經給予補充調節。

（3）奇經與肝、腎等臟及女子胞、腦、髓等奇恒之腑的關係比較密切，它們在生理上與病理上都有聯係。

The Eight Extraordinary Vessels

1. The Concept of the Eight Extraordinary Vessels

"The Eight Extraordinary Vessels" are a general term for the Governing Vessel, Conception Vessel, Penetrating Vessel, Girdling Vessel, yin heel vessel, yang heel vessel, yin link vessel, and yang link vessel. They are called "Extraordinary Vessels" because their distribution is less regular as those of the twelve channels, and because they have neither direct relationship with the internal organs, nor exterior-interior coordination between them.

2. The Functions of the Eight Extraordinary Vessels

The eight extra channels crisscross the path of the twelve primary channels, and function in the following ways:

(1) To further strengthen the connection of the twelve primary channels. For example, the Governing vessel governs the yang channels, and the Conception vessel is called the sea of the yin channels.

(2) To regulate the qi and blood of the twelve primary channels. When the amount of blood and qi inside the twelve primary channels is so full that it overflows, the excess will be stored in the eight extraordinary vessels. Conversely, when the amount of blood and qi in the primary channels is insufficient, it will be supplemented from what is stored in the eight extraordinary vessels.

(3) The eight extraordinary vessels are closely related to the Liver, Kidney and other regular internal organs, and also to the uterus, brain, marrow and extraordinary organs. They communicate with them physiologically and pathologically.

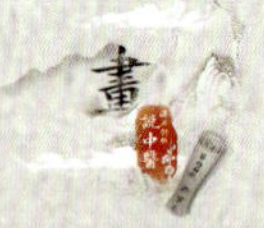

3. 循行與功能概況

表 4-5　奇經八脈循行與功能概況表

經名	循行部位	功能
督脈	胞中→會陰→脊柱内→頂部（入顱絡腦）→頭頂→額、鼻、上唇	總督一身之陽經，爲"陽脈之海"，並與腦、脊髓和腎有密切聯係
任脈	胞中→會陰→陰阜→腹、胸正中綫→咽喉、下頜、口唇、面頰→目眶下	總任一身之陰經，爲"陰脈之海"又與孕育有關，稱爲"任主胞胎"

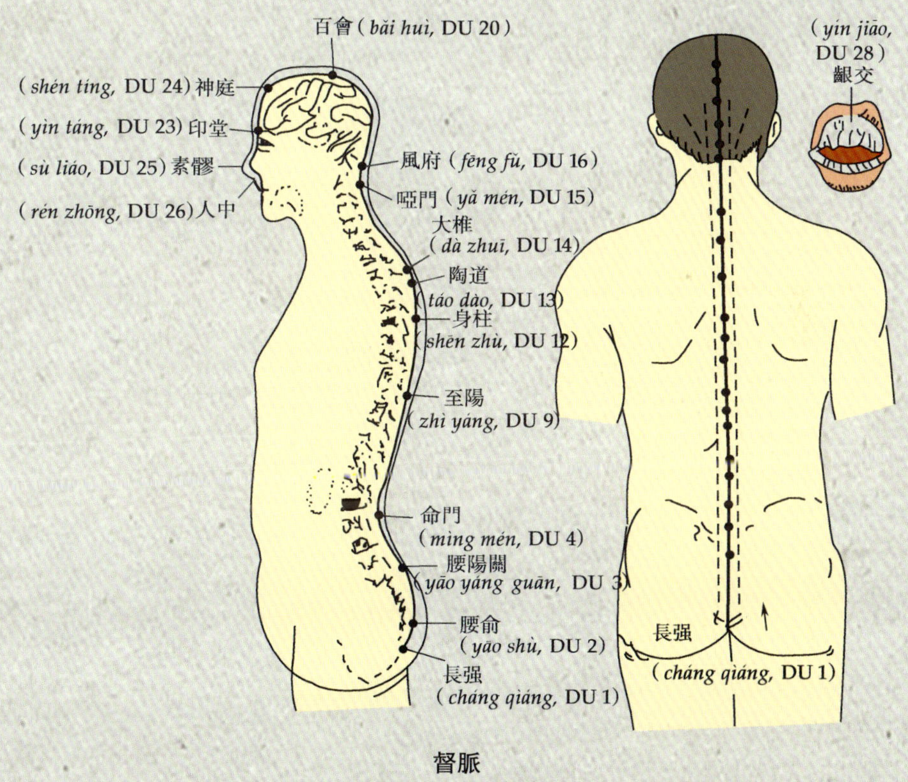

督脈

Governing vessel

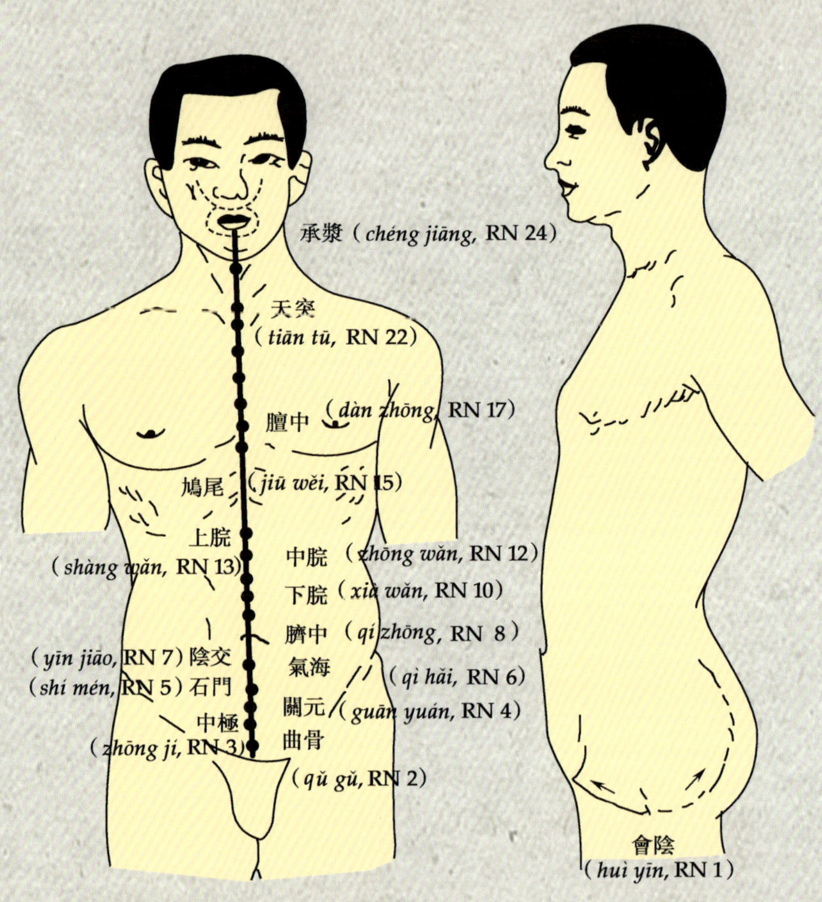

任脈

Conception vessel

3. The Route of Their Flow and Functions

Table 4-5 The Route of Their Flow and Functions

Extraordinary Vessel	Vessel course	Function
Governing vessel	Lower abdomen—perineum—inside the spinal column—nape—vertex forehead—nose & upper lip.	It governs the yang channel, therefore is named the sea of yang channels. It has a close relationship with the brain, marrow, Kidney.
Conception vessel	Lower abdomen—perineum — anterior—pubic region—midline of the abdomen and chest—throat, chin, lips & cheek—infraorbital region.	It governs all the yin channels of the whole body, therefore is named the sea of all the yin channels. In addition, it is said, "the Conception vessel is in charge of pregnancy" .
Penetrating vessel	① Placenta— front wall of abdomen—spinal column ② placenta— back wall of abdomen—chest—throat—round the lip—the medial malleolus— dorsal foot— big toe ③ placenta—perineum— medial aspect of thigh--plantar	The Penetrating vessel flows upward to the head and downward to the foot, and connect with the whole body .It is also responsible for regulating the qi and blood of the twelve primary channels, therefore it is also called "the sea of the twelve primary channels." Also it is sometimes termed "the sea of blood" for it is related with menstruation.
Girdling vessel	Hypochondrium—GB 26 (*dài mài*), around the waist—superior—iliac crest—the lower abdomen.	It wraps around the waist similar to a girdle, and binds together all the channels.
Yin heel vessel	Under malleolus—medial malleolus—medial posterior aspect of lower limbs—front genitals—abdomen, chest, ST 12 (*quē pén*), tonsils—inner canthus.	It controls the yin of the left and right sides of the whole body, and also nourishes the eyes, controls the opening and closing of the eyelids and the motion of the lower limbs.
Yang heel vessel	Malleolus external malleolus lateral lower limbs—posterior-lateral aspect of the abdomen and chest—lateral aspect of the shoulder and neck—corner of the mouth—inner canthus—hairline behind the ears.	It controls the yang of the left and right sides of the whole body, and also nourishes the eyes, controls the opening and closing of the eyelids and the motion of the lower limbs.
Yin link vessel	The medial aspect of shin (connects with SP 6, *sān yīn jiāo*) —medial aspect of lower limbs—abdomen (where it travels with the Spleen channel) —costal region—throat (where it connects with the Conception vessel).	It maintains and communicates with all the yin channels of the body.
Yang link vessel	Below the lateral malleolus—lateral aspect of lower limbs—posterior- lateral trunk—posterior armpit, shoulder, neck, posterior aspect of the ears, forehead—sides of the head, posterior side of nape.	It maintains and communicates with all the yang channels of the body.

經名	循行部位	功能
衝脈	①胞中→腹腔後壁→脊柱内 ②胞中→腹腔前壁→挾擠、布胸中→喉→環口唇→内踝→足背→大趾 ③胞中→下出會陰→股内側→足底	貫串全身，爲氣血要衝，能調節十二經氣血，稱“十二經脈之海”，與月經有關，又稱“血海”
帶脈	季脅←帶脈穴、繞腰一周→前下方→髂骨上緣→少腹	圍腰一周，猶如束帶，能約束縱行諸脈

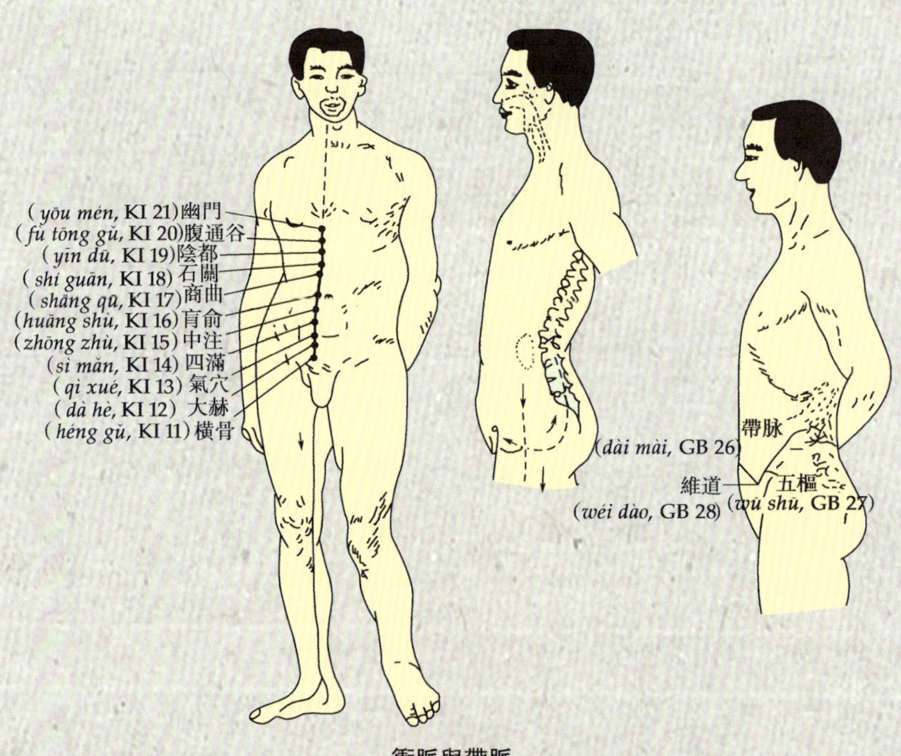

衝脈與帶脈

Penetrating vessel & Girdling vessel

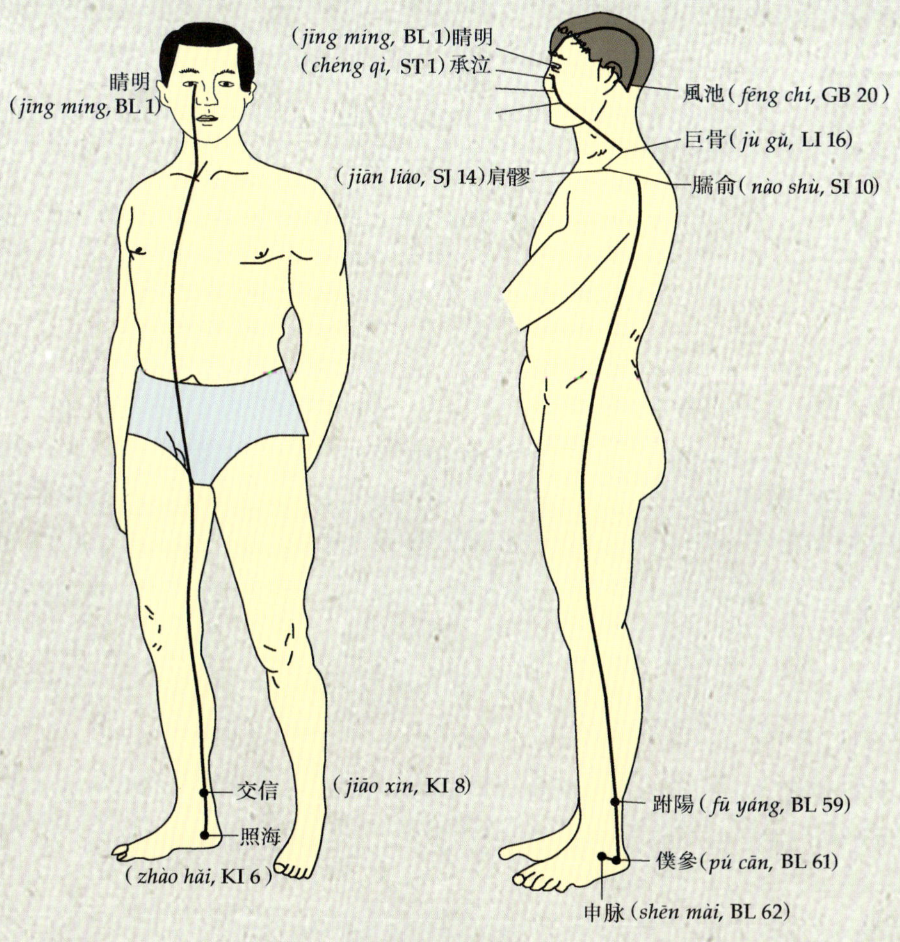

陰蹺脈與陽蹺脈

Yin heel vessel & Yang heel vessel

經名	循行部位	功能
陰蹺脈	足踝下→內踝→下肢內側後方→前陰→腹、胸、缺盆、結喉旁→目內眦	主一身左右之陰，又主濡養眼目，司眼瞼開合，下肢運動。
陽蹺脈	足踝下→外踝→下肢外側→腹部、胸部後外側→肩、頸外側→挾口角→目內眦→發際耳後	主一身左右之陽，又主濡養眼目，司眼瞼開合，下肢運動。

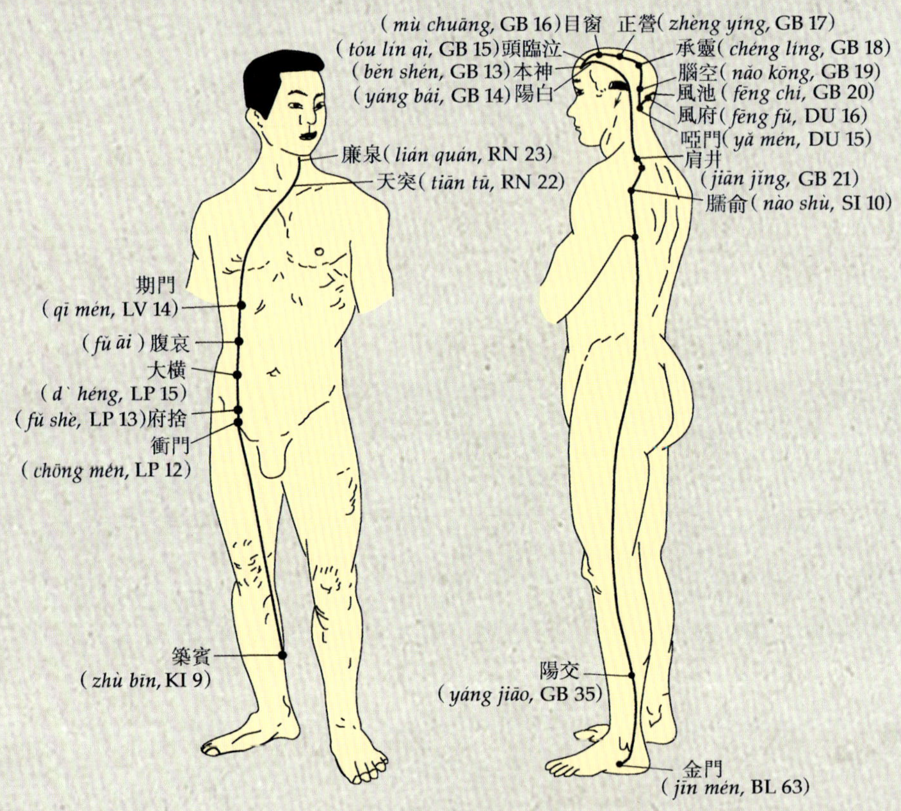

陰維脈與陽維脈

Yin link vessel & Yang link vessel

經名	循行部位	功能
陰維脈	小腿内側(足三陰交會處)→下肢内側→腹部(與脾經同行)→脅部→咽喉(會任脈)	維係諸陰經
陽維脈	外踝下→下肢外側→軀幹後外側→腋後、肩、頸、耳後、額→頭側、項後(會督脈)	維係諸陽經

四、經絡的生理功能及經絡學説的應用

The Physiological Functions of the Channels and Application of Channel Theory

1. 經絡的生理功能

（1）聯係作用

主要體現在聯係臟腑器官，溝通上下内外。人體是由五臟六腑、五官九竅、四肢百骸、皮肉筋骨等組成的，它們雖各有不同的生理功能，但又共同進行着有機的整體活動，這種有機配合，相互聯係，主要是依靠經絡係統的聯絡、溝通作用實現的。

1. The Physiological Functions of the Channels and Collaterals

(1) Connection

The channels connect the Zang-fu organs and link the body's exterior with its interior and its upper region with the lower. The human body consists of the five Zang-organs and six Fu-organs, five sense organs and nine orifices, four limbs and joints, skin, muscles, tendons, vessels and bones. Although there are differences in different body parts' physiological functions, they all cooperate together in integrated activities. This interrelationship and cooperation are built upon the connection and linking functions of the channels and collaterals.

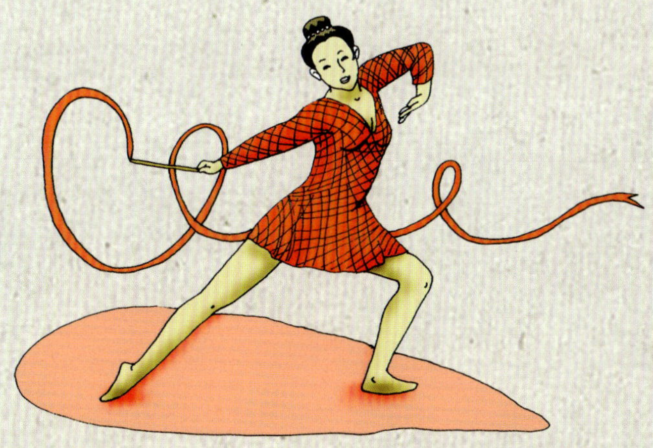

（2）濡養作用

主要體現在通行氣血。氣血通過經絡循環貫注通達全身，發揮其營養臟腑組織器官、抗御外邪保衛機體的作用。

(2) Nourishing

This function is mainly performed by the circulation of qi and blood. The qi and blood circulate within the whole body to nourish the Zang-fu organs and tissues, and to protect the body against exterior evils.

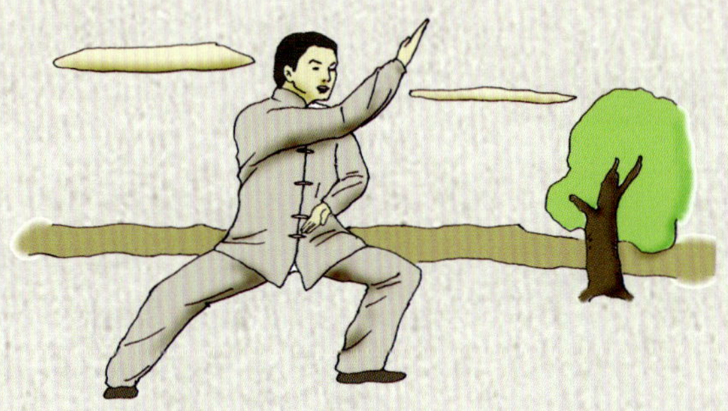

（3）感應作用

經絡是人體各組成部分之間的信息傳導網。當肌表受到某種刺激時，刺激量就沿着經脈傳於體内有關臟腑，使該臟腑的功能發生變化，從而達到疏通氣血和調整臟腑功能的目的。臟腑功能活動的變化亦可通過經絡而反應於體表。經絡循環四通八達而至機體每一個局部，從而使每一局部成爲整體的縮影。

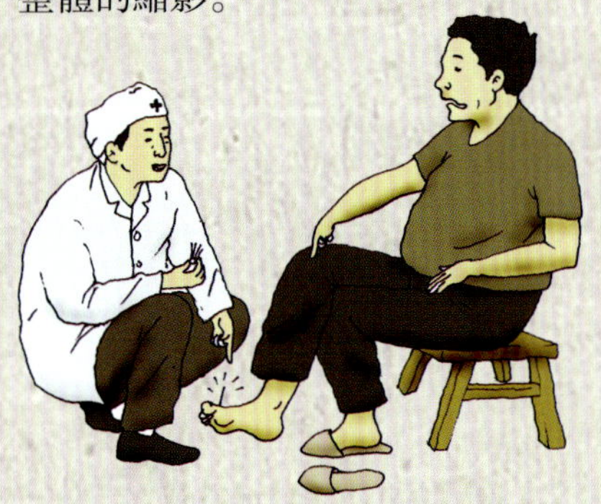

(3) The Sensory Function

Channels and collaterals form a network for transmitting information to all parts of human body. When the muscular striae are excited, the stimulation goes along the channels and collaterals to their related organs, where they cause changes in the function of these organs, which are transmitted in the circulation of qi and blood, and also adjust the functional objectives of the Zang-fu organs. In turn, the functions of the organs can be reflected by the channels and collaterals. Because the circulation of the channels and collaterals reaches every part of the body, a part of the body can be seen as a representative of the whole body.

（4）調節作用

經絡能運行氣血和協調陰陽，使人體機能活動保持相對的平衡。當人體發生疾病時，出現氣血不和及陰陽偏勝偏衰的證候，可運用針灸等治法以激發經絡的調節作用，即原來亢進的可使之抑製，原來抑製的可使之興奮。

2. 經絡學説的應用

（1）闡釋病理變化

1）經絡是外邪由表入裏的途經：

如外邪侵襲肌表，初見寒熱頭痛等癥，若外邪循經内傳於肺，則可出現咳喘、胸痛、胸悶等肺病癥狀。

(4) Regulating the Balance

The channels and collaterals circulate qi and blood and coordinate yin and yang to keep a relative balance in the body's activities. When disease occurs in the body, the symptoms of qi and blood disharmony, and an excess or deficiency of yin and yang emerge; this can be treated by acupuncture and moxibustion therapy to stimulate the channels and regulate their functions, in fact by using hyperfunction to cause inhibition, and inhibition to cause its agitation.

2. The Application of Channel and Collateral Theory

(1) To Explain Pathological Changes

1) The channels and collaterals are the pathways along which exogenous evils enter the internal organs from the body surface. For example, when external evils attack the body surface, symptoms of fever or headache are manifested early. Cough, pain or stuffiness in chest are caused by external evils as they pass through the channels and collaterals, and finally travel into the Lung.

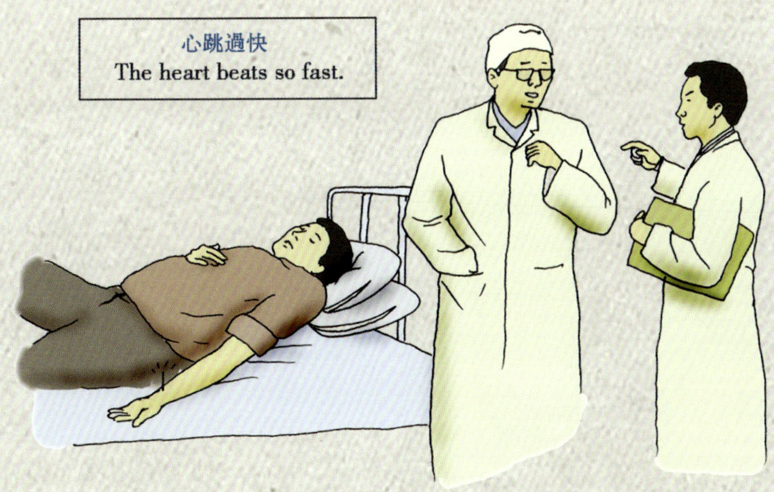

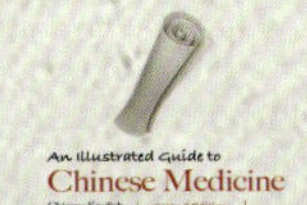

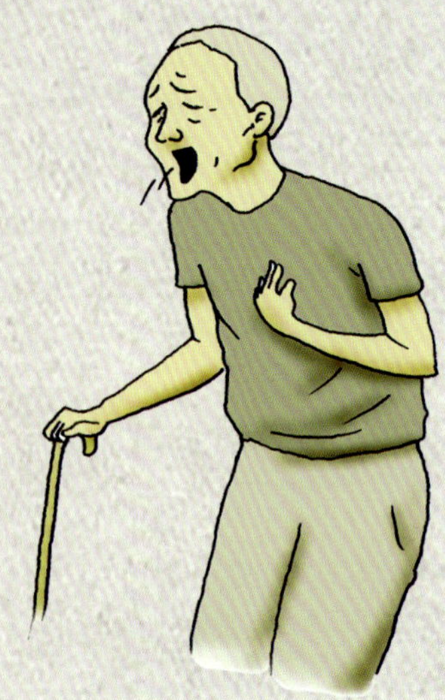

2）經絡是内臟病變反應於體表的途徑：内臟病變通過經絡傳導，反映於體表的某些特定部位及官竅．如：肝病可見兩脅或少腹疼痛。

2) The channels and collaterals are the routes of the pathological changes arising between the Zang-fu organs and the tissues of the body surface. Pathological changes of the internal Zang-fu organs can be reflected on the surface of the body, having been conducted by the channels and collaterals and manifested at special locations or at the corresponding orifices. For example, Liver disease may manifest as distention and pain in both hypochondriac regions and lower abdomen.

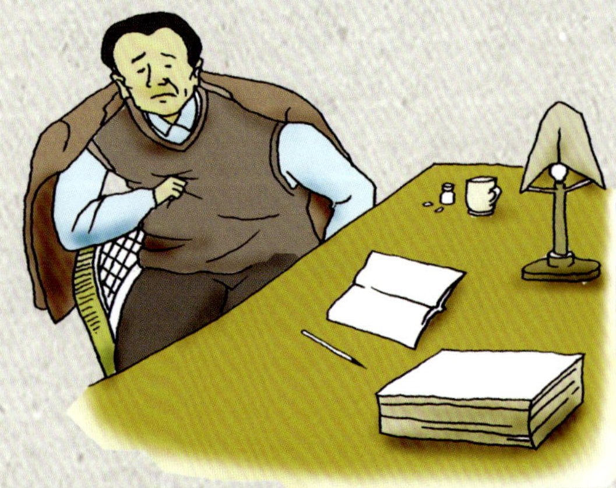

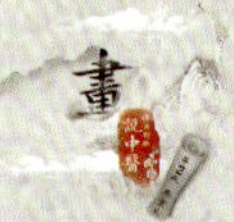

3）經絡是臟腑病變相互傳變的途經：互爲表裏臟與腑病變之間的傳變。如心火循經下移小腸；非表裏關係的臟腑病變的傳變。如肝失疏泄可影響脾胃運化。

（2）指導疾病的診斷

1）循經辨癥，判斷病位：由於經脈有一定的循行部位和絡屬臟腑，因此，臨床根據疾病癥狀出現的部位，可提示病在何經、何臟、何腑。如腰部疼痛多與腎有關；兩脅疼痛多爲肝膽疾病。

3) The channels and collaterals are the pathways of transmission of pathological changes to the Zang-fu organs. Interiorly and exteriorly, the Zang organs and fu organs influence each other's pathology. For example, Heart fire may descend to the Small Intestine. There is also transmission between Zang-fu organs which is not interior-exteriorly related: for example, if the Liver fails to govern the free coursing, the function of transformation and transportation of the Spleen and Stomach will be affected.

(2) Directing the Diagnosis of Disease

1) Diagnosing the disease by the channel, and accurately determining the area involved. As the channels differ in their courses and pertaining organs, diagnosis and determining the channel or organ where pathological changes take place can be inferred from the analysis of the location of symptoms and signs. For example, lumbar pain indicates Kidney disease, hypochondriac pain may indicate Liver or Gallbladder involvement.

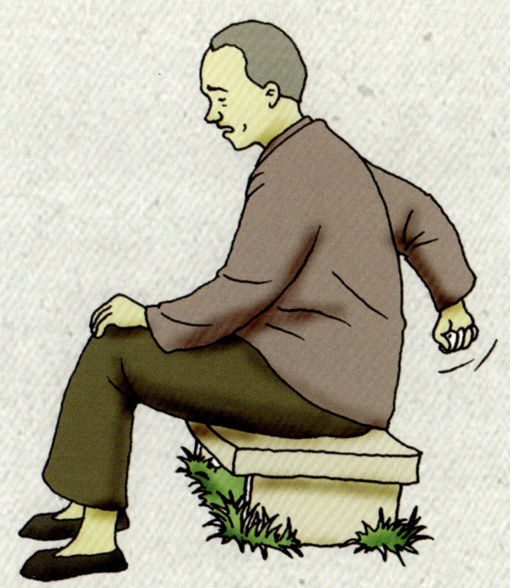

2）按察俞穴判斷病位：俞穴是經氣聚集的地方，臟腑病變時，病氣常可在特定的俞穴部位出現反应，或表現爲壓痛，或呈現爲結節狀、條索狀的反映物，或局部出現一些形態變化等。因此，根據這些病理反映，可幫助進行診斷。如胃病患者在胃俞穴及足三裏穴多會有明顯的痛覺異常。

2) Diagnosing the location of disease according to the shu-points

Shu-points are the sites through which qi accumulates in the channels. When pathological changes take place in the Zang-fu organs, there is always a reaction at a certain shu-point or reactive changes such as tenderness, tubercles and cord-like lumps or other changes in a certain part of the body. Therefore, these pathological reactions can be some help to diagnosis. For instance, a patient with Stomach disease may have obvious pain in BL 21 (*wèi shù*) and ST 36 (*zú sān lǐ*).

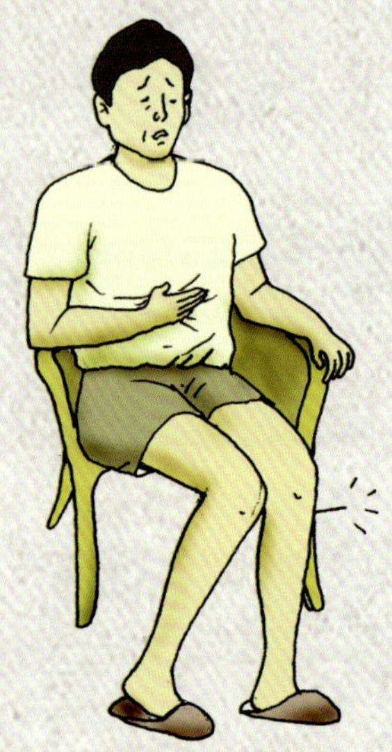

（3）指導疾病的治療

1）循經取穴

針灸和推拿療法，主要是針對某一經或某一臟腑的病變，在其病變的鄰近部位或經絡循行的遠隔部位上取穴，通過針灸或按摩，以調整經絡氣血的功能活動，從而達到治療的目的。而穴位的選取，首先必須按經絡學説來進行辨證，斷定疾病屬於何經後，再根據經絡的循行分布路綫和聯係範圍來選穴。

(3) Guiding the Treatment

1) Selecting Points along the Channels

To obtain good therapeutic effect when treating pathological changes in certain channels or Zang-fu organs, acupuncture and tui na methods use local points, near the affected area, or distal points along the channels, in order to regulate the functional activities of qi and blood of the channels. To choose the right points, one must first follow the guidelines of channel theory and differentiation.

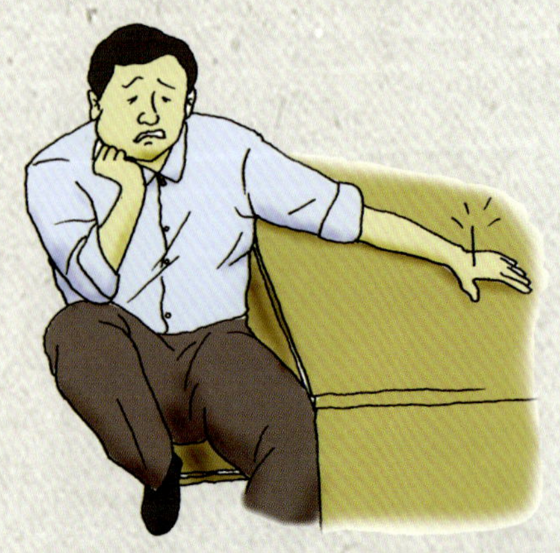

2）分經用藥

藥物治療也是以經絡爲渠道，通過經絡的傳導轉輸，使藥達病所，發揮其治療作用。古代醫家根據某些藥物對某一臟腑經絡所具有的特殊選擇性作用，創立並形成了“藥物歸經”理論。還根據經絡學説，創立了“引經報使”理論。如治頭痛，屬太陽經的可用羌活，屬陽明經的可用白芷，屬少陽經的可用柴胡，因羌活、白芷、柴胡不僅分別歸手足太陽、陽明、少陽經，且能作爲他藥的向導，引導他藥歸入上述各經而發揮治療作用。

2) Herbal Therapy also Relies on Channel Theory

The herbs take effect through the channels, through which they are delivered to the affected part. Based on long-term clinical practice, ancient doctors formed a theory called the "channels entered". This concerns itself with the specific selectivity of herbs for one or more of the channels, as well as the foundation of channel guiding action theory. To treat headache, *qiāng huó* (Rhizoma et Radix Notopterygii) can treat taiyang channel headache; *bái zhǐ* (Radix Angelicae Dahuricae) can treat yangming channel headache, and *chái hú* (Radix Bupleuri), can treat shaoyang channel headache. These three herbs not only pertain to the taiyang, yangming, and shaoyang channels respectively of the hand and foot, but can also guide other herbs through these channels in order to achieve a better therapeutic effect.

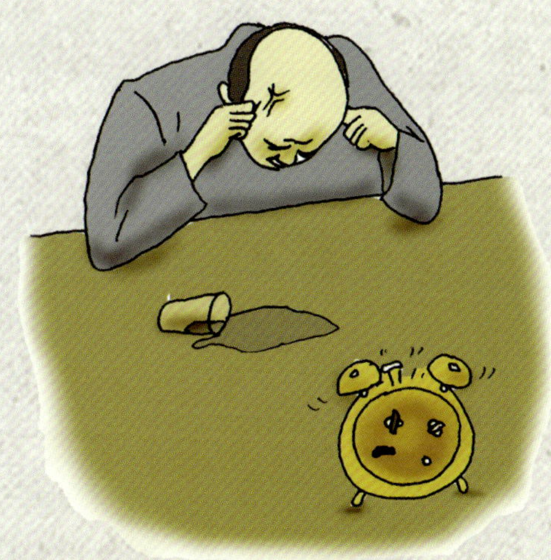

第五章 體質 Chapter 5 Constitution

人的體質是千狀萬態，重視人的體質及其差異性是中醫學的一大特點。

Chinese medicine emphasizes the concept that different people have different constitutions.

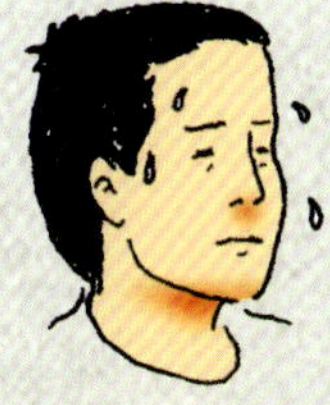

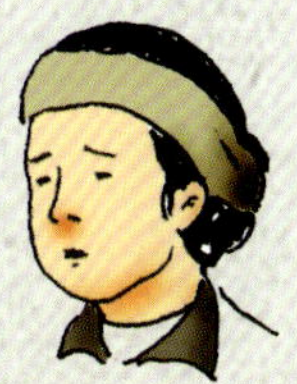

一、體質的概念

The Concept of Constitution

體質，是指人類個體在生命過程中，由先天因素和後天因素等所決定的表現在形態結構、生理功能和心理活動等方面綜合的相對穩定的特性。就是人群在生理共性的基礎上，不同個體所具有的身心特殊性。

Physical constitution refers to a person's physical structure during the course of her life. Congenital and acquired factors determine the manifestations of the body structure, physiological functions and psychological activities reflected in one's constitution as integrated and relatively stable characteristics. Namely, this means the specific physical and mental characteristics that each individual has based on common human physiological features.

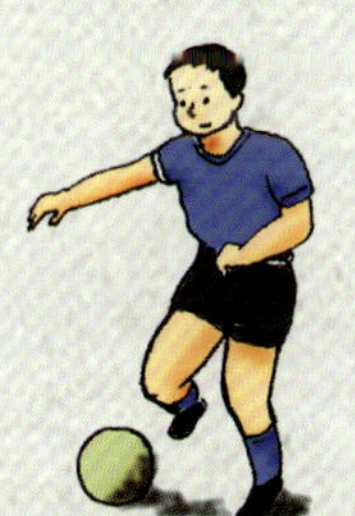

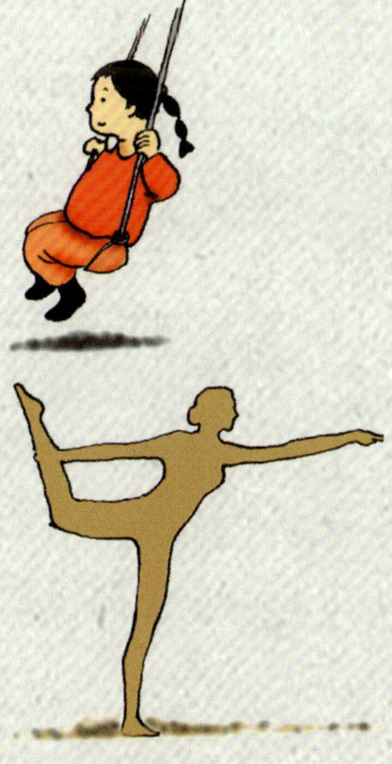

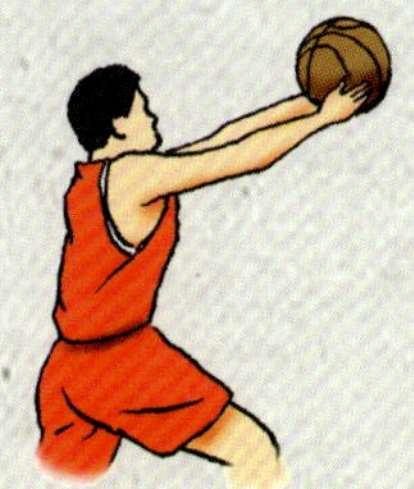

二、體質的形成

人之體質的形成，往往受到諸多因素的影響，但歸納起來主要有以下幾個方面。

1. 先天因素

先天，又稱稟賦，是指嬰兒出生之前在母體內所稟受的一切特徵。先天因素是體質形成的基礎，父母生殖之精氣的盛衰，常決定着子代體質的强弱。

The Formation of Constitution

The formation of constitution is affected by many factors.

1. The Congenital Factors

Congenital constitution, also called natural endowment, refers to all the characteristics inherited from the mother before birth. The congenital factors are the foundation of forming one's constitution. The waning and waxing of the parent's reproductive essence qi determines the strength and weakness of their children's constitution.

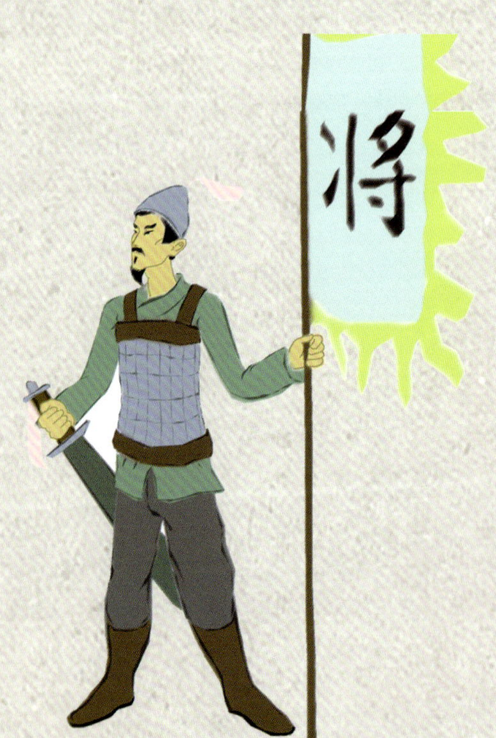

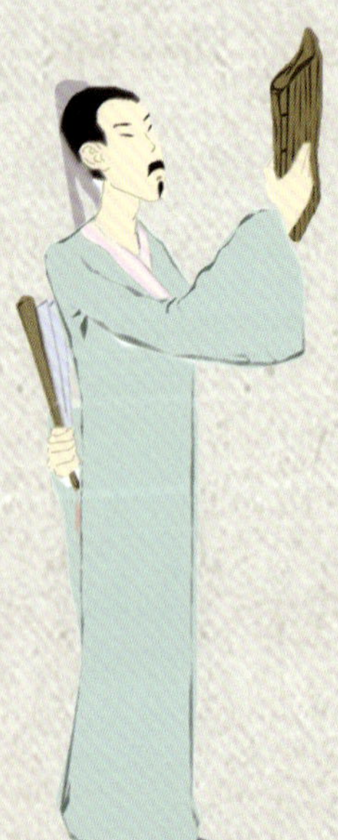

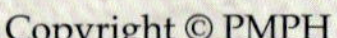

2. 後天因素

後天，是指人從出生到死亡之前的生命歷程。後天因素可分爲機體内在因素和外界環境因素。機體内在因素包括飲食、勞逸、婚育、鍛煉、疾病、情誌變化等；外界因素是指人們所處的環境，包括人們賴以生存的基本條件，如物質生活條件、勞動條件、衛生條件、氣候條件、社會製度、生態環境及教育水準等。

（1）飲食

飲食營養是決定體質强弱的重要因素。合理的膳食結構，科學的飲食習慣，對維護和增强體質十分有益。反之，長期營養不良或營養不當，以及偏食嗜某些食物，均會影響個體體質的變化。如嗜食肥甘可助濕生痰，形成痰濕（多偏胖）體質；嗜食辛辣則易化火灼津，形成陰虚火旺（多偏瘦）體質。

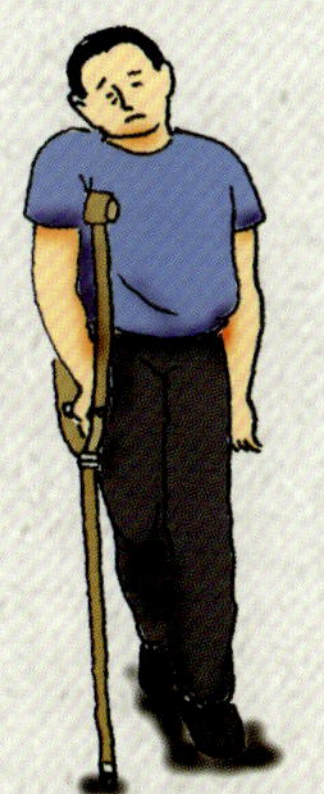

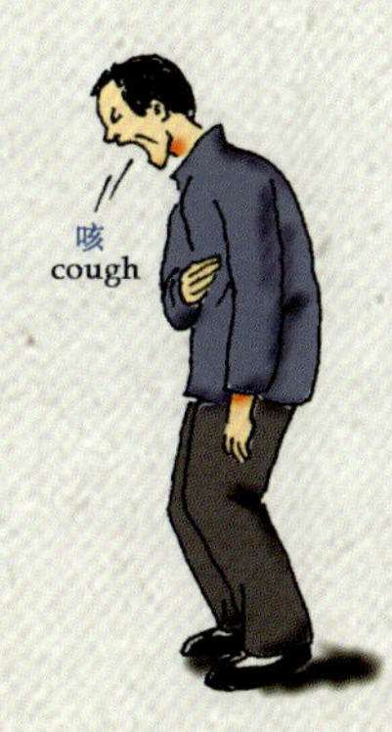

2. The Acquired Factors

Acquired constitution refers to the life processes of a person from birth to death. These are divided into internal and environmental. The internal factors include diet, work & rest, marriage & procreation, physical exercise, diseases and emotional changes. Environmental factors refers to where people live, and include basic living and working conditions, hygiene, climate, social rules, ecological environment and education standards.

(1) Diet

The nutrition gained from food is an important factor which decides the constitutional strength and weakness. Adequate diet and good eating habits benefit maintaining the constitution's strength. On the other hand, long term poor diet, improper diet, or the desire to eat only certain kinds of food can affect and change the constitution. For example, overeating of fatty and sweet foods may cause dampness accumulation, resulting in phlegm, which lead to a phlegm-damp constitution (fat body), overeating of spicy foods can easily produce fire which scorches fluids and leads to yin deficiency constitutional hyperactivity of fire (and usually a thin body).

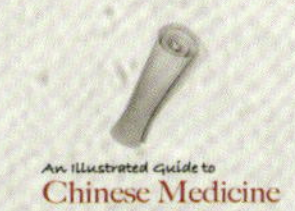

（2）勞逸

勞，即勞動，包括體力勞動和腦力勞動；逸，指休閑、無所事事的行爲狀態。但若過度勞累（包括勞力過度、勞神過度、房勞過度等），對人們的體質都將產生不利影響。而過度安逸，也可導致氣血運行遲緩，臟腑功能減弱，而致體質虛弱多病。

（3）鍛煉

"生命在於運動"，體育鍛煉是增强體質的法寶。體育鍛煉可以改善血液循環，促進新陳代謝，疏通經絡氣血，增强肌肉力量，提高抗病能力。

（4）婚育

"男大當婚，女大當嫁。"房事（性生活）是正常的生理活動之一，長期戒絶房事，身心欲望得不到滿足，心情久鬱，可致氣血不暢，體質下降，甚至發生疾病。反之，房事過度則精氣大傷，腎精腎氣受損，也可致體質下降。

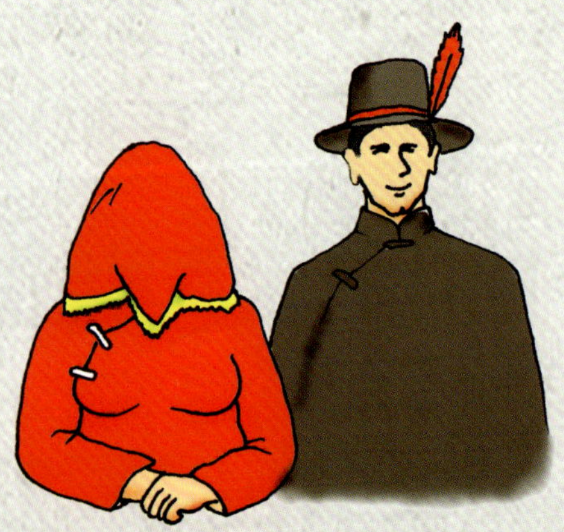

(2) Work and Rest

Work includes both physical and mental work. Rest means the cessation of work, exertion, or activity. Overworking (which could be physical, mental, or sexual) harms one's constitution. Resting too much can cause the slowed flow of qi and blood, and decline of the Zang-fu organs' functions, thus leading to a weak constitution and many diseases.

(3) Physical Activities

A Chinese saying says that "Life depends on movement". Physical exercise is a magic formula for building a strong constitution. Additionally, it improves blood circulation, promotes metabolism, regulates blood, qi, and the meridians, strengthens muscles, and improves the body's resistance to diseases.

(4) Marriage & Procreation

A Chinese saying says that "Every grownup man and woman should marry". Sexual life is a normal physiological activity. Lack of sexual activity over a long time can result in unsatisfied physical and mental desires and bad mood, which result in the abnormal flow of qi and blood, constitutional decline, and may even cause sickness. On the other hand, excessive sexual activity can damage the essential qi and consume the Kidney essence and qi, and also result in constitutional decline.

（5）情誌

精神狀態對體質的影響更爲重要。精神愉快，氣血通暢，正氣旺盛，邪氣難以侵犯人體，情誌不暢，精神異常，氣機逆亂，臟腑經絡功能紊亂，則正氣減弱而易於發病。鬱悶寡歡的“肝鬱質”，易誘發癌瘤。因此保持良好的心情和精神，對人的體質十分有益。

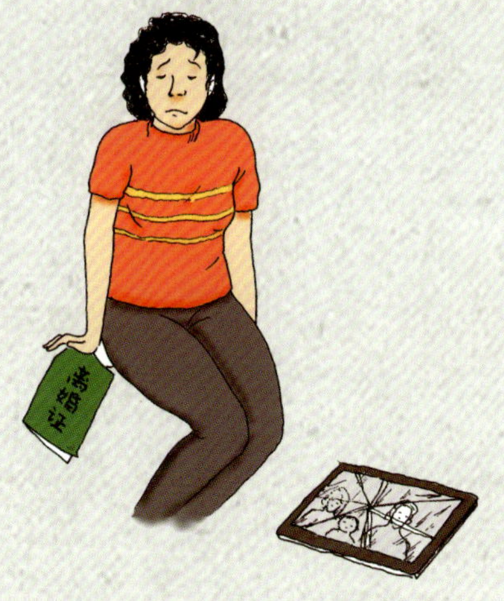

（6）疾病

疾病往往也是導致體質改變的一個重要因素。一般情況下，機體將在病愈之後逐漸地自我修複，不會影響體質。然而，某些重病、久病以及慢性消耗性疾病和營養障礙性疾病，對體質的影響非常明顯，使氣血陰陽的損傷變爲形成穩定性體質的因素。如肺痨病人，多爲“陰虛質”；慢性肝炎久病不愈者，多爲“濕熱質”。

(5) Emotions

The mental state has an important impact on the constitution. A happy state of mind maintains the normal circulation of blood and qi, and also sufficient right qi so that evil qi will be less able to attack the body. On the other hand, restrained emotions can give rise to abnormal mental state, chaotic counterflow of the qi dynamic, and disorder of the Zang-fu organs and meridians; weakened right qi can give rise to diseases. A depressed mood, called liver-constraint constitution, can easily lead to cancer. Maintaining a good state of mind benefits to the body.

(6) Disease

Diseases are an important factor in constitutional changes. Under normal circumstances, the body can gradually restore itself after recovering from illness and the constitution is unaffected. However, some severe, chronic, and consumptive diseases, and also undernourishment have very definite effects upon the constitution. Therefore, damage to qi, blood, yin and yang form steady constitutional factors. For example, patients with tuberculosis are mostly yin-deficiency constitutional types, and those with chronic unremitting hepatitis are damp-heat constitutional types.

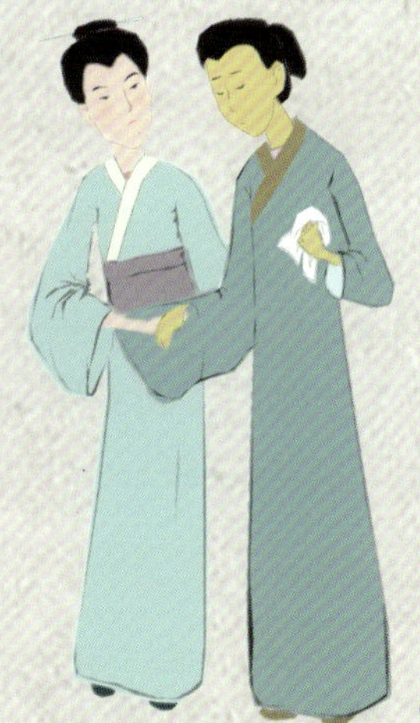

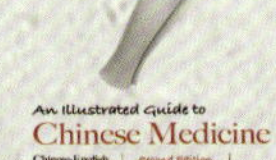

3. 其它因素

（1）環境因素

不同的地理環境，其水土性質、氣候特點、生活習俗有所不同，最終導致人的體質出現地區性的差異。如不同國家的人有不同的體質特點，同一國家不同地區的人也存在着明顯的體質差異。

（2）年齡因素

人的體質都有一個隨年齡增加而逐漸成熟、定型和演變的發展變化過程。在這一過程中，臟腑精氣由弱到强，又由强到弱。青春期和更年期是人生健康保養中最重要的兩個階段。14～18 歲青春期，是人體內機能與結構急劇變化的時期，體內各種生理活動進行着整體性調整，是人生中第一個轉折時期；50 歲左右的婦女和 55～60 歲左右的男子進入了更年期，是從成年期轉入老年期。

3. The Miscellaneous Factors

(1) Environmental Factors

Differences in the elements of one's physical environment, such as water, soil and climate, as well as differences in life style can cause people to develop different constitutions. This can vary not only from country to country, but also within the same country.

(2) Age Factor

As time goes by, the human body develops, changes, and matures. During this process, the essential qi of the Zang-fu organs change from weak to strong and back again to a weak state. The two most important phases of health maintenance are adolescence and climacteric period. Adolescence (fourteen to eighteen years old) is the period of the most rapid changes in the body's structure, physiological activities, and function of the organs. In the years of 50, or 55 to 60, women and men enter a stage of climacteric period respectively.

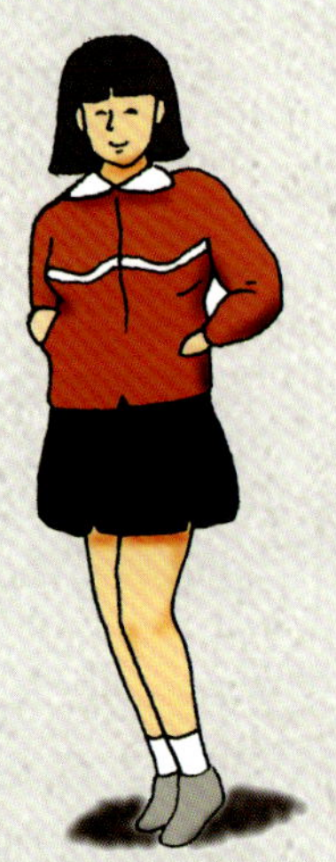

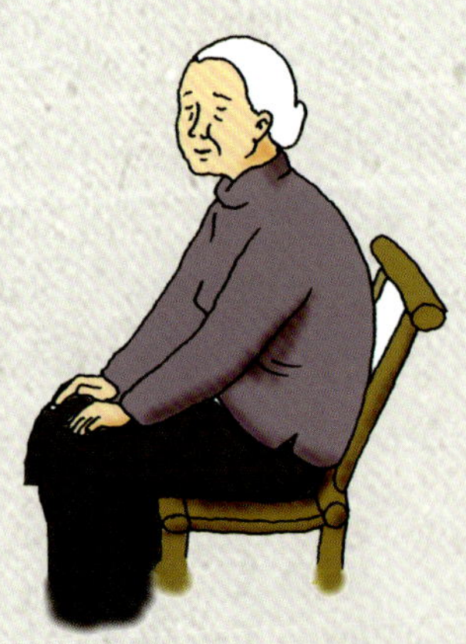

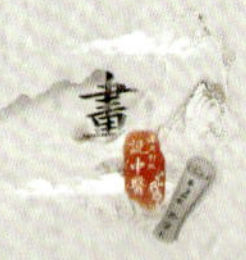

（3）性别因素

男女體質有着各自的特點。男爲陽，多禀陽剛之氣；女爲陰，常具陰柔之質。一般而言，男子體格高大健壯有力，好動而粗獷；女子體型小巧苗條而柔和，喜静而穩健。

(3) Sexual Activity Factor

Males and females have different characteristics in their constitutions. Males pertain to yang and endowed by firm qi; females pertain to yin and have a gentle quality. In general, men are tall, masculine, rough and dynamic; women are gentle, quiet, calm, and physically smaller.

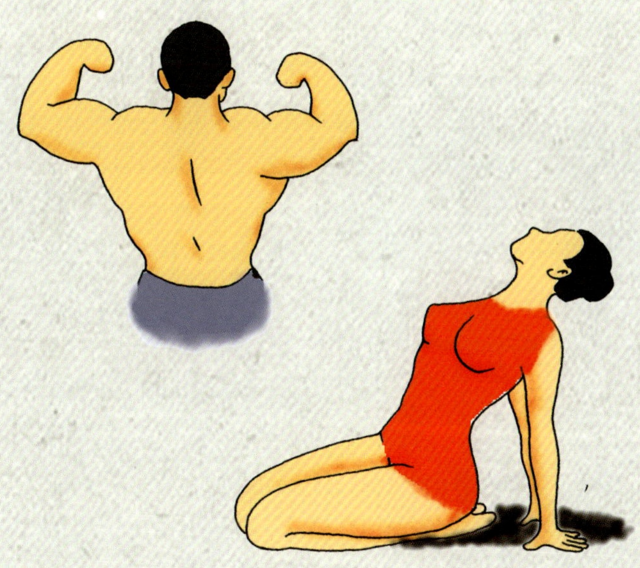

三、體質學説的應用

The Application of Constitution Theory

1. 體質與發病

體質健壯，正氣旺盛，則邪氣難以致病；體質虛弱，正氣内虛，則易於發病。

1. The Constitution and the Occurrence of Diseases

If the constitution is strong and the right qi is sufficient, evil qi will be less able to attack the body. If the right qi is deficient and the constitution is weak, diseases can easily occur.

2. 體質與養生

善養生者，應兼顧個體的體質特點。如在飲食調養方面，體質偏陽者，飲食宜涼而忌熱；體質偏陰者，飲食宜溫而忌寒；形體肥胖者，食宜清淡而忌肥甘；陰虛火旺者，食宜涼潤而忌辛熱。在精神調攝方面，抑鬱質之人，應注譩情誌的調節，消除其不良情緒。在體育鍛煉方面，也要因人而異，不同體質的人，應根據自身的體力和愛好，選擇適宜的鍛煉方法和强度。

2. The Constitution and Health Care

Self-awareness of one's constitutional type is important. People of yang-constitutional type should follow cool diets rather than hot ones. People with yin-constitutional type should follow warm diets rather than cold. Obese people should eat light foods instead of fatty and sweet foods. People with yin-deficiency and hot-excess constitutional types should have cool and moistening foods instead of spicy and hot foods. Depressed people should pay attention to regulate their emotions. As for physical exercise, since different people have different constitutions, each person should choose the suitable type of exercises according to her or his physical strength.

四、中醫體質的分型

Classification of Constitutions

1. 氣虛質

（1）特徵表現

氣虛質的人，肌肉鬆軟。和別人爬同樣層數的樓，氣虛的人就氣喘吁吁的。這種類型的人，講話的聲音低弱、性格内向、情緒不穩定、膽小，老是感到自已上氣不接下氣，氣不夠用，容易出汗，只要體力勞動的強度大就容易感到累，身體防禦能力下降，易感冒。

1. Qi Deficiency Type

(1) Symptoms

Individuals who belong to qi deficiency type tend to have flabby muscles and often present with shortness of breath when climbing stairs. They always speak with feeble voice and are introvert and timid in personality. They often feel out of breath and sweat easily. As long as they do intensive physical work, they are liable to get tired; the ability of the immune system of the body wears down and they catch cold easily.

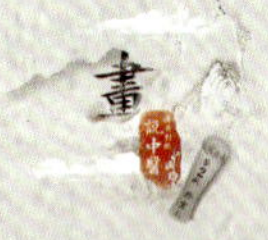

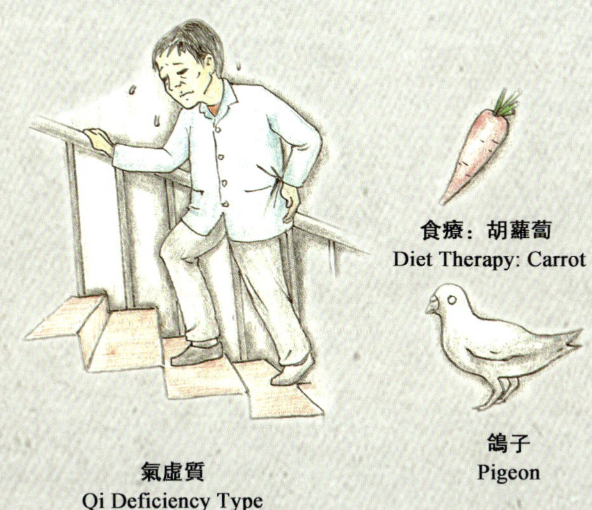

食療：胡蘿蔔
Diet Therapy: Carrot

鴿子
Pigeon

氣虛質
Qi Deficiency Type

（2）氣虛質食療——益氣健脾

1）鴿子

鴿子具有滋腎益氣、祛風解毒、補氣虛、益精血、暖腰膝、利小便作用。

2）胡蘿蔔

胡蘿蔔營養齊全，可以健脾和中、調節脾虛，益氣效果相當顯著。建議每天喝一碗胡蘿蔔粥。

2. 陽虛質

（1）特徵表現

陽虛質的人，多形體白胖，肌肉不健壯，常常感到手腳發涼，胃脘部、背部或腰膝部怕冷，衣服比別人穿得多，夏天不喜歡吹空調，不耐受寒邪，耐夏不耐冬，喜歡安

(2) Diet Therapy—Tonifying Qi and Strengthening the Spleen

1) Pigeon

It has the function of benefitting qi and nourishing kidney, expelling wind and removing toxin, tonifying qi, reinforcing essence and blood, warming waist and knee, and promoting urination.

2) Carrot

It is a kind of comprehensive nutritional food and has remarkable effect on strengthening the spleen and stomach, regulating the spleen deficiency, and tonifying qi. Having a bowl of carrot porridge every day is a good choice.

2. Yang Deficiency Type

(1) Symptoms

Individuals of this type usually have plump physique and weak muscles. They often have cold hands and feet, cold feeling in stomach, back, waist or

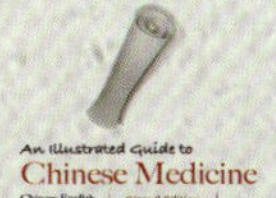

靜，吃或喝涼的東西總會感到不舒服，容易大便拉稀，小便顏色清而量多。性格多沉靜、內向。

（2）陽虛質食療——溫補氣血

1）羊肉

羊肉含有豐富的蛋白質，中醫認為可以補腎壯陽、暖中祛寒，陽虛的人可以每週喝一次當歸生薑羊肉湯。

2）茴香

茴香辛甘溫，具有溫陽補火和散寒理氣的作用，可以自製五香粉，做菜時加一點，就成了藥膳菜。

knee. They always wear more clothes than others and dislike air conditioning during summers. They cannot endure the cold and often feel uncomfortable after eating cold foods. They are susceptible to health problems such as diarrhea and have clear and copious urine. They are always quiet and introvert in personality.

(2) Diet Therapy—warm-tonification of Qi and Blood

1) Mutton

Mutton is rich in protein. It has the function of tonifying kidney and strengthening yang, warming the stomach and expelling the cold. The people who are of yang deficiency can have Angelica, Ginger and Mutton Soup once a week.

2) Fennel

The nature of fennel is sweet-warm and has the function of warming yang and nourishing fire, expelling cold and regulating qi. It can be made into five-spice powder or put into dishes to make medicinal diet.

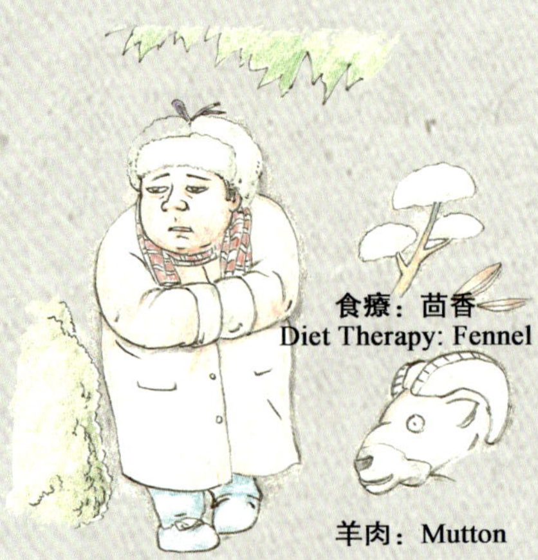

陽虛質
Yang Deficiency Type

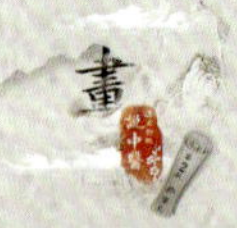

3. 陰虛質

（1）特徵表現

陰虛質的人體形多瘦，經常感到手腳心發熱，臉上冒火，面頰潮紅或偏紅，耐受不了夏天的暑熱，常感到眼睛幹澀，口幹咽燥，總想喝水，皮膚幹燥，經常大便幹結，容易失眠，性情急躁，外向好動，舌質偏紅，苔少。

（2）陰虛質食療——滋補腎陰

1）甲魚

甲魚可以滋補腎精，補益陰虛，可以做枸杞甲魚湯。

2）石榴

石榴味甘酸澀，生津止渴，有助於消化、緩解身體疲勞。

3. Yin Deficiency Type

(1) Symptoms

Individuals of this type usually have a thin physique. They always suffer from heat effusion in the face and the heart of the palms and soles, have flushed cheeks and cannot endure the summer heat. They often complain about dry eyes, mouth and throat dryness, eager to drink water, dry skin, and dry stools. They are susceptible to insomnia and are outgoing and impatient in personality. Their tongue is reddish and the tongue coating is less.

(2) Diet Therapy—Nourishing Yin and Tonifying the Kidney

1) Turtle

It can nourish kidney essence and tonify yin deficiency. We can use it to make Chinese Wolfberry (*gǒu qǐ zǐ*) and Turtle Soup.

2) Pomegranate

It's sweet and sour in taste and has functions such as promoting the secretion of saliva and quenching thirst, helping digestion, and relieving the physical fatigue.

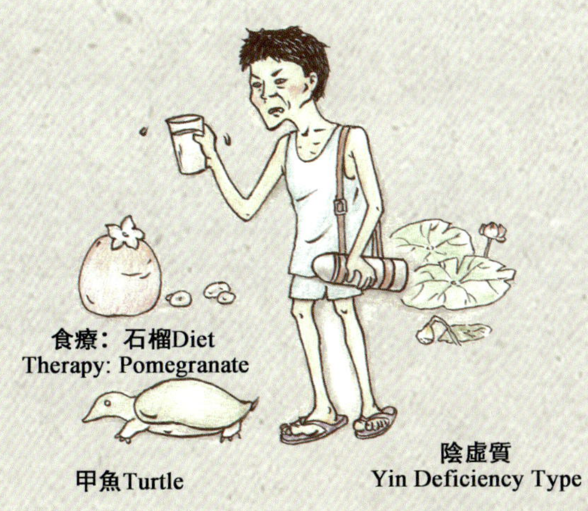

4. 痰濕質

（1）特徵表現

痰濕質的人，體形肥胖，腹部肥滿而鬆軟。容易出汗，且多黏膩。經常感到肢體酸困沉重、不輕鬆。經常感覺臉上有一層油。嘴裡常有黏黏的或甜膩的感覺，嗓子老有痰，舌苔較厚。性格比較溫和，多善於忍耐。

（2）痰濕質食療——平衡脾胃

1）白蘿蔔

白蘿蔔可清熱生津、涼血止血，痰濕體質的人可以經常做蘿蔔絲餅，當做主食食用。

2）絲瓜

絲瓜清熱化痰、涼血解毒，對脾胃異常、身體水腫有相當好的調理作用。

4. Phlegm & Dampness Type

(1) Symptoms

Individuals of this type are usually overweight and have paunchy belly. They often present with sticky sweat, fatigue or heaviness of the body, oily face, sticky or sweet taste in the mouth, phlegm in the throat, and a thick tongue coating. They have a mild temper, steady and patient personalities.

(2) Diet Therapy—Balancing the Spleen and Stomach

1) Radish

It can remove heat and promote fluid, and also can cool blood to stop bleeding. The people who are of phlegm &dampness can often take radish strips cake as the staple food.

2) Luffa

It has the effects of removing heat and eliminating phlegm, cooling blood and removing toxic material from the body, and regulating the discomfort of stomach and spleen and the edema of the body.

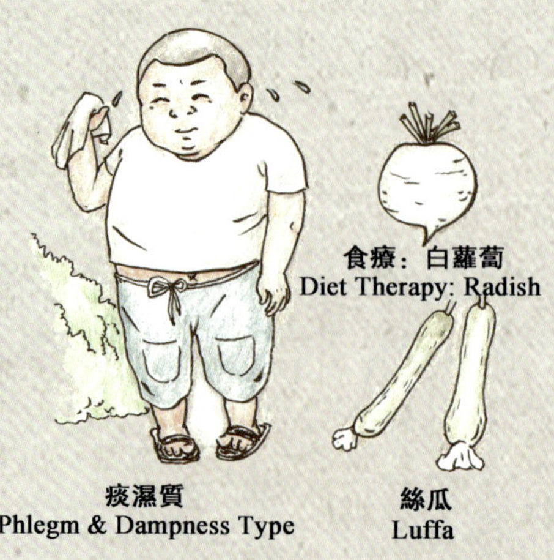

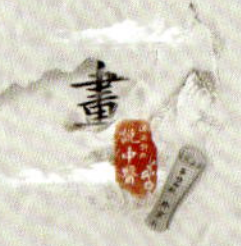

5. 濕熱質

（1）特徵表現

濕熱質的人，形體偏胖或蒼瘦，面部和鼻尖總是油光發亮，臉上容易生粉刺，皮膚容易瘙癢，常感到口苦、口臭或嘴裡有異味，大便黏滯不爽，小便有發熱感，尿色發黃，女性常帶下色黃，男性陰囊總是潮濕多汗，脾氣比較急躁。

（2）濕熱質食療——排濕清熱

1）薏苡仁

具有健脾、益胃、清熱、祛濕功效，濕熱體質的人可以做薏苡仁紅豆湯飲用。

2）綠豆

綠豆清熱解毒、利水消腫，可以美膚美顏、清口臭，喝綠豆湯，能幫助身體排濕、解熱。

5. Damp-heat Type

(1) Symptoms

Individuals belong to this type are either with a full-figured or thin physique. They often present with an oily face that erupts acne or pimple frequently, itchiness on the skin, a bitter or stink taste in the mouth, sticky stool, burning sensation when urination, yellow urine, yellow excessive vaginal discharges in female, wet scrota in male. They tend to be irritable and short-tempered.

(2) Diet Therapy—Removing Dampness and Eliminating Heat

1) Coix Seed

It has the effects of strengthening the spleen, reinforcing the stomach, removing heat and eliminating dampness. People who are of damp-heat type can often drink Coix Seed and Red Bean Soup.

2) Mung Bean

It has the effects of removing heat and toxic material from the body, inducing diuresis to alleviate edema, improving the conditions of skin, and removing the stink in the mouth. Drinking mung bean soup can help the body removing heat and eliminating dampness.

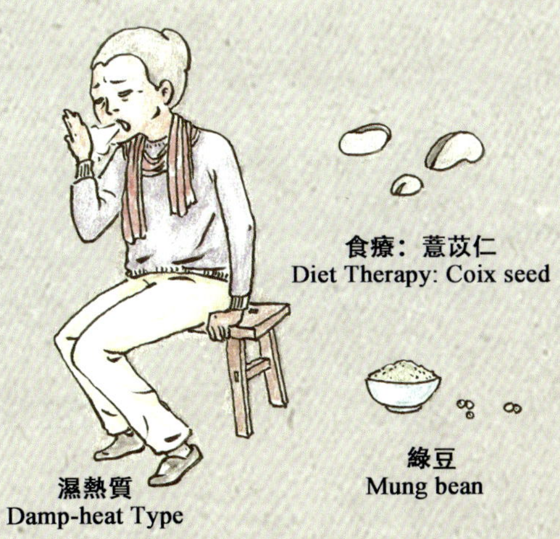

6. 瘀血質

（1）特徵表現

血瘀質的人，面色偏暗，嘴唇顏色偏暗，舌下的靜脈瘀紫。舌質黯有點片狀瘀斑，皮膚比較粗糙，有時在不知不覺中會出現皮膚瘀青。眼睛裡的紅絲很多，刷牙時牙齦容易出血，容易煩躁、健忘，性情急躁。

（2）血瘀質食療——活血化瘀

1）山楂

山楂有消食健胃、活血化瘀的作用，可以經常吃一些用山楂做的小零食，例如山楂梨絲。

2）苦丁茶

苦丁茶能生津、消食、化瘀，可以每天喝苦丁蜂蜜茶。

6. Blood Stasis Type

(1) Symptoms

Individuals of this type often present with a dull complexion, dark-red lips, dark-purple sublingual vein, lusterless or rough skin, unknown bruise on the body surface, and red blood in the eyes. They are susceptible to gingival bleeding when brushing the teeth. They tend to be impatient, forgetful and irritable.

(2) Diet Therapy—Promoting Blood Circulation to Remove Blood Stasis

1) Haw

It has the effects of improving digestion and promoting blood circulation to remove blood stasis. We can have some haw snacks such as haw and pear slips during our daily life.

2) Kudingcha (Broadleaf holly leaf)

It has the effects of promoting fluid, improving digestion and removing blood stasis. We can drink some Kudingcha and honey tea every day.

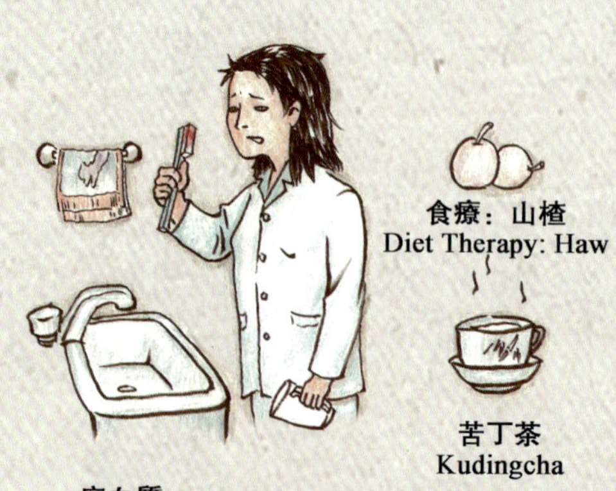

瘀血質
Blood Stasis Type

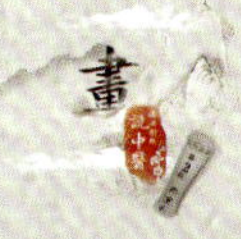

7. 氣鬱質

（1）特徵表現

氣鬱質的人，體形偏瘦的較多，常感到悶悶不樂、情緒低沉，容易緊張、焦慮不安，多愁善感，感情脆弱，敏感多疑，容易感到害怕或容易受到驚嚇，常感到乳房及兩脅部脹痛，常有胸悶的感覺，經常無緣無故地歎氣，咽喉部經常有堵塞感或異物感，容易失眠。

（2）氣鬱質食療——醒神解鬱

1）蓮藕

蓮藕有清熱生津、緩解心情煩躁的作用，晚餐可以經常炒一些蓮藕食用。

2）金橘

金橘可理氣、解鬱、化痰，經典的食用方法是製作金橘飲，作爲茶飲。

7. Qi Stagnation Type

(1) Symptoms

Individuals of this type are mostly thin, and tend to be depressed, nervous or anxious, melancholy, sensitive, suspicious and timid. They often present with distention and pain in the breasts and ribs, chest distress, frequent sighing, and congestion or foreign-body sensation in the throat. They are susceptible to insomnia.

(2) Diet Therapy—Refreshing the Mind and Relieving Qi Stagnation

1) Lotus Root

It has the effects of removing heat, promoting fluid and relieving irritability. We can often take fried lotus root for dinner.

2) Kumquat

It has the effects of regulating qi, relieving qi stagnation and eliminating phlegm. We often make it into kumquat tea.

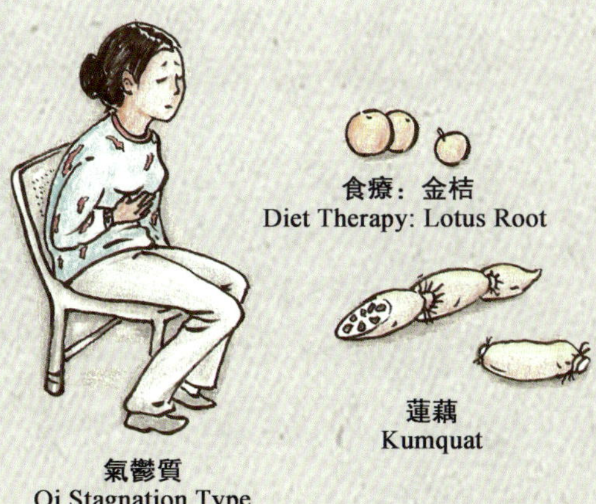

氣鬱質
Qi Stagnation Type

8. 特禀質

（1）特徵表現

特禀質就是一類體質特殊的人群。其中：過敏體質的人，有的即使不感冒也經常鼻塞、打噴嚏、流鼻涕，容易患哮喘，容易對藥物、食物、氣味、花粉、季節過敏，有的皮膚容易起蕁麻診，皮膚常因過敏出現紫紅色瘀點、瘀斑，皮膚常一抓就紅，並出現抓痕。

（2）特禀質食療——益氣固表

1）蜂蜜

蜂蜜能益氣固表、促進身體新陳代謝，可經常食用。

2）大棗

大棗能抗過敏，促進身體排毒代謝，建議特禀質體質的人可經常喝黨參紅棗茶。

8. Special Constitution Type

(1) Symptoms

People of this type refers to a group of sensitive people with special constitution. Some often develop nasal congestion, sneezing, runny nose, panting without catching cold. Some are very sensitive to drugs, foods, smells, pollen or seasons. Some often suffer from urticaria, purple spots or patches under the skin, and scratches on the skin after scratching.

(2) Diet Therapy—Tonifying Qi for Consolidating Exterior

1) Honey

It has the effects of tonifying qi for consolidating exterior, and improving metabolism. It can be drunk frequently.

2) Chinese-date

It has anti-allergic effects and can improve detoxification and metabolism. It is recommended that people of special constitution type can often drink Ginseng and Red Date Tea frequently.

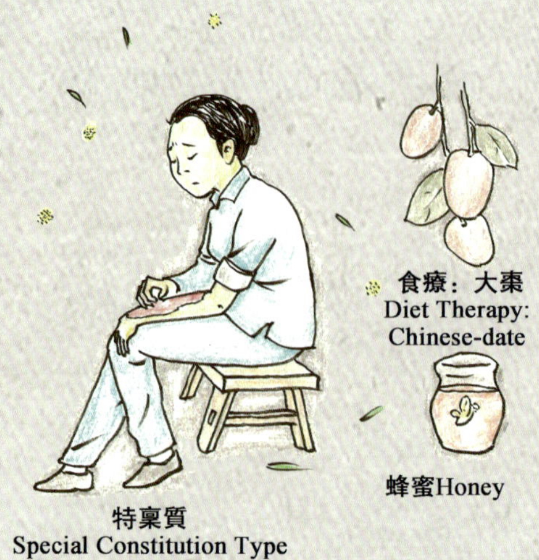

特禀質
Special Constitution Type

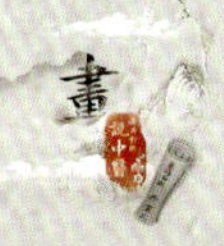

9. 平和質

（1）特徵表現

平和質是生命力旺盛的表現，這類人體形勻稱健壯，面色、膚色潤澤，頭髮稠密有光澤，目光有神，唇色紅潤，嗅覺通利，不容易疲勞，精力充沛，睡眠、食欲良好，大小便正常，性格隨和開朗，平時患病較少，對自然環境和社會環境適應能力較强。

（2）平和質食療——食物平衡

1）紅薯

紅薯含有大量的維生素，有補益氣力的功效。最好的食用方法是蒸食。

2）小米

小米入脾、胃、腎經，可以健脾和胃、滋陰養血，每天早晨最好喝一碗小米粥。

9. Neutral Type

(1) Symptoms

People of this type usually present with exuberant vitality. Individuals have a strong and fit physique. They often present with smooth and glossy complexion, lustrous and dense hair, bright eyes, red and moisture lips, proper senses of smell, uneasy to feel fatigue, full of energy, good sleep and appetite, normal bowel and urinary habits, being optimistic. They are adaptable to natural and social environmental changes.

(2) Diet Therapy—Balancing Diet

1) Sweet Potatoes

It is rich in vitamins and has the effects of enhancing the physical strength. The best way is to steam it for eating.

2) Millet

It enters the spleen, stomach and kidney meridians according to TCM theory and has effects of strengthening the spleen, regulating the stomach, and nourishing yin and blood. It is recommended to have a bowl of millet porridge every morning.

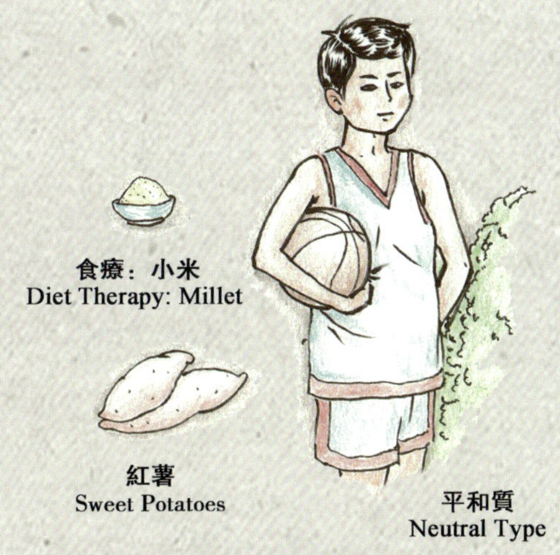

第六章 病因 Chapter 6 Etiology

病因，又稱致病因素，就是引起疾病的原因。中醫病因學説以整體觀爲指導思想，其認識方法具有鮮明的特點。一是“問診求因”，即通過詢問發病的經過及相關情況，以推斷其病因，如感受自然界的風、寒、暑、濕，强烈的精神刺激，飲食不節，跌僕金刃，蟲獸傷等，這些都是可見、可感知的病因，可通過問診而得知。二是“取象比類”，認識病因，它把疾病的性質和致病特點，例如把游走不定、變化多端、動摇不定的臨床表現比作風；把黏滯、重濁、趨下的臨床表現比作濕等等。三是“辨證求因”，這是中醫認識病因的特有方法和主要手段。一切疾病的發生，都是某種致病因素作用於機體的結果。如根據患者出現身體某部刺痛、舌有紫斑等，就可判斷爲瘀血致病。

中醫學中的病因主要包括六淫、癘氣、七情、飲食、勞逸、外傷、痰飲、瘀血、結石、寄生蟲、中毒、藥邪、醫過以及胎傳等。

Etiology is the explanation of how pathogenic factors cause diseases. Chinese medicine's theory of etiology uses the concept of the "whole body" as its guiding principle, and has a distinct method to determine the disease's characteristics. Firstly, in order to decide the pathogenic factors the doctor inquires about the course of the disease. For example, a question is whether the patient was affected by natural forces (wind, cold, summer-heat, dampness), emotionally upsetting situations, improper diet, traumatic injuries, and parasites. All these disease factors are visible and can be revealed by inquiry. Secondly, Metaphor is recognizing the pathogenic factors by analogy. For example, the clinical manifestations characterized by wandering location, instability and trembling are similar to wind; fluids which are sticky, heavy, turbid and which might manifest in the lower part of the body are similar to dampness. Thirdly, "determining pathogenic factors based on symptoms and signs differentiation" is a unique method to classify the pathogenic factors in Chinese medicine. All occurrences of disease rise from and reflect pathogenic factors affecting the human body. For example, blood stasis manifests as purple macula on the tongue or as stabbing pain.

Chinese medicine etiology includes six climatic influences, epidemic pathogenic factors, seven emotions, diet, imbalance of work and rest, traumatic injury, phlegm and fluid retention, blood stasis, stones, parasites, toxins, medical mistreatment as well as congenital factors.

一、外感病因

The Exogenous Pathogenic Factor

外感病因是指來源於自然界，多從肌表、口鼻侵入人體，引起外感性疾病的致病因素。外感病因包括六淫、癘氣等。

1. 六淫

是風、寒、暑、濕、燥、火六種外感病邪的統稱。淫，有太過、浸淫之謚，引申爲不正、異常。

（1）風

風爲陽邪，其性開泄。風邪具有向上（升），向外（散）等陽性特性。風邪傷人常侵襲人體上部（頭、面）和肌表，使皮毛腠理開泄而出現頭痛、汗出、惡風等癥狀。

The pathogenic factors which come from nature include the six external and epidemic pathogenic factors which penetrate into the body through the skin, mouth and nose.

1. The Six Exogenous Factors

Six exogenous factors: wind, cold, summer-heat, dampness, dryness and fire are actually a general term for the six abnormal climatic influences.

(1) Wind

Wind is a pathogenic factor characterized by discharging and opening actions, and upward and outward moving, which shows its yang nature. It usually attacks the upper part of the body, head and face, and skin and muscle. The most common symptoms are headache, aversion to wind and sweating.

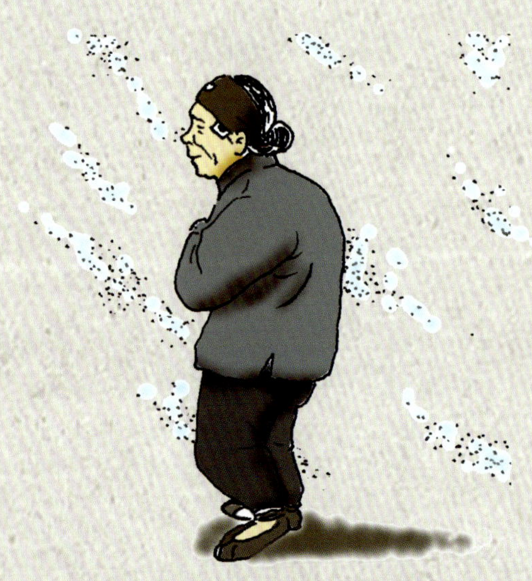

風善行而數變。善行是風邪具有病位游移，善行不居的特性。如風痹中的游走性關節疼痛。數變是指風邪具有變幻無常和發病迅速的特性，如風疹時隱時現。

Wind pathogenic factor, like wind in nature, is moving and changing. Diseases caused by the wind pathogenic factor are characterized by its easy movement from one area to another, like the wandering pain of wind bi; and quick onset and irregular changes, such as sporadic attacks of hives.

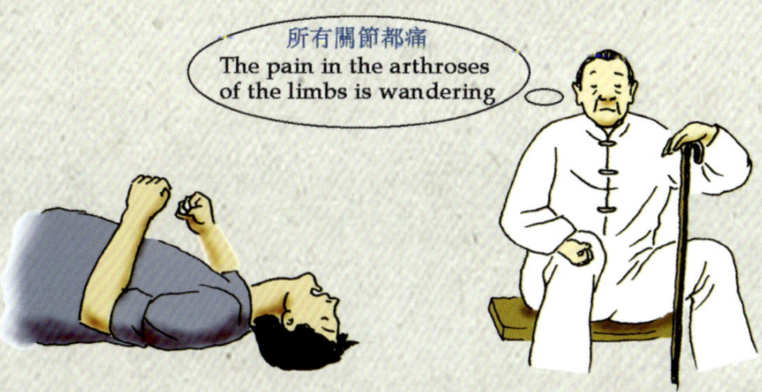

風爲百病之長、善合他邪致病。風爲六淫病邪中的主要因素，常是外邪致病的先導。

Among the six pathogenic factors, wind is the most common one; it can carry other pathogenic factors with it, and it plays a leading role in producing external syndromes.

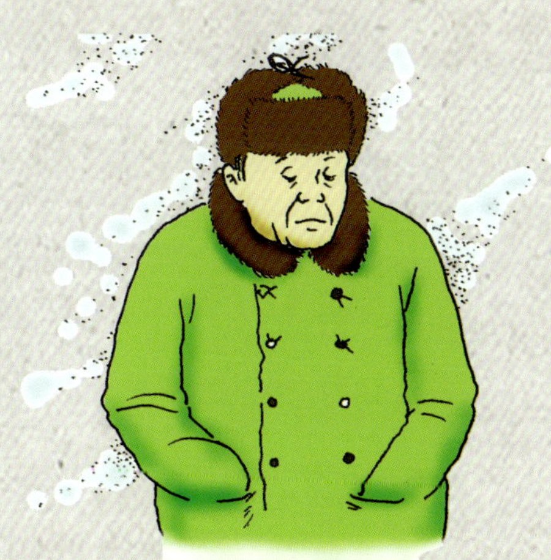

（2）寒

寒爲陰邪，易傷陽氣。從而使陽氣失去正常的溫養氣化作用，出現寒證兼陽傷的徵象，如外寒侵襲肌表，衛陽被遏，就會惡寒。

寒性凝滯。寒邪外侵，阻礙了陽氣的溫煦推動作用，致氣血阻滯而疼痛，如寒痹肢體疼痛，中寒腹痛等。

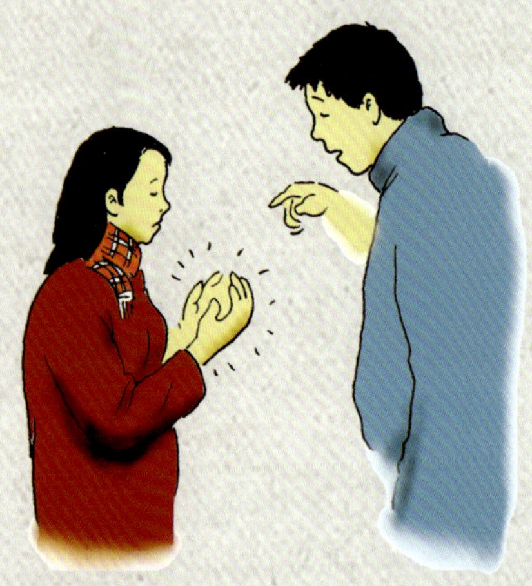

寒性收引。寒邪侵襲人體、可使氣機收斂，腠理、筋脈收縮而攣急，可見無汗、肢體屈伸不利等。

(2) Cold

Cold is a yin pathogenic factor that can easily damage the yang qi and cause its failure to warm, nourish and transform qi. For example, if cold invades the skin and muscle, the movement of defensive yang is arrested, and then the symptoms of aversion to cold will appear.

Cold is characterized by congealing and stagnating. The invasion of external cold causes the dysfunction of yang qi in warming and promoting movement, resulting in pain due to stagnation of qi and blood. For example, with cold bi there is pain of limbs and body, and with cold in the middle burner there is abdominal pain.

Cold is characterized by contracting and shrinking. The invasion of external cold into the body may restrain the qi mechanism, resulting in the closing of the pores, spasming of the tendons and vessels, and be manifested by lack of sweating and difficult movement of the limbs.

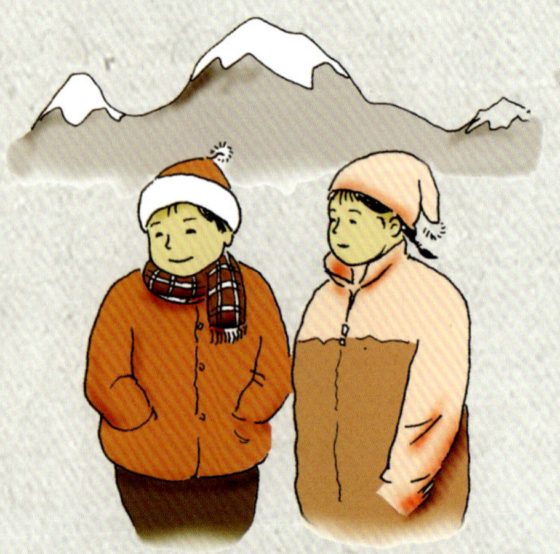

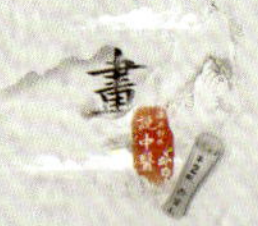

(3) 暑

暑爲陽邪，其性炎熱。暑邪侵害人體，多見陽熱證候，如高熱、肌膚灼熱、煩渴、汗出、脈洪數等。

暑性升散，易傷津耗氣，暑邪傷人，可使腠理開泄而大汗，大量汗出致津液耗傷，因而出現煩渴，尿短赤等癥，在大汗的同時，氣隨津泄而致氣虛，出現氣短乏力，甚至突然昏倒、不省人事。

(3) Summer-heat

Summer-heat is a yang pathogenic factor, it is hot in nature. Heat syndrome is commonly seen with the attack of summer-heat. Symptoms include high fever, burning sensation of the skin, thirst, sweating, and a pulse that is surging and rapid.

Summer-heat is characterized by ascending and scattering, and can easily hurt the body fluids and consume the qi. Summer-heat may cause the pores to open, causing profuse sweating and resulting in the impairment of body fluids. If symptoms such as thirst, scanty and yellow urine appear simultaneously with consumption of qi and loss of body fluids, this will result in shortness of breath, lassitude and even sudden fainting and loss of consciousness.

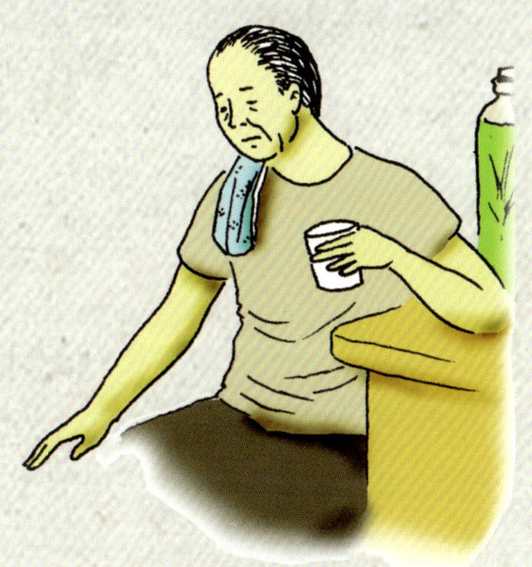

暑多挾濕。暑季炎熱，多雨而潮濕。熱蒸濕動，故在發熱煩悶的同時，常兼四肢疲倦，胸悶嘔惡、大便溏瀉不爽等濕阻的癥狀。

Summer-heat is often with dampness pathogenic factor. The summer heat season is rainy, damp and very hot. When summer heat is combined with dampness, the common symptoms are fever, chest oppression, vexation, heavy limbs, stifling sensation in the chest, vomiting, nausea and watery stool.

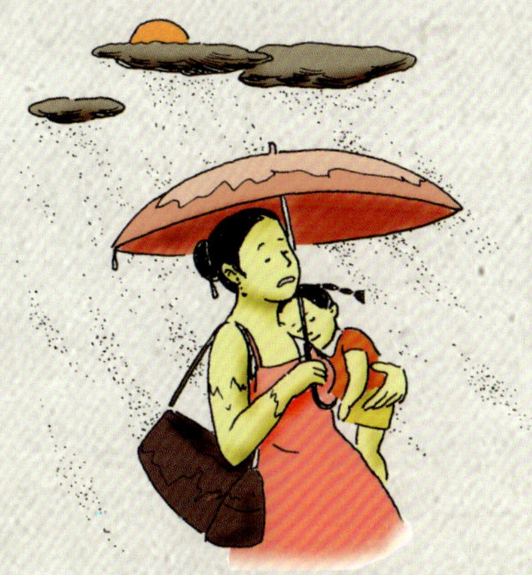

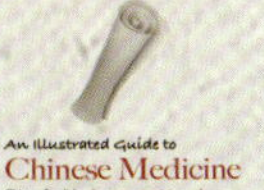

（4）濕

濕爲陰邪，易阻遏氣機，損傷陽氣。濕邪爲病，易使氣機升降出入失常，常出現胸悶脘痞、小便短澀、大便不爽等癥。濕常易困脾，而使脾陽不振，發爲水腫、腹瀉、尿少等癥。

(4) Dampness

Dampness is a yin pathogenic factor, that easily obstruct the qi mechanism and damage the yang qi. Damp disease impairs the normal qi mechanism of ascending, descending, exiting and entering resulting in symptoms such as a feeling of oppression in the chest, glomus, scanty and difficult urination, and uncomfortable, incomplete defecation.

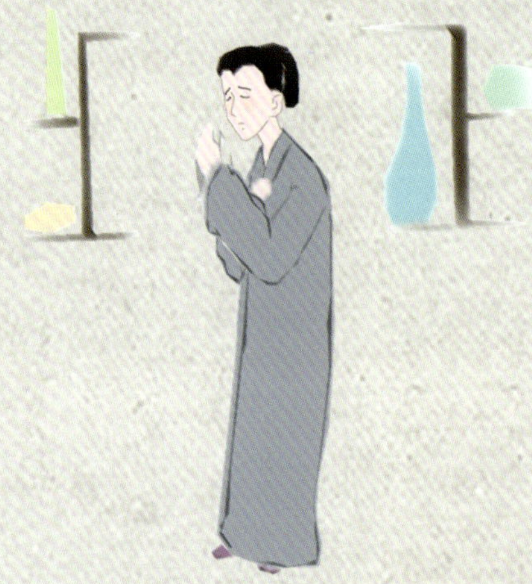

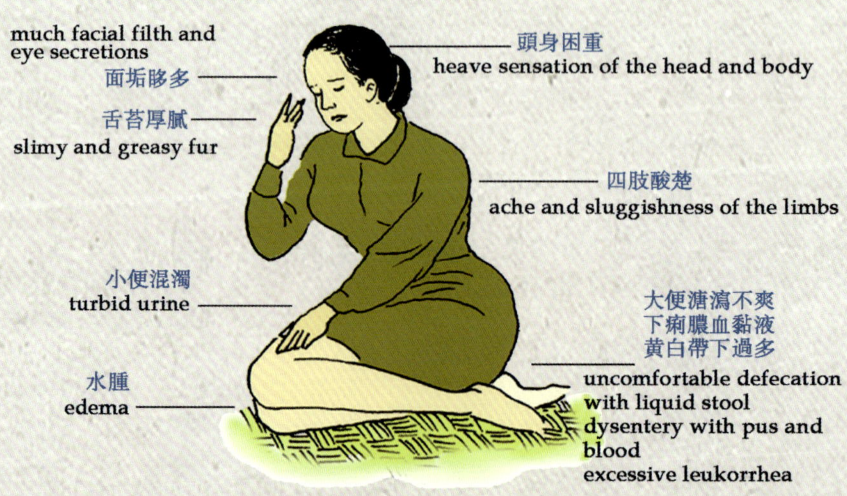

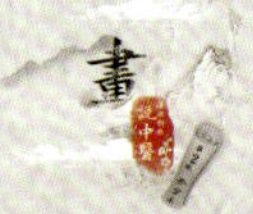

濕性重濁趨下。重即沉重、重著。濁即穢濁，濕邪致病可出現多種穢濁癥狀，濕邪爲病多趨於下部。

濕性粘滯。主要表現：一是濕病癥狀多粘滯而不爽，如排出物及分泌物多滯澀而不暢；二是指濕邪爲病多纏綿難愈，病理較長或反複發作，如濕痹、濕疹、濕溫病等。

Dampness is characteristically heavy, turbid and descending. Dampness disease symptoms are turbid and dirty and usually occur in the lower part of the body.

Dampness is also characterized by stickiness and stagnation therefore damp diseases tends to accumulate; damp diseases are persistent, lingering, frequently recur and are difficult to cure; for example damp bi, eczema and warm damp disease.

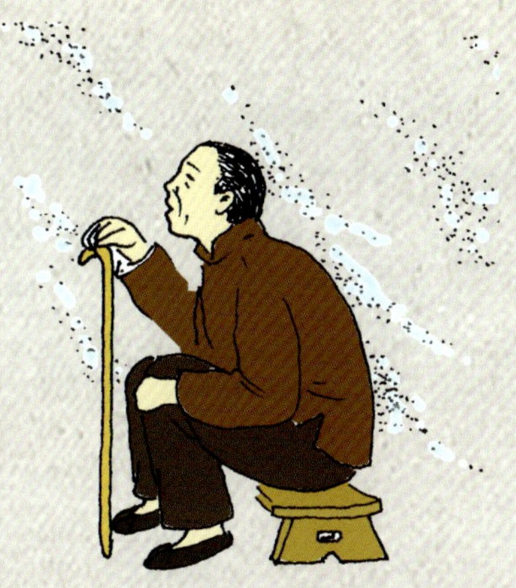

（5）燥

燥性幹澀，易傷津液。致陰津虧虛，見有口鼻幹燥，咽幹口渴、皮膚幹澀、毛發不榮、小便短少、大便幹結等癥。

(5) Dryness

Dryness is characterized by drying and parchedness, and easily consumes and damages the body fluids. Common symptoms are dryness in the mouth, nose and throat; thirst, dry and rough skin, malnourished hair, scanty urine and dry and hard stool.

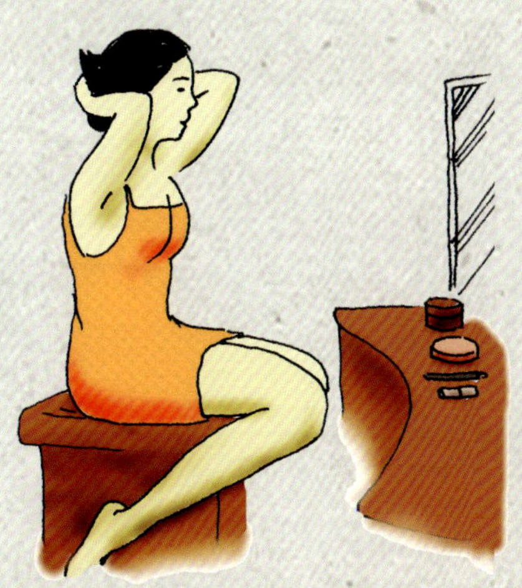

燥易傷肺，且最耗傷肺津，從而出現幹咳少痰，或痰粘難咯，或痰中帶血，或喘息胸痛等癥。

（6）火

火熱爲陽邪，其性炎上。故火熱傷人，多見高熱、煩渴、汗出、脈洪數等陽盛癥狀，且常上擾神明出現心煩、狂躁妄動、神昏譫語等癥。

Dryness easily impairs the Lung and consumes the lung fluids. The symptoms are dry cough with little phlegm, sticky phlegm that is hard to expectorate, sputum with blood, asthma and chest pain.

(6) Fire

Fire is a yang pathogenic factor characterized by upward flaming. When fire pathogenic factor attacks the body, it may give rise to high fever, thirst with restlessness, sweating and the pulse is surging and rapid. When heat flames upwards it will disturb the mind and cause vexation, mania, reckless behavior, coma and delirious speech.

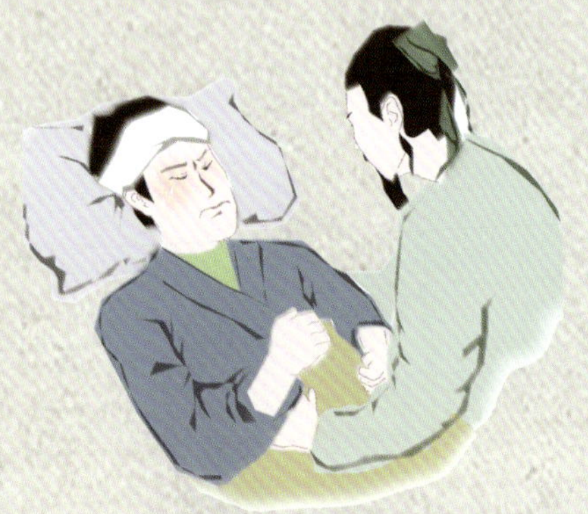

火易耗氣傷陰，火邪爲病，或直接損傷正氣，或因津傷而致氣傷。如火熱熾盛，在壯熱、汗出、渴引等津傷的同時，又可出少氣懶言，肢體乏力等氣虛之癥。

Fire easily consumes the qi and damages the yin and either directly damages the right qi, or indirectly damages it by consuming the body fluids. High fever in conjunction with sweating and thirst, which damages the yin, signs of qi deficiency such as decreased energy, laziness of speech and weakness of the four limbs will appear.

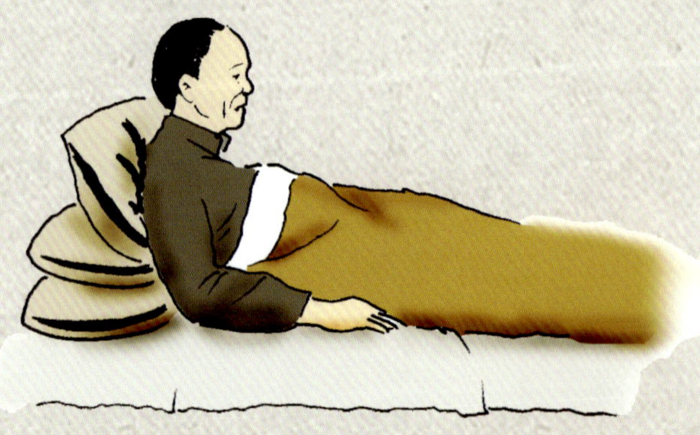

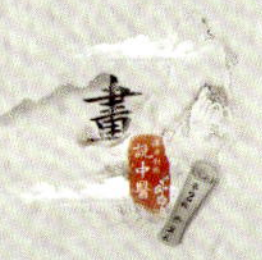

火易生風動血。火邪灼傷津液，筋脈失養，可致肝風内動，出現高熱，神昏、抽搐、角弓反張等。火熱之邪入於血絡、迫血妄行，導致出血證，如吐血、衄血、便血、尿血、皮膚發斑等。

Fire readily generates wind and stirs up the blood; it also consumes the body fluids, causing lack of nourishment in tendons and vessels. It could also result in internal wind from the Liver stirring the wind, causing high fever, coma, spasm and opisthotonus (spasm of the body where the head and heels are bent backward and the body is bowed forward). The fire pathogenic factor can damage the blood vessels by heating them so that the blood leaves its course, leading to various kinds of bleeding such as vomiting blood, nosebleed, blood in the stool or urine and purpura.

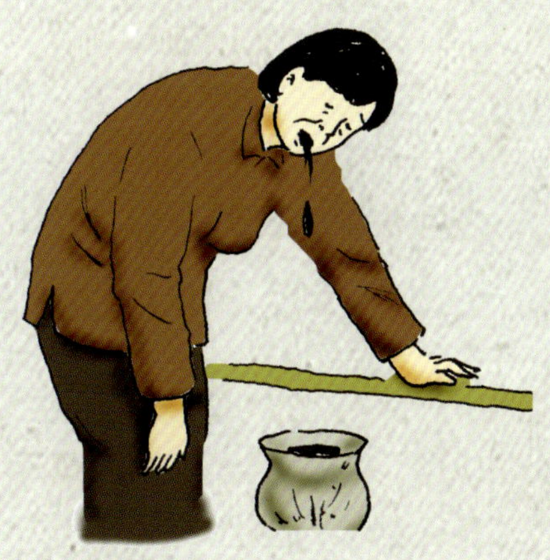

火易致腫瘍，火熱之邪入血分，且可聚於局部，腐觸血肉，而發爲癰腫瘡瘍。

When fire pathogenic factor penetrates the blood level, it can stagnate in a particular area, erode the blood and flesh and lead to sores and ulcers.

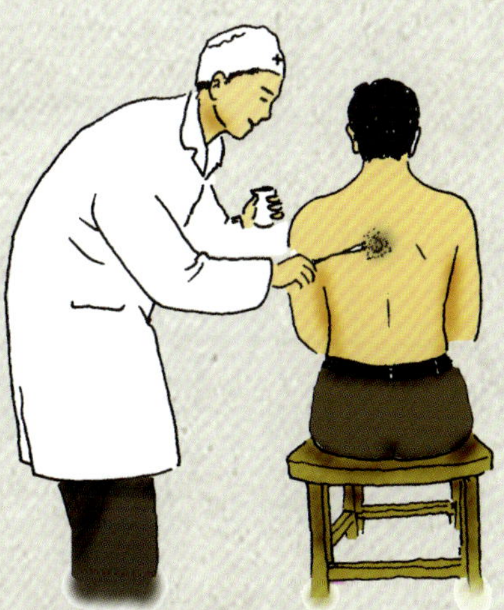

2. 癘氣

癘氣，是一種具有强烈傳染性的外邪。常引起傳染病的流行。

癘氣的形成和疫病流行的因素：一是氣候因素，自然氣候的反常，如久旱酷熱、水澇、濕霧瘴氣等，均可滋生癘氣而導致疾病的發生；二是環境和飲食衛生，如水源、空氣污染、食物污染也可引起癘病發生；三是預防隔離措施不力，往往會使疫病發生或流行；四是社會因素如戰亂和災荒，社會動蕩不安，人們的工作環境惡劣，生活極度貧困，衛生防疫條件落後等，則疫病易於發生和流行。

2. The Pestilential Pathogenic Factors

Pestilential pathogenic factor is an external disease with high contagious characteristics that spreads rapidly. Reasons for this kind of epidemic disease include:

Firstly, climatic factors: abnormal changes in climate such as lasting drought, extremely hot weather, waterlogged environments, dampness, fog and miasma.

Secondly, environment, diet and hygiene: air pollution, dirty water or food.

Thirdly, is ineffective prevention and isolation of contagious disease.

Last one is social factors, such as war, famine disaster, social upheaval, very poor working and living conditions, and undeveloped facilities for disease prevention.

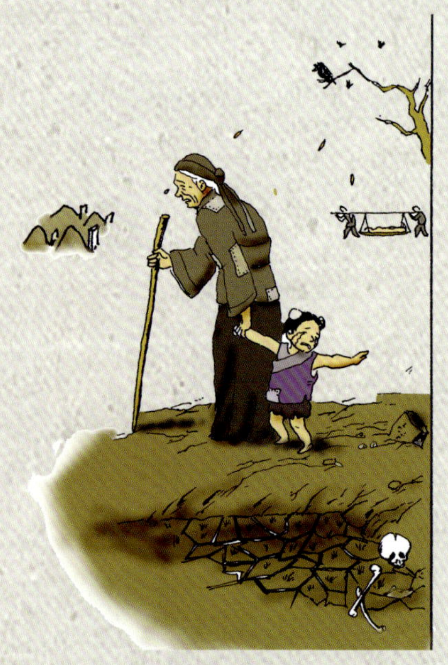

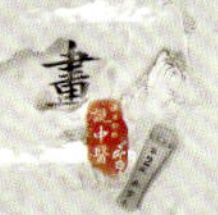

二、内傷病因

內傷病因是與外感病相對而言。它包括飲食失宜、七情、過勞、過逸等。

1. 飲食失宜

飲食是人體攝取食物，轉化爲水谷精微及氣血，維持生命活動的最基本條件，但是飲食失宜，又可爲致病因素，飲食失宜包括饑餓失常，飲食不潔和飲食偏嗜三個方面。

飲食饑飽失常。過饑則氣血生化之源缺乏，久則氣血衰少而爲病弱。過飽，或暴飲暴食，超過脾胃的消化吸收能力，則會出現腹脹、厭食、吐瀉等癥。

Disease Causes due to Internal Injury

The opposite of external pathogens, this includes improper diet, the seven emotions, over work and too much rest.

1. Improper Diet

Diet is very important for maintaining normal health because it is the basis for transforming food and drinks into essence, qi and blood. Improper diet is a common pathology; its meaning includes excessive hunger, overeating, consuming unclean food and drinks or only one kind of flavor, temperature or type.

Excessive hunger and overeating can lead to qi and blood deficiency; after a long time, disease will arise. Eating and drinking too many damages the Spleen and Stomach (digestive system), causing abdominal distension, loss of appetite, vomiting and diarrhea.

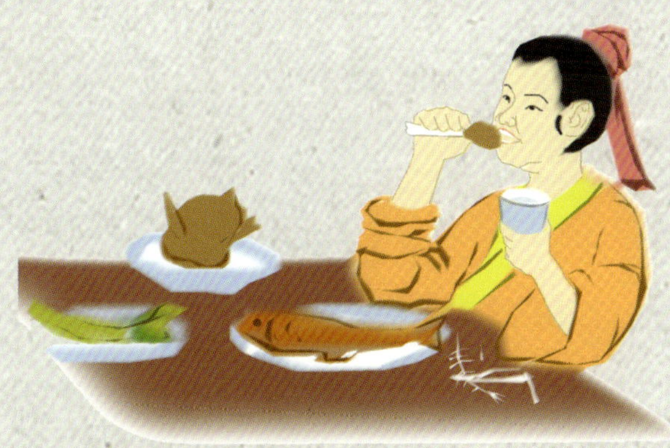

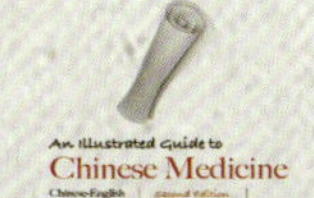

飲食不潔，可引起多種胃腸道疾病，出現腹痛、吐瀉、痢疾等或引起寄生蟲病。

飲食偏嗜也會致病。偏食生冷（如冷飲等），易於損傷脾陽，使寒濕內生，發生腹痛、泄瀉等癥，偏食辛溫燥烈（如辣椒等），可便胃腸積熱引起便秘或痔瘡等癥。

Eating and drinking unclean food and drinks can result in many kinds of diseases of intestines and Stomach with symptoms such as abdominal pain, vomiting, diarrhea, dysentery and even parasitic diseases.

Preference for raw or cold food and drinks can damage the Spleen yang qi, leading to internal cold dampness syndrome with symptoms such as abdominal pain and diarrhea. Preference for hot, spicy and dry food like peppers, can lead to heat accumulation in the Stomach and intestines with symptoms such as constipation or hemorrhoids.

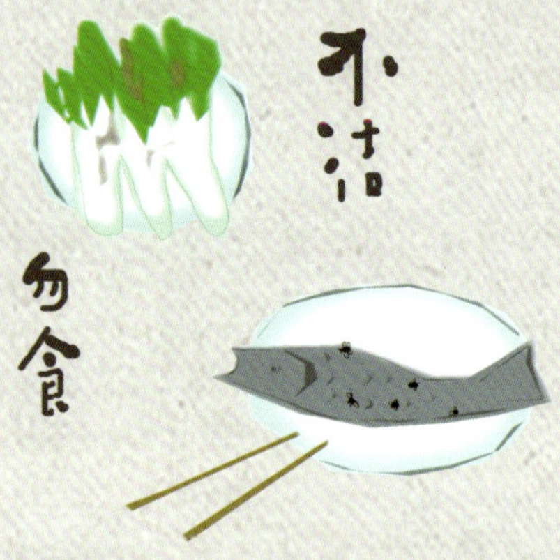

過食肥甘厚味，易化生內熱，甚至引起癰疽瘡毒等癥。若飲酒過度，可致酒毒攻心，神識昏迷等。

Preference for greasy, rich and sweet food can easily lead to internal heat which can cause toxic abscess, ulcer or sores. Drinking too much alcohol will lead to a state of alcohol poison which attacks the heart and manifests in unconsciousness.

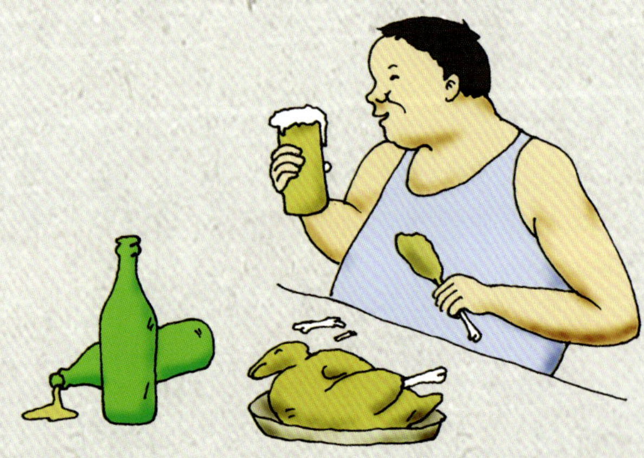

2. 七情内傷

七情是指人的喜、怒、憂、思、悲、驚、恐七種情誌變化。在正常情況下，七情是人體的正常情感反應，是人體正常的機能狀態，不會使人發病。衹有當突然的、强烈的或持久的不良情誌刺激，如暴怒、狂喜、悲哭、大驚、猝恐、思慮、憂愁等，超過了人體心理承受和調節能力，引起臟腑氣血功能紊亂，才會導致疾病的發生。此時的七情便爲致病因素。

喜則氣緩。喜爲心之誌，若過度狂喜，可致心氣渙散，精神不能集中，甚則失神狂亂。

2. Internal Injury by Seven Emotions

The seven emotions are joy, anger, worry, pensiveness, sorrow, fright and fear. Under normal conditions, the seven emotions represent normal feelings and reactions and do not cause diseases. When there is emotional upset which is sudden, strong or over a long term, the seven normal emotions will change to excessive joy, rage, melancholy, excessive thinking, grief, severe fright and sudden fear. These emotions can surpass a person's physiological endurance, disturb the function of the Zang and Fu organs and become the seven pathogenic factors.

Joy relates to the Heart organ and slows the qi down; excessive joy scatters the Heart qi, this manifest as an inability to concentrate and mania in severe cases.

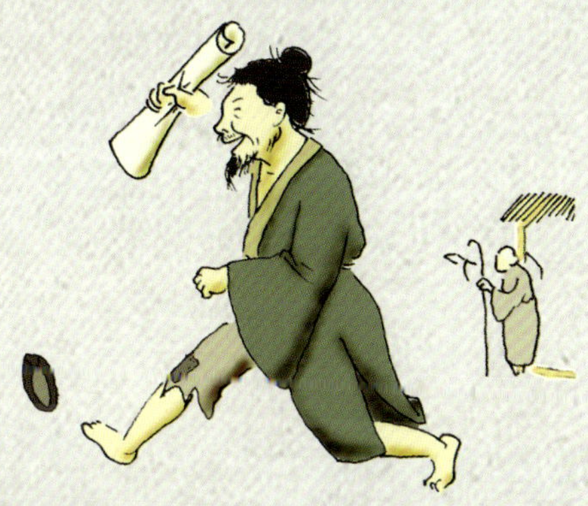

怒則氣上。怒爲肝之誌。過於憤怒，可使肝氣横逆上衝，血隨氣逆，蒙蔽清竅引起昏厥。

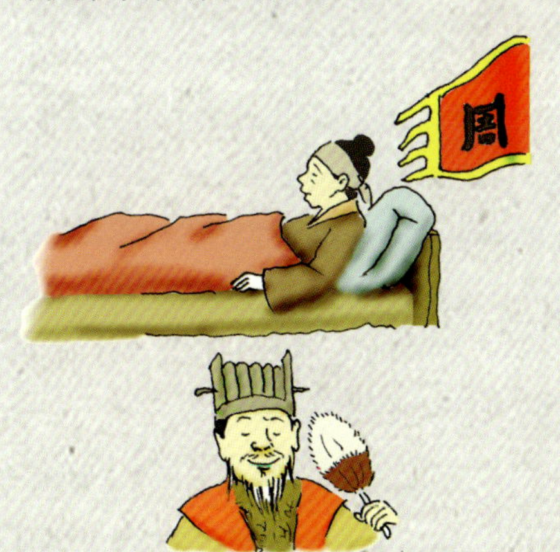

Anger relates to the Liver organ and makes the qi rise; rage can make the qi and blood goes upwards where they block the upper orifices and cause coma.

思則氣結。思爲脾之誌。思慮勞神過度，傷心損脾，出現心驚健忘、失眠多夢、胃納呆滯、脘腹痞塞等。

Pensiveness relates to the Spleen and stagnates the qi, excessive thinking damages both the Heart and Spleen, which manifests as palpitations, forgetfulness, insomnia, many dreams, indigestion, poor appetite and abdominal distension.

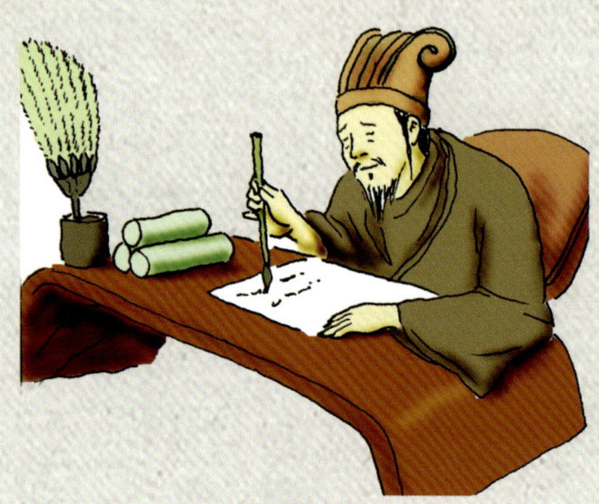

悲則氣消、悲爲肺之誌。悲哀太過，往往耗傷肺氣，可見胸悶氣短，精神萎靡，乏力等。

恐則氣下，恐爲腎之誌。長期或突然的過度恐懼，可使腎氣不固，而致二便失禁，遺精滑泄等。

驚則氣亂，突然受到驚恐，則心氣紊亂、氣血失調，以致心無所依、驚慌失措等。

Sorrow relates to the Lung and disperses the qi; melancholy consumes the Lung qi, which manifests as chest oppression, shortness of breath, dejection and fatigue.

Fear relates to the Kidney and makes the qi descend; sudden or prolonged fear may cause the Kidney qi not consolidate, manifested as incontinence of urinary and fecal, seminal emissions and frequent diarrhea.

Fright puts the qi in chaos; sudden fright disturbs the Heart qi, and causes disharmony between qi and blood which can manifest as panic.

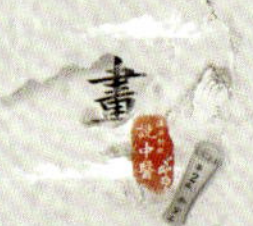

3. 勞逸過度

正常的勞動有助於氣血流通，增强體質；而必要的休息可以消除疲勞，恢複體力和腦力。勞動與休息的合理調節，是保證人體健康的必要條件。但若長時間的過度勞累或過度安逸，都可能成爲致病因素而使人發病，勞力過度，是指較長時期的過度用力。勞力過度則傷氣，氣傷則氣少力衰、神疲、消瘦、四肢困倦、懶言懶動、動則氣喘。

3. Overwork and Too Much Rest

A normal amount of work and physical exercise can help the circulation of qi and blood, and result in good health. Rest restores both physical and mental strength. Proper balance between work and rest is important for maintaining health. However, overwork or too much rest (physical or mental) over a long time will cause diseases. Physical overwork refers to overstrain from physical labor over a long period of time, it can damage the qi and lead to deficiency which manifests as lack of strength, mental weakness, weight loss, heavy fatigued limbs, no desire to speak, laziness and shortness of breath after physical exercise.

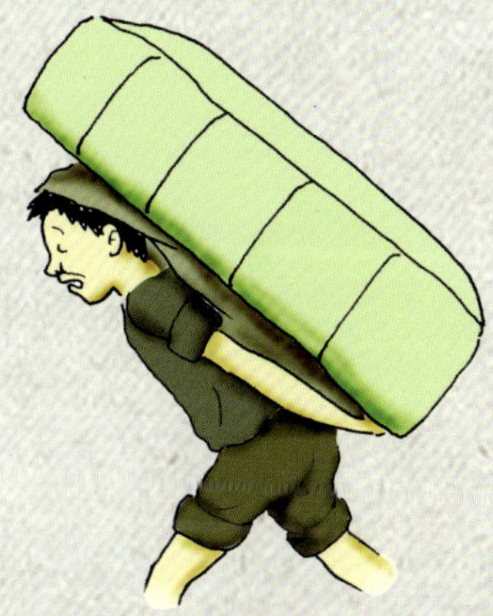

勞神，是指思慮太過，暗傷心血、損傷脾氣，分別出現心悸、健忘、失眠、多夢等心神失常及納呆、腹脹、便溏等脾不健運的癥狀。

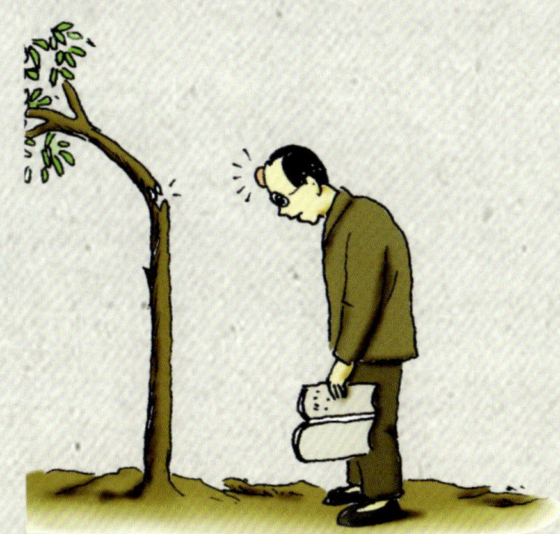

Excessive mental work refers to over-thinking, which cause damage to the Heart blood and the Spleen qi. The symptoms related to the Heart are palpitations, amnesia, insomnia, many dreams; the Spleen related symptoms are indigestion and loss of appetite, abdominal distension and loose stools.

房勞過度，是指性生活不節製，房事過度。房勞易傷腎精，出現腰膝酸軟、眩暈、耳鳴、精神萎靡、性機能減退或遺精、早泄、陽痿等癥。

Excessive sexual activity can easily damage the Kidney essence. The related symptoms are pain and weakness in the lumbar back and knees, dizziness, tinnitus, dejection, impotence, reduced seminal amount, nocturnal emission and premature ejaculation.

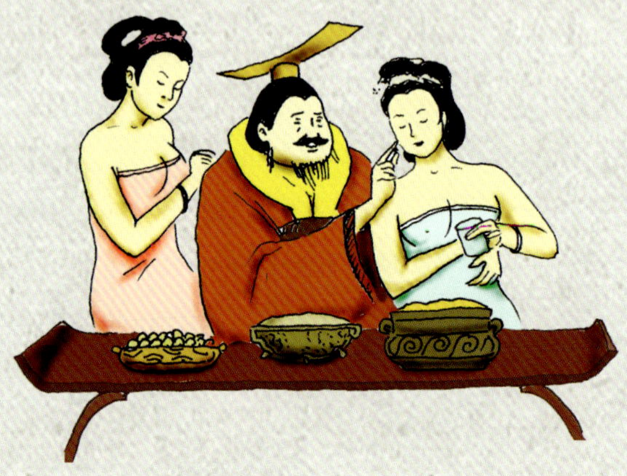

過度安逸，易使氣血運行不暢，脾胃功能減退，可出現食少乏力、精神不振、肢體軟弱或發胖臃腫，動則心悸、汗出、氣喘等表現。

Too much resting can easily cause abnormal flow of qi and blood, resulting in weakened function of the Spleen and Stomach and will manifest as poor appetite, fatigue, mental depression, weak limbs, weight gain, palpitations, shortness of breath and sweating.

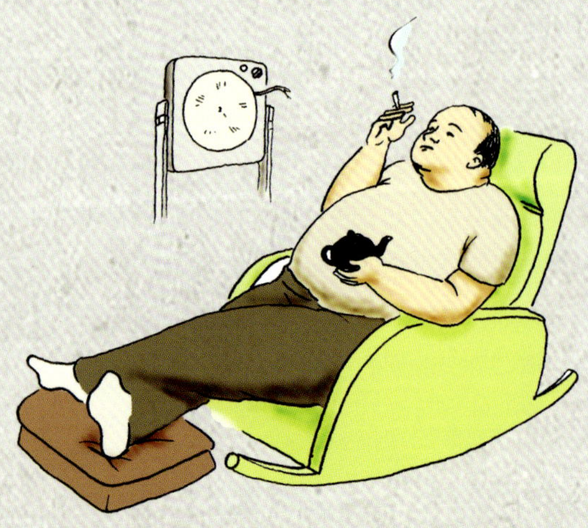

三、病理產物性病因

Causes of Disease due to Pathological By-products

在疾病過程中形成的病理產物，又可成爲新的病證發生的病因，此稱爲病理產物性病因，常見有“痰飲”、“瘀血”、“結石”三大類。

1. 痰飲

痰飲是由於多種致病因素作用於人體後，引起機體水液代謝障礙所形成的病理產物。它又可作用於機體，阻滯經絡，阻礙氣血，影響臟腑功能，導致各種新的病證出現。

痰和飲是機體水液代謝障礙所形成的病理產物。一般來説，稠濁者爲痰，清稀者爲飲。

痰作爲致病因素，可分爲有形之痰和無形之痰。有形之痰指視之可見、觸之可及、聞之有聲的痰而言。所以不單指咳吐出來的痰液，還包括瘰癧、痰核等停滯於體內而未被排出的類似痰液。

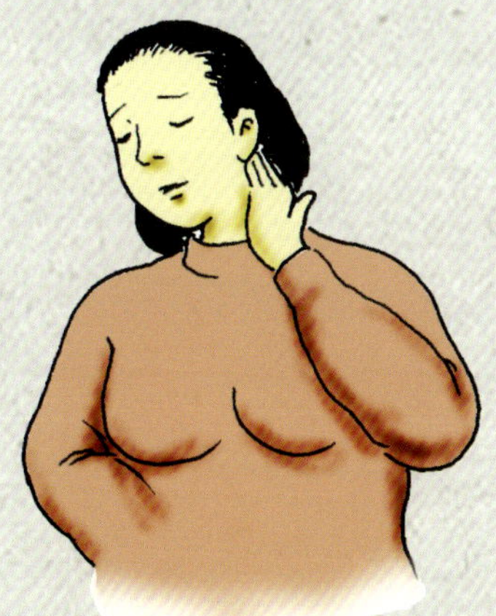

The pathological by-products are formed during the process of disease and themselves can cause new disease. There are three categories: phlegm and fluid, blood stasis and stones.

1. Phlegm and Fluids

Phlegm and fluids are pathological by-products. They are produced by many types of disease factors which affect the body and cause problems with water metabolism, resulting in blockage of the channels, qi and blood, and impaired function of the Zang-fu organs.

Generally, phlegm is thick and turbid while the fluids are thin and clear.

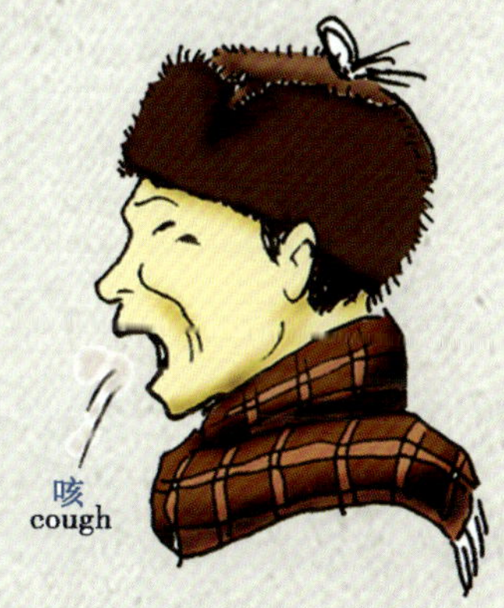

Phlegm is classified into two forms: visible and invisible. The visible form can be heard and touched. Phlegm not only comes out from the body, such as coughing up sputum, but it can also remain inside the body in the form of scrofula and nodules.

無形之痰是指視而不見、觸之不及的痰而言。痰隨氣機降全身無處不到。常見頭暈、目眩、心悸氣短、惡心嘔吐、神昏譫語等。因而有“百病多由痰作祟”、“怪病多痰”之説。

Invisible phlegm cannot be touched, it follows the qi mechanism and can be anywhere in the body. Common symptoms are vertigo, dizziness, palpitation, shortness of breath, nausea, vomit and delirium speech. There are two famous saying: "Many diseases are caused by phlegm" and "Strange diseases are phlegm".

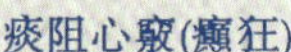

痰阻心竅(癲狂)
Phlegm in the orifico of the heart
(maniac)

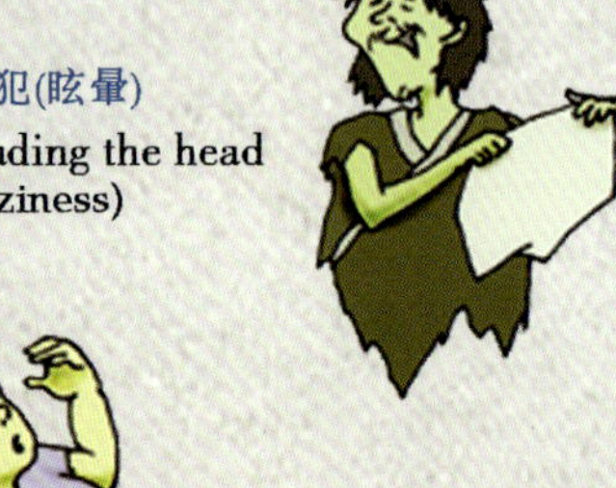

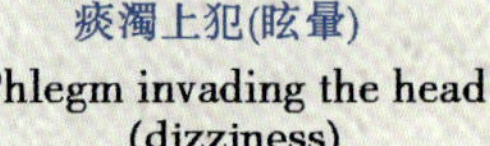

痰濁上犯(眩暈)
Phlegm invading the head
(dizziness)

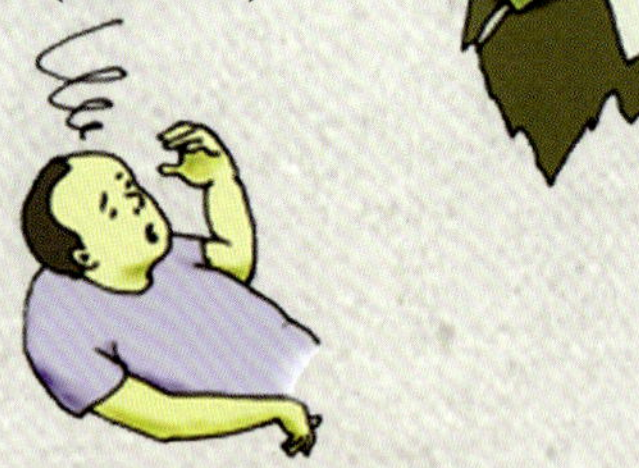

痰阻經絡(中風)
Phlegm in the channels and collate rals
(apoplexy)

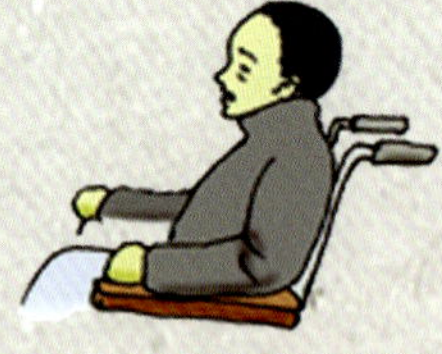

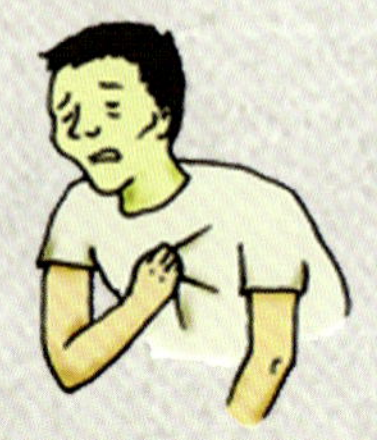

痰瘀心脉(心絞痛)
Phlegm in the heart channel
(angina)

瘀蒙清竅(昏迷)
Phlegm in seven orifices
(coma)

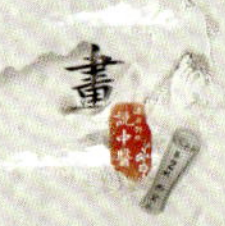

飲是水液停留於人體局部的病證，一般分爲四種。飲在腸間，則腸鳴瀝瀝有聲，稱痰飲；飲在胸脅，則胸脅脹滿，咳唾引痛，稱懸飲；飲在胸膈，則胸悶、喘咳不能平卧，稱支飲；飲溢肌膚，則見肌膚水腫、無汗、身體疼痛，稱溢飲。

Rheum (fluid retention) refers to diseases due to water accumulation in a certain part of the body, and includes four types: fluid retention in the intestines causes borborygmus (intestinal sounds), and is called phlegm-rheum. Rheum at the chest and hypochondrium, causes distention and fullness, and pain when coughing up saliva; it is called suspended rheum. Rheum at the chest and diaphragm, causes stifling sensation in the chest, asthma and orthopnea (difficulty in breathing when lying down), and it is called propping rheum. Rheum in the muscles and skin, causes edema, anhidrosis (absence of sweat), and body pain, and it is called spillage rheum.

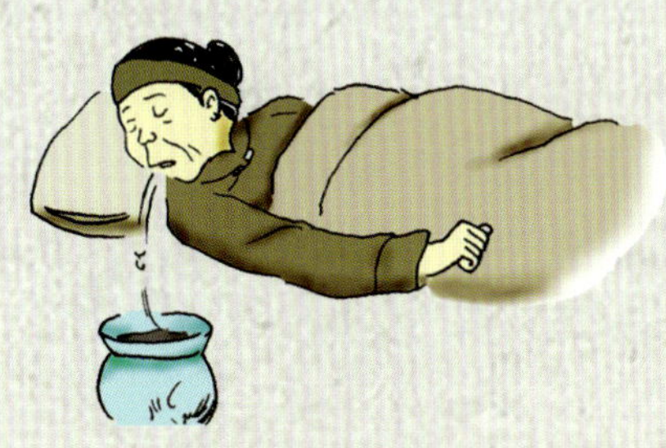

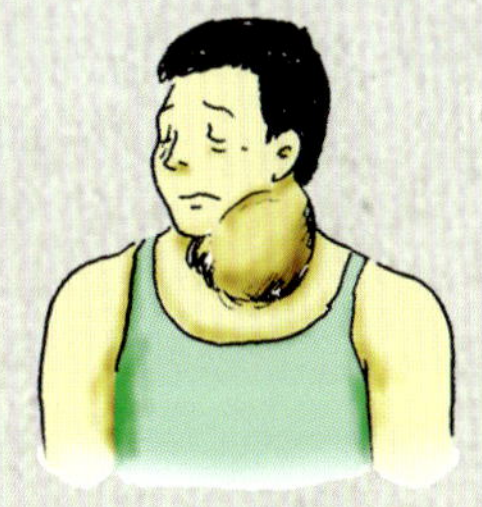

2. 瘀血

瘀血，泛指體内血液停滯，包括離經之血積存體内及血液運行不暢而阻滯於經絡臟腑。形成因素：一是因氣虚、氣滯、血寒、血熱等原因，使血行不暢而凝滯。二是由於内外損傷，氣虚失攝或血熱妄行等原因造成血離經脈，積存於體内而形成。

2. Blood Stasis

Blood stasis is stagnation of the blood circulation in the body and can be found outside and inside the meridians, and also in the viscera. The formative factors of stagnant blood may be firstly, that blood circulation is disturbed due to qi deficiency, qi stagnation, and cold or heat in the blood. Secondly, hemorrhage due to qi deficiency and inability to hold the blood in the meridians and vessels or bleeding caused by heat in the blood.

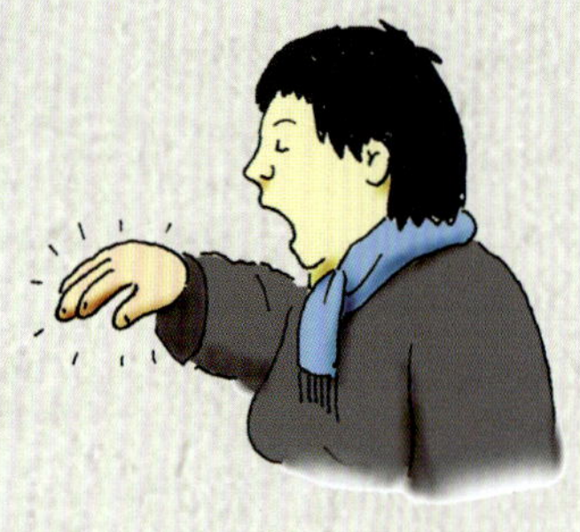

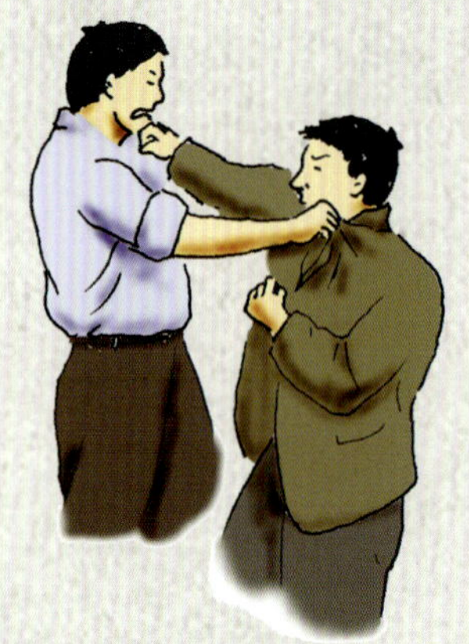

（1）瘀血的致病特點

1）易於阻滯氣機

氣捨於血中，賴血的運載而達全身。瘀血形成之後，不但失去濡養作用，反而阻滯於局部，影響氣的運行，故說"血瘀必兼氣滯"。

2）阻礙血脈運行

瘀血爲有形實邪，可導致局部和全身的血液運行失常，使臟腑功能發生障礙，如瘀阻心脈，可致胸痹心痛；瘀積於肝，可致脅痛包塊；瘀阻胞宮，可致痛經閉經等。

（2）瘀血的病證特點

瘀血的臨床表現有以下幾個特點：

(1) Pathogenic Features of Blood Stasis

1) Blood stasis easily blocks the qi movement; the qi relies on the blood to be transported to the whole body. After blood stasis has been formed, not only does qi fail to nourish the body but also blood stasis obstructs certain parts of the body and influences the flow of qi, hence the saying "Blood stasis must be accompanied by qi stagnation".

2) Blood stasis obstructs the circulation of blood, it is an excessive pathogenic factor with form. It can cause disorder of blood transportation in certain parts of the body or in the whole body and obstruct the normal function of the viscera. For example, blood stasis at the Heart causes chest Bi and chest pain; at the Liver, it causes hypochondriac pain and lumps; at the uterus, it causes dysmenorrhea and amenorrhea.

(2) Symptoms Characteristics of Blood Stasis

The clinical manifestations of blood stasis can be summed up as follows:

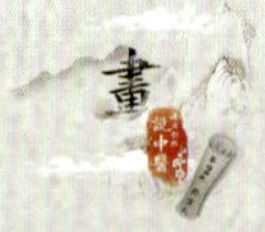

1）疼痛

一般表現爲刺痛，痛有定處，拒按。

2）腫塊

積於體表者可見青紫腫脹，積於體内者則成腫塊。

3）出血

血色多呈紫暗，或夾有瘀血塊。

4）望診特點

面色、口唇、肌膚、爪甲青紫；舌質紫暗，或舌質有瘀點、瘀斑，或舌下絡脈曲張青紫等。久瘀者則可見面色黧黑，或肌膚甲錯。

5）脈象特點

常見細澀、沉弦或結代等脈象。

1) Pain, usually stabbing, fixed pain, with aversion to pressure.

2) Lumps may be blue or purple color, due to accumulation of blood in the body.

3) Bleeding, the blood's color is dark purple and there could also be blood clots.

4) Character of Inspection

Complexion, lips, skin, nails and tongue, all are blue or purple color due to the blood stasis; in addition, there are stasis speckles, stasis macules on the tongue or sublingual veins, which are all purple or blue color. Blood stasis over a long time manifests as a dark complexion and dry skin.

5) The pulse is usually thready and rough, deep and wiry, or knotted and intermittent.

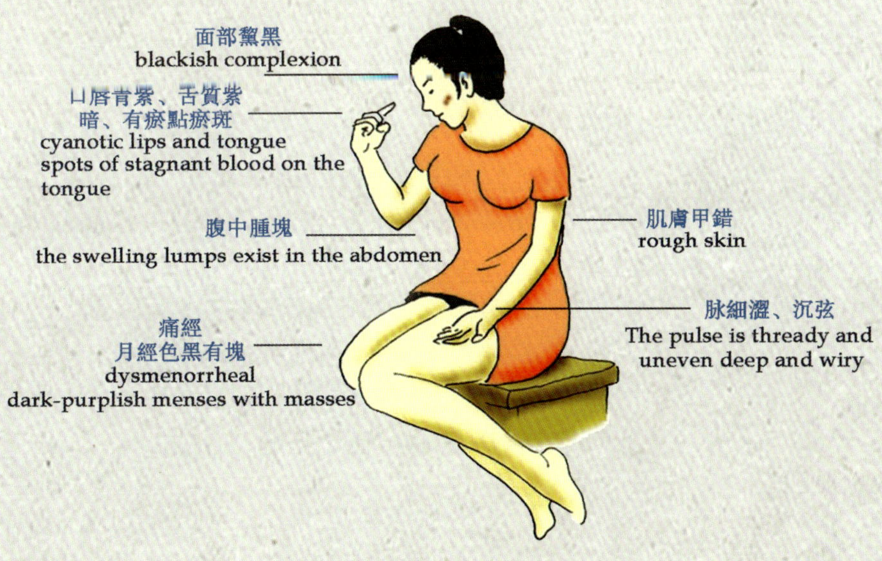

3. 結石

結石是體内濕熱濁邪蘊結不散，煎熬而形成的砂石樣的病理產物。常見的結石有肝、膽結石，腎、膀胱結石，胃結石等。

結石的形成原因：一是飲食不節，偏嗜肥甘厚味（高糖高脂肪類食物）；二是情誌内傷，使肝失疏泄，膽氣不達，膽汁蘊結；三是服藥不當，長期服用鈣、鎂、鉍等藥物，與濁物、水濕、熱邪相合，釀成結石。

結石的致病特點：一是多發於空腔性臟器，如膽囊、膽管、腎盂、輸尿管、膀胱及胃腔等；二病程較長，癥狀不定；三是易阻滯氣機，損傷脈絡；四是疼痛，具有間歇性特點，發作時劇痛難忍，而緩解時如常人。

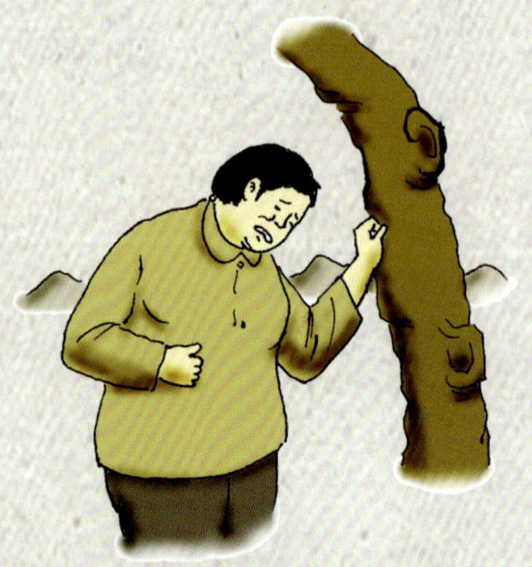

3. Stones

Stones are pathological by-products, generated from internal prolonged retention of damp heat and turbid pathogenic factors. Common organs where stones can be found are the Liver, Gallbladder, Kidney, Bladder and Stomach.

Stone formation is caused by: improper diet, overeating fatty, sweet and greasy foods, internal injury from imbalance in the emotions will cause irregular flow of the Liver qi, deficiency of Gallbladder qi will affect its ability to disseminate and accumulate Gallbladder bile, and, improper medicine use. Prolonged consumption of calcium, magnesium and bismuth, or other pathogenic factors like turbid matters, water-dampness and heat, can also lead to the formation of stones.

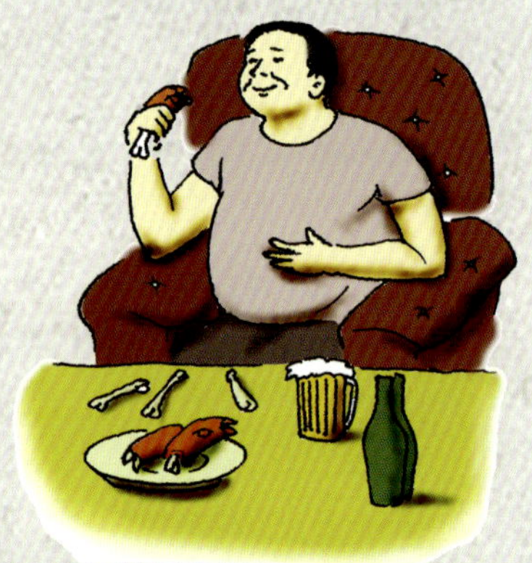

The pathogenic features of stones are that they frequently appear in the cavity of the viscera such as gallbladder, bile duct, renal pelvis, ureter, urinary bladder and stomach. They have a long course of disease and diverse range of symptoms, they easily lead to stagnation of the qi dynamic and injury to the collaterals and vessels. They cause intermittent pain, so that when the symptoms appear. The pain is severe and difficult to bear but when they are relieved, the patient feels healthy.

四、其它病因

在中醫病因學中，除六淫、癘氣、七情内傷、飲食失宜、勞逸過度病理産物之外還有外傷、蟲獸傷、寄生蟲、藥邪、醫過、先天因素等致病因素。

The Miscellaneous Pathogenic Factors

In Chinese medical etiology, besides the six climatic influences, epidemic pathogenic factors, internal injury by the seven emotions, improper diet, overwork and too much rest, there is also trauma, mistreatment, injury by animals, parasites, poisons and congenital factors.

第七章 病機 Chapter 7 Pathogenesis

一、發病

人體自身及其與外界環境之間，始終維持着相對的動態平衡，即所謂“陰平陽秘”。如果“陰陽失調”就是疾病的發生。

疾病的發生和變化，總體上不外邪正兩方面，正是指正氣，是人體的機能活動和抗病、康復的能力。

邪，是指邪氣，泛指各種致病因素，疾病的發生和發展就是邪正相互鬥爭的反映。

Pathogenesis

Between humans and nature, there is a constant dynamic balance, called the equilibrium of yin and yang. If yin and yang are in disharmony, disease will occur.

The disease occurrence and changes involves two factors: *zhèng* and *xié*. *Zhèng*, called the right qi, refers to human physical functions as well as its resistance to disease and ability to recover.

Xié, called the evil qi, refers to various kinds of pathogenic factors. The occurrence and development of disease is the struggle between the right qi and the evil qi.

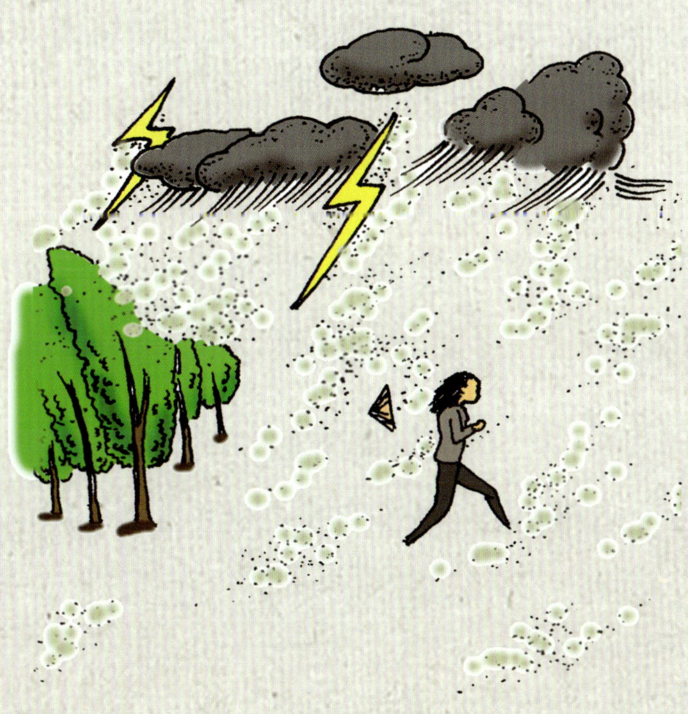

正氣不足是發展的内在依據。一般説來，衹有在正氣相對虚弱，不足以抵抗病邪時，邪氣才能乘虚入侵而致病。

Right qi deficiency is the basic internal cause of disease development. Generally, only when the right qi is relatively weak and fails to resist the attack of the evil qi, does the evil qi take advantage of this weakness and invade the body, causing disease.

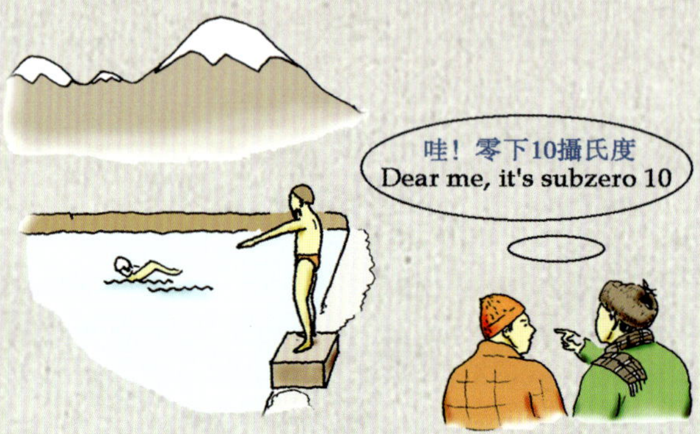

邪氣是發病的重要條件。中醫學强調正氣在發病學上的主導地位，但不排除邪氣致病的重要作用，因爲正氣抗邪是一定限度的，在邪毒特强的情况下可使正氣很快損傷而受邪發病。如疫癘之邪傷人可在短期内使很多人同時發病。

Evil qi is an important cause of disease occurrence. Chinese medicine emphasizes the right qi and its leading role in pathogenesis, yet it does not rule out the important influence of the evil qi in causing disease. When the evil qi is in a state of extreme predominance, the right qi is easily damaged, causing disease. For example, epidemic pathogenic factor (evil qi), in a short period of time, can simultaneously cause disease in a lot of people.

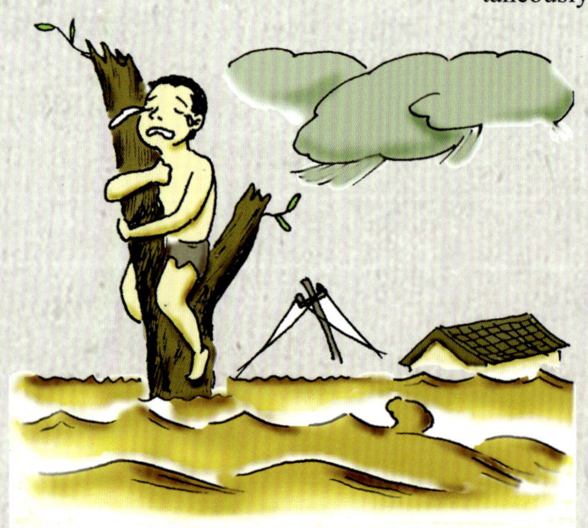

邪正鬥爭的勝負，決定發病與不發病以及疾病的轉歸。正勝邪退，則疾病趨於好轉而痊愈；邪勝正衰，則疾病趨於惡化甚至死亡。

The struggle between the right qi and the evil qi determines the prognosis and the recovery of the disease. If the right qi is stronger than the evil qi, the prognosis is good and the disease will be cured; if the evil qi is stronger than the right qi, the prognosis is bad and the patient might even die.

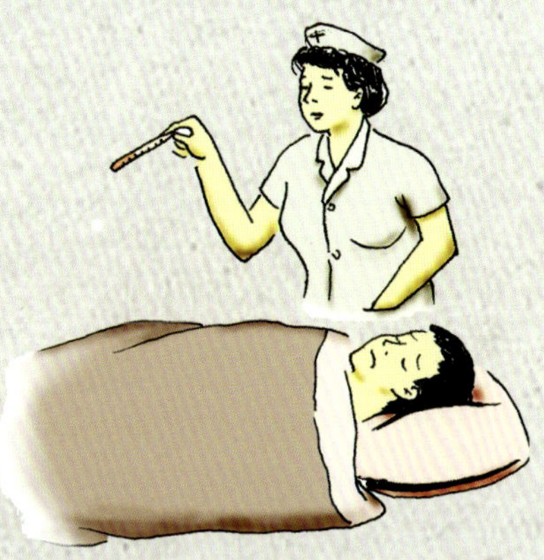

疾病發生與外環境密切相關。很多疾病的發生或某些慢性病的複發多與季節有關。如春季多風病，夏季多暑病，長夏多濕病，秋季多燥病，冬季多寒病等。

Disease occurrence is closely related with the environment. The occurrence of many diseases and relapse of certain chronic diseases are related to seasons. In the spring, diseases are related to wind. In the summer, diseases are related to summer-heat. In the autumn, diseases are related to dryness. And in the winter, diseases are related to cold.

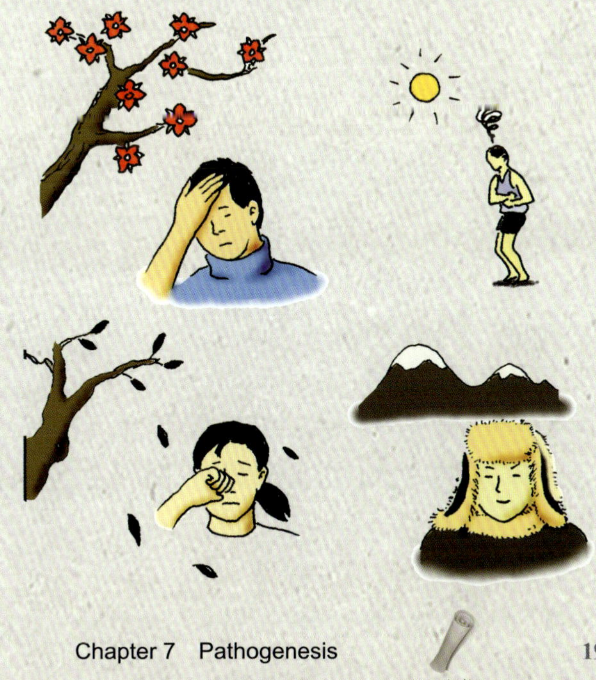

不良的生活環境，如工業廢氣、廢物、廢水等，都能污染環境、水源，從而直接或間接地損害人體、影響正氣。

Poor living environment, such as industrial wastes, gases and waste water, cause pollution of the environment and the water resources, which directly or indirectly damages the right qi of the body.

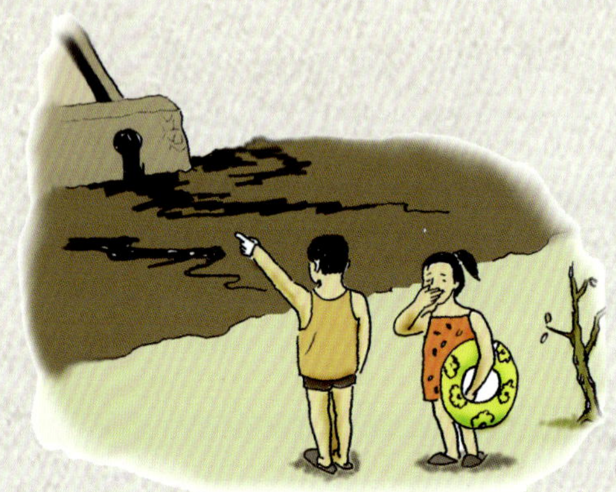

二、基本病機

Fundamental Pathogenesis

基本病機是指機體在致病因素作用下所產生的基本病理反映，是疾病發生的病變本質變化的一般規律。在此，主要闡述基本病機中的邪正盛衰和陰陽失調。

Fundamental pathogenesis refers to the fundamental pathological reaction of the human body when affected by pathogenic factors. This general principle reflects the change of nature of the disease. The two main parts of the pathogenesis are the excess and deficiency of the right qi and the evil qi, the imbalance of yin and yang, are to be discussed as follows:

1. 邪正盛衰與疾病的虛實變化

1. The Relationship between the Struggle of the Right Qi and the Evil Qi and the Deficiency and Excess Changes of a Disease.

（1）實證

(1) Excess Syndrome

在疾病發展過程中，邪正雙方力量對比的盛衰，決定著病證的虛實變化。實性病機主要是指邪氣亢盛，是以邪氣盛爲主要矛盾的一種病理反映。因爲邪氣亢盛，

During the disease process, the struggle

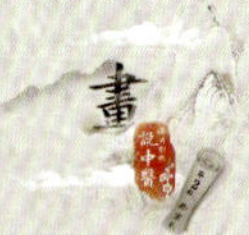

正氣未衰（相對的），邪正劇烈相爭，臨床表現爲一係列以亢奮、有餘、不通爲特徵的實性病理變化，［如同敵方（邪氣）氣勢洶洶，我方（正氣）奮勇殺敵，雙方交戰，炮聲隆隆，硝烟彌漫］。實證多見於外感病的初、中期階段，一般病程較短。臨床表現如壯熱，狂躁，聲高氣粗，腹痛拒按，二便不通，脈實有力等。

between the right qi and evil qi (pathogenic factors) determines the disease condition and change (deficiency or excess). Excess syndrome primarily indicates an excess of evil qi. If the right qi is relatively strong when the evil qi is attacking the body, the struggle between them will be intense. Clinically, during this excess condition, there are a series of pathological reactions like hyper-function, surplus and obstruction. The evil qi is like an aggressive enemy that attacks the body (the right qi), which fights back. When these two sides are fighting, it is as if the guns are roaring and a cloud of smoke floats above them. This type of excess syndrome is mostly seen in the early or middle stages of an external pathogenic disease, generally lasting a short period of time. The clinical manifestations are high fever, mania, loud voice and rough breathing, abdominal pain with aversion to pressure, urine retention, constipation and a pulse that is powerful and in excess.

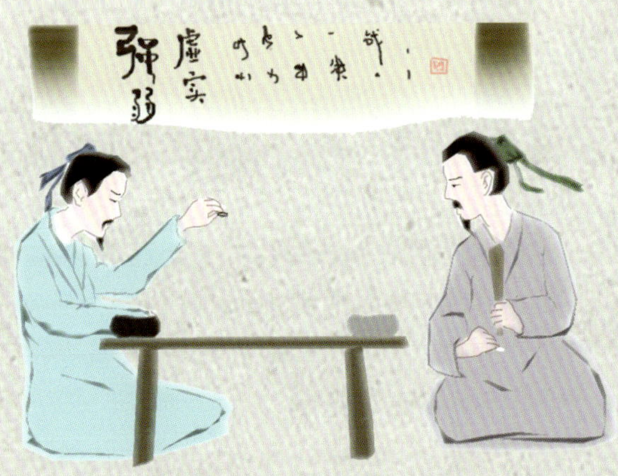

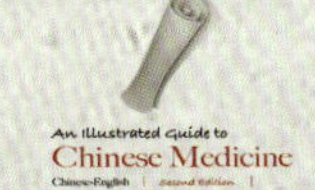

（2）虛證

虛性病機主要是指正氣不足，是以正氣虛損、抗病能力減弱爲矛盾主要方面的一種病理反映。因正氣虛弱，抗病力低下，一般邪氣也不盛，正邪不能激烈相爭，難以出現較爲劇烈的病理反映，[如同敵我大戰之後。我方（正氣）疲憊，敵方（邪氣）戀戰。雙方力量均已消耗對峙]。在臨床上出現一係列以衰退、虛弱、不固爲主要特徵的虛性病理變化。臨床表現如神疲體倦，面容憔悴，心悸氣短，自汗盜汗，畏寒肢冷，脈虛無力等。

(2) Deficiency Syndrome

Deficiency syndrome is mainly due to insufficiency of right qi. When the right qi is deficient, its ability to resist disease decreases. Generally, in a deficiency condition, the evil qi is not in excess, therefore the fight between the right qi and the evil qi is not so intense. It resembles after a war, where the two sides (evil qi and right qi) are exhausted. Clinically, during this deficiency condition, there are pathological reactions like decline, weakness and insecurity, for example, lassitude of the spirit and fatigue, pale complexion, palpitation and shortness of breath, spontaneous perspiration, night sweats, cold limbs, and a pulse that is deficient and weak.

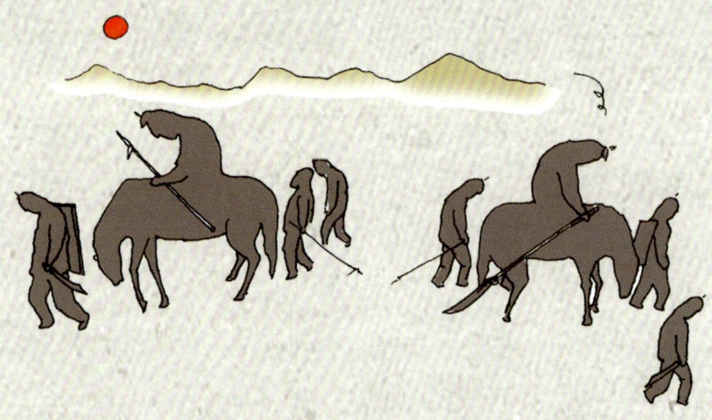

2. 陰陽失調

即陰陽之間失去平衡協調的病理狀態。

（1）陰陽偏勝

（2）陽偏勝

陽偏勝是指機體在疾病過程中出現的一種陽氣偏盛、功能亢

2. Imbalance of Yin and Yang

When the balance and coordination between yin and yang is lost, the term "yin and yang in equilibrium" becomes a pathological condition.

(1) Relative Dominance of Yin or Yang

(2) Yang Dominance

During the process of disease there is a pathological condition when the yang-qi is in excess,

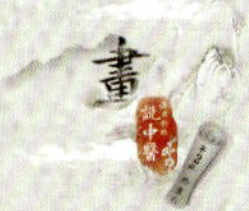

奮、機體反應性增强、陽熱過剩的病理狀態。陽熱亢盛（如高熱患者）的病變可見高熱、面紅等陽熱現象，還可見到口咽幹燥、小便短少、大便幹結（陰液損傷）現象。

thus the body is hyper-functioning, and the heat is in surplus. Common symptoms are high fever, red face, dry throat and thirst, scanty urine, constipation (damage to the yin fluids).

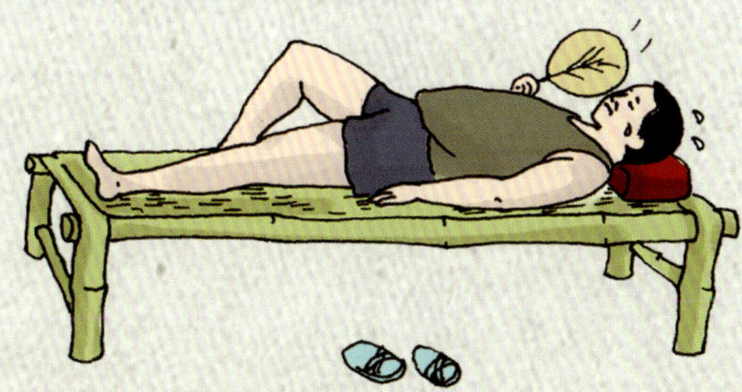

（3）陰偏勝

陰偏勝是指機體在疾病過程中所出現的一種陰氣偏盛，功能障礙或减退，産熱不足，以及陰寒性病理産物積聚的病理狀態。如陰盛（嚴冬劇寒）的病變，陽氣也會不同程度的受損。因此，在陰寒盛出現腹部或肢體冷痛的同時，常兼見神疲倦怠、畏寒、四肢欠溫（陽氣不足）的癥狀。

(3) Yin Dominance

During the process of disease there is a pathological condition when the yin-qi is in excess, which manifests as functional disorder of the internal organs, not enough energy is generated, and accumulation of yin-cold products. For example, the transforming of the excess of yin (like the cold of severe winter) will result in the damage of the yang-qi. Therefore, when the excess of yin occurs, there is abdominal or limb pain and cold, and at the same time there is also lassitude of the spirit, fatigue, aversion and cold limbs (yang-qi insufficiency).

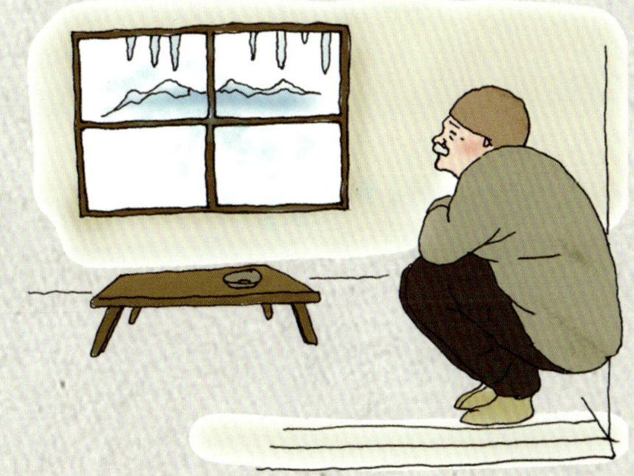

3. 陰陽偏衰

（1）陽偏衰

即是陽虛，是指機體陽氣虛損，功能活動減退或衰弱，溫煦功能減退（熱能不足）的病理狀態，現爲畏寒喜暖，神疲乏力，四肢不溫，舌淡脈遲等癥。（如年高體弱者多怕冷肢涼）

（2）陰偏衰

陰偏衰即偏衰是指機體的精、血、津液等物質虧損，滋養功能減退（陰液不足），表現爲五心煩熱，潮熱盜汗，面紅升火，消瘦，舌紅脈細數等癥（如婦女更年期常出現此證）。

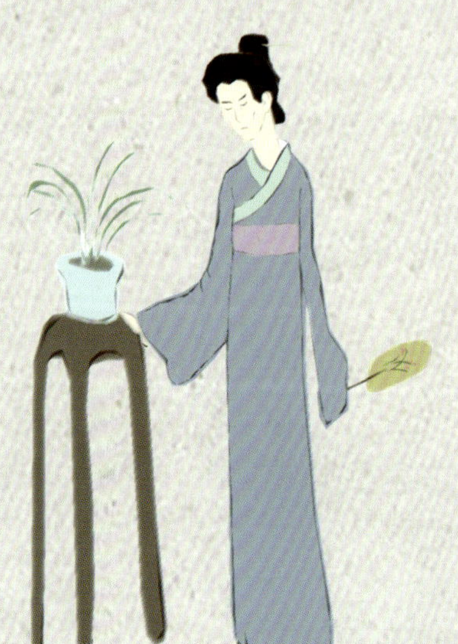

3. Relatively Weakness of Yin or Yang

(1) Deficiency of Yang

Relative weakness of yang indicates a pathological condition in which the yang-qi is insufficient, therefore the body functions decline, and there is a preference for warmth. Clinically, the symptoms are aversion to cold and preference to warmth, lassitude of the spirit, fatigue, cold limbs, pale tongue, and slow pulse. For example, elders with weak body, often fear cold and have cold limbs.

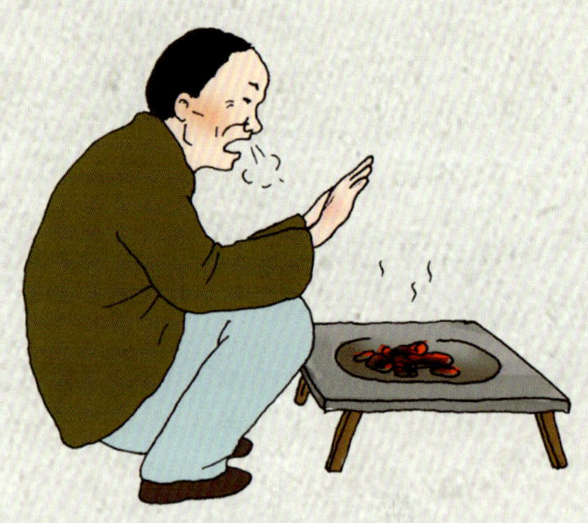

(2) Deficiency of Yin

Relative weakness of yin indicates loss of essence, blood, body fluids, and decrease in the function of nourishing (yin-fluid insufficiency). The common symptoms are five palm heat (sensation of heat in the chest, palms and soles), tidal fever, night sweats, red face, emaciation, red tongue with thin coating thready and rapid pulse (Often see in menopausal stage).

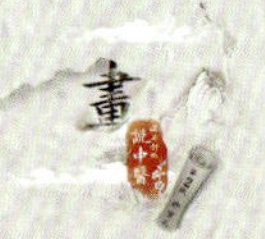

第八章 養生及防治原則

Chapter 8 Health Care and Principles of Prevention and Treatment

一、養生原則

養生，即保養生命之謂。養生就是採取各種方法保養身體，增强體質，預防疾病，增進健康，延緩衰老。可歸納爲以下幾個方面：

1. 順應自然

就是要求人的生命活動，要遵循自然界的客觀規律，順應自然界的運動變化而主動地採取各種養生措施，達到避邪防病，保健延年的目的。

2. 形神共養

中醫養生學主張，静以養神，動以養形。静以養神，就是通過清静養神、修性怡神、氣功練神等方法，保持樂觀安静、心平氣和的精神狀態。動以養形是指通過形體鍛煉、勞動、散步、導引、按摩等，以運動形體，疏通經絡，促進氣血流暢。

The Principles of Health Care

Health care means life maintenance, which adopts various methods to preserve the body, strengthen constitution, prevent diseases, improve health and prolong life. It includes the following aspects:

1. Correspondence with Nature

All life activities of the body follow natural objective laws and changes. Taking various actions can achieve the prevention of disease, health protection and prolong life.

2. Preserving the Body and Spirit

Chinese medicine believes that quiet nourishes the spirit, while motion nourishes the body. Relaxation and the practice of qi gong can maintain a peaceful and happy state of mind. Physical exercise, movement, walking, working and massage can dredge the meridians and promote qi and blood circulation.

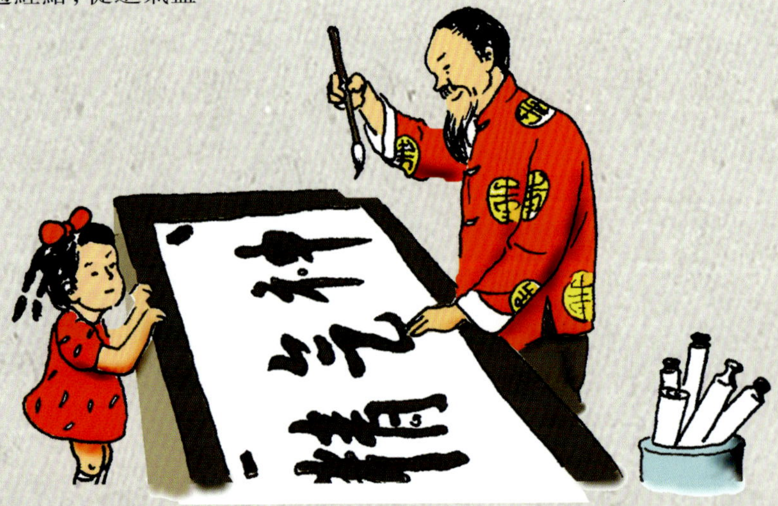

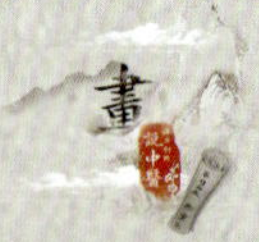

3. 調養脾胃

脾胃强弱是决定人之健康和健康長壽的重要因素。調養脾胃的關鍵是飲食調節，做到寒熱適中，饑飽有度，營養全面，清潔衛生。既保護脾胃功能不受侵害，又保證人體所需營養物質充足平衡。

4. 保精護腎

精是構成人體和促進人體生長發育的基本物質。精、氣、神乃人身“三寶”，爲健康長壽的根本，也是養生保健的關鍵。因此，保精重在保養腎精。保護腎精的關鍵在於房事有節，不妄作勞，從而使腎精充盈，氣足神旺，以利於身心健康。

3. Regulate Nourish Spleen and Stomach

The state of the strength or weakness of the Spleen and Stomach is an important factor in health and longevity. The key to regulate and nourish Spleen and Stomach is to balance the amount and temperature of foods, and to have an understanding of nutrition and hygiene. In order to keep Spleen and Stomach properly functioning, it is necessary to eat sufficient and balanced foods.

4. Protect the Essence and Guard the Kidney

Essence is a basic substance for development. Essence, qi and spirit are the three treasures, the root of health, longevity and the key of health protection. Thus, protecting the essence relies on protecting the Kidney essence. The key to protect Kidney essence is to avoid excessive sexual activity. Normal sexual life can lead to abundance of Kidney essence and sufficient qi and spirit, which will benefit the body and mind.

二、預防原則

預防，是指採取一定的措施來防止疾病的發生與發展。《内經》中的“治未病”預防思想，對後世預防醫學的發展做出了極大的貢獻。“治未病”是中醫學的重要預防思想和治療思想。未病先防，就是在疾病未發生之前，採取各種措施來防止疾病的發生。邪氣侵入是導致疾病發生的重要條件，正

The Principles of Prevention

Disease prevention is the measures taken in order to stop disease occurrence and development. *The Yellow Emperor's Classic of Internal Medicine* <*Huáng Dì Nèi Jīng*> states that the preventive treatment of disease contributed to the development of preventive medicine in later generations. In Chinese medicine, the concept of preventive medicine is an important principle of treatment. Prevention is taking measures to avoid disease before they occur. Disease occurs due to attacks by evil qi at the

氣不足則是疾病發生的内在根據。因此，預防疾病，除了要避免病邪入侵之外，更重要的是提高正氣，增强抗病能力。

exterior or insufficient right qi at the interior. Therefore, strengthening the right qi and improving the body's resistance to disease is even more important than preventing attacks of evil qi.

1. 提高正氣，增强抗邪氣能力

正氣的强弱，由體質所决定。一般來説，體質壯實者，正氣充盛；體質虛弱者，正氣不足。因此，增强體質是提高正氣抗邪能力的關鍵。增强體質要注譩調攝精神，調理飲食起居，鍛煉身體，適應自然規律以及適當的藥物預防等。

1. Strengthen the Right Qi and Body's Resistance to Evil Qi

The right qi's state of strength or weakness depends on the constitution. Generally, the right qi of healthy and strong people is abundant, and weak people have insufficiency of right qi. Therefore, strengthening the body is a key to increasing the right qi and the body's ability to resist evil qi. In order to build up the body's resistance to disease, it is important to maintain a balanced diet, daily life activities, normal emotional state and physical exercise to live by the laws of nature, and to take suitable herbs to prevent diseases.

（1）重視調攝精神

中醫學認爲人突然、强烈或反複持久的精神刺激，可使人體氣機逆亂，氣血陰陽失調而發病。情誌刺激還可導致正氣不足，招致外邪致病。因此，保持愉快舒暢的良好心情，減少不良的精神刺激和過度的情緒波動，從而使機體的氣機調暢，氣血和平，正氣充沛，抗邪有力，防止疾病的發生。

(1) Normal Emotional State

Chinese medicine believes that sudden, strong and repeated mental stimulation can cause disturbance of the qi mechanism, leading to disorder of yin, yang, qi and blood, and gives rise to diseases. Mental stimulation can also lead to insufficient right qi, and can allow external evils to penetrate. Therefore, maintaining a state of happiness can decrease the occurrence of bad mental stimulation and excessive emotional changes. Lively physiological functions and balanced qi and blood, leads to an abundance of right qi and a strong ability to resist evil qi. All these can prevent the occurrence of diseases.

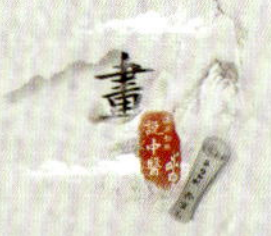

（2）注譩飲食起居

生活保持一定的規律性，做到飲食有節，起居有常，勞逸有度，是預防疾病發生的措施。在飲食方面要注譩饑飽適度，五味調和，衛生清潔，不可饑飽無常、暴飲暴食、偏飲偏食，以免損傷脾胃。在起居方面要順應四時氣候變化來安排作息時間，培養有規律的起居習慣，盡力做到定時睡眠，定時起床，定時工作或學習，定時體育鍛煉等，提高對自然環境變化的適應能力，以防止外邪的入侵。

（3）加强身體鍛煉

經常鍛煉身體，可以增强體質，提高人體的抗病能力。中國傳統的“太極拳”、“氣功”、“易筋經”、“八段錦”等多種健身活動，不僅能增强體質，預防疾病，而且對許多疾病還有一定的治療作用。

(2) Diet and Daily Life Activities

The measures to prevent disease occurrence are to regulate daily life activities, diet and work. Regulating the diet means to eat and drink suitable amounts of food and beverages, to eating all five flavors and to maintain good food hygiene. Eating excessively or insufficiently, and excessive consumption of one flavor can damage the Spleen and Stomach. Daily activities should be coordinated with the changing four seasons. A fixed time for sleeping, waking, working, studying, resting and exercising can improve the ability to adjust to nature's changes and to prevent evil qi attacks.

(3) Physical Exercises

Physical exercises can strengthen the constitution and improve resistance to diseases. Chinese traditional health-improving exercises, such as "tai ji", "qi gong", "yi jin jing", and "ba duan jin" not only strengthen the constitution and prevent diseases, but also treat many diseases.

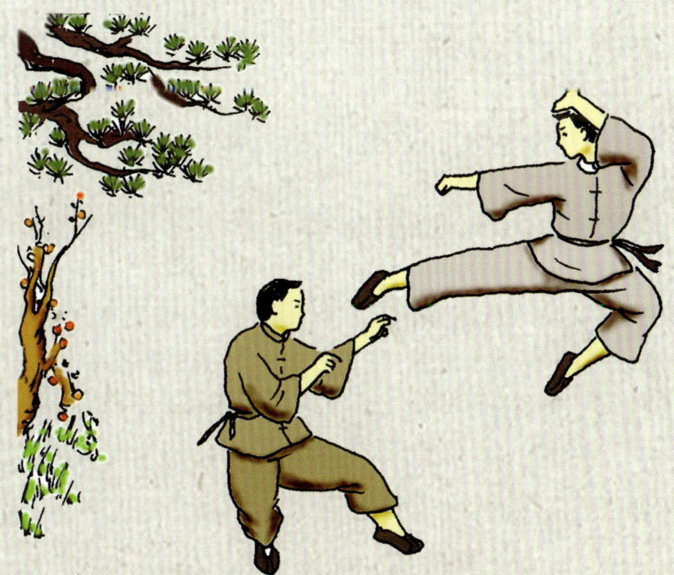

（4）人工預防免疫

人工免疫，是增强人體正氣，提高免疫能力，預防傳染病的重要手段。如接種疫苗、菌苗、類毒素等，使人體產生主動免疫，從而提高了抗邪能力，預防某些疾病的發生。

(4) Immunity

Immunity is an important method of strengthening the right qi, and preventing infectious diseases. Vaccination can improve resistance to evil qi and prevent diseases.

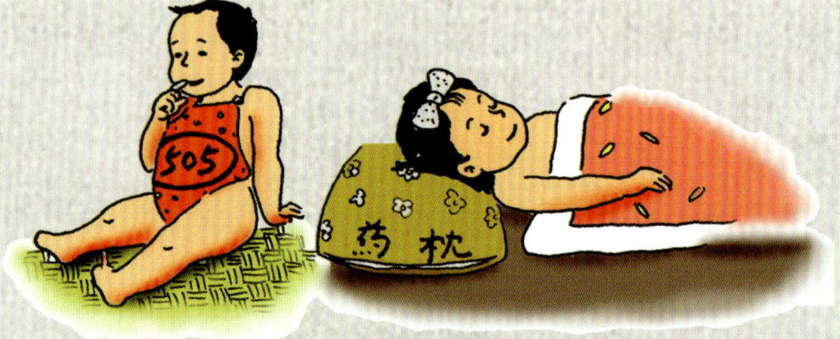

2. 避其邪氣，防止病邪侵害

（1）避其邪氣

未病先防必須注譩防止邪氣侵害。包括講究衛生，保護環境、水源、食物等不被污染，適應氣候變化而及時調節冷暖，還要防範外傷、蟲獸傷及有毒的傷害等。

2. Prevent Evil Qi Attacks, Prevent Disease Occurrences

(1) Prevent evil qi attacks

It is first necessary to avoid evil qi attacks, which include keeping good hygiene, protecting the environment, having clean water and food, dressing properly and according to weather, avoiding external injuries, insect or animal bites or poison.

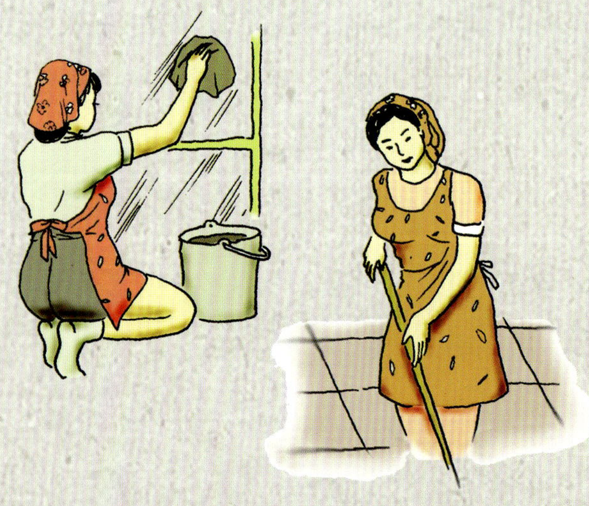

（2）藥物預防

早在《内經》中就有藥物預防傳染病的記載，目前在臨床上也常用中草藥物來預防傳染性疾病，如用板藍根、大青葉、貫衆等預防流感、流腦、非典，用茵陳、梔子等預防肝炎，用大蒜、馬齒莧等預防菌痢等。也可以用藥物來殺滅或驅除病邪，如燃燒烟熏法、藥囊佩帶法、浴敷塗擦法等。這些都是簡便易行、行之有效的方法。

(2) Preventative Medicinals

The Yellow Emperor's Classic of Internal Medicine <*Huáng Dì Nèi Jīng*> states that herbs can prevent infectious diseases. Nowadays in clinic, herbs are used in the same way. For example, *bǎn lán gēn* (Radix Isatidis) and *dà qīng yè* (Folium Isatidis) are used to prevent influenza, epidemic cerebrospinal meningitis and SARS, *yīn chén* (Herba Artemisiae Scopariae) and *zhī zǐ* (Fructus Gardeniae) are used to prevent hepatitis, *dà suàn* (Bulbus Allii [1985]) and *mǎ chǐ xiàn* (Herba Portulacae) are used to prevent dysentery. Herbs can also eliminate diseases, and such methods as herbal fumigation, medicine bag and medicinal bath with rubbing technique are easy to apply.

三、治療原則

The Treatment Principles

治則，也稱治療原則，是治療疾病必須遵循的基本法則，是在中醫學整體觀念和辨證論治理論指導下製定的治療方法的總則，對臨床治療立法、處方、用藥等，具有普通指導諡義。

1. 中醫治療觀

（1）治病求本

治病求本，是中醫治療學的主導思想，治病求本的核心就是要在複雜的疾病病理變化中，善於透過現象看本質，辨清病因病機，並以有效的治療解决疾病的主要矛盾。

Treatment principles are the basic rules of disease treatment. They are formulated under the concept of integrity and syndrome differentiation and treatment. These rules are the common guiding principles in clinic, for the use of prescriptions, herbs and so forth.

1. The Perspectives of Chinese Medical Treatment

(1) Treating the Root

Treating the root is a guiding principle in Chinese medicine. Its core is to look past the disease appearance to its true nature, and to distinguish the etiology and pathological mechanism in the process of complicated disease pathological changes. At the same time, it is to effectively resolve the main contradictory features of the diseases.

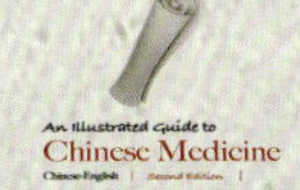

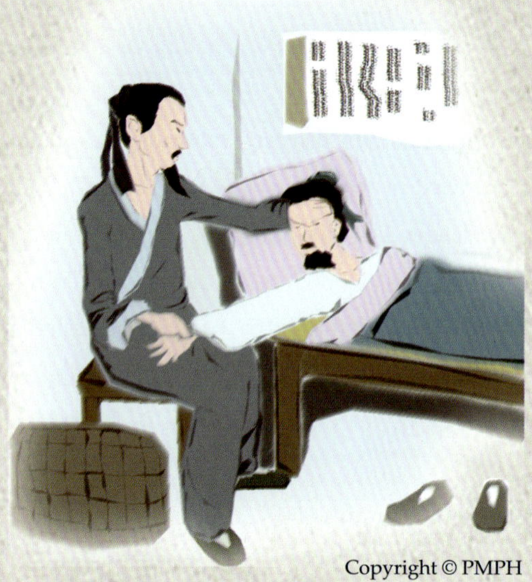

（2）不治已病治未病

1）未病先防

就是在疾病未發生之前，做好預防工作以防止疾病的發生，其主要方面一是增强體質，提高抗病能力，二是注譩防止病邪的侵襲與傷害。人體如果處於亞健康狀態，就要加强保健與預防措施。

(2) Preventive Treatment of Disease

1) Disease Prevention

Taking preventive measures to avoid disease previously is by strengthening the constitution and improving disease resistance, and paying attention to evil qi attacks and injuries. If the body is not healthy, one should strengthen one's health and take preventive measures.

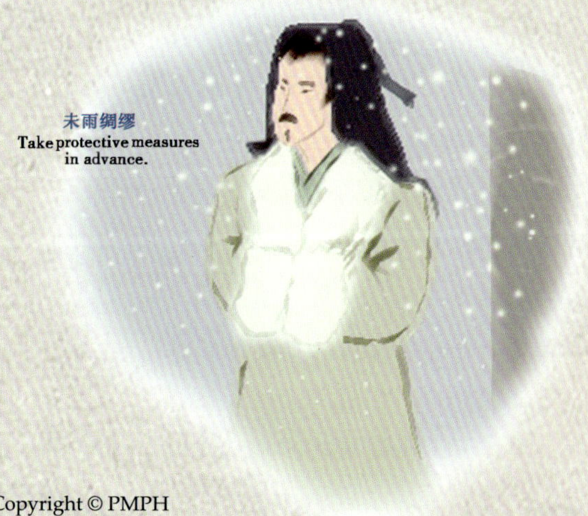

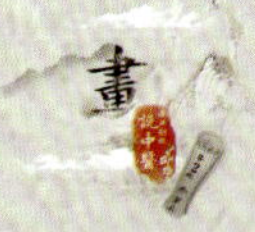

2）既病防變

如果疾病已經發生，則應爭取早期診斷，早期治療，並根據不同疾病的發展變化規律，採取相應的治療措施，以防止疾病的發展與傳變。

（3）治病先治神

治神，常常採用精神療法，也叫情誌療法、心理療法，它是通過醫者的言、行、情、誌等影響病者的認知、情感和行爲，以達到治療目的方法。以達到寬慰病人情懷，調整心身機能，促進疾病康複的目的。

（4）以平為期

健康即陰陽的協調平衡，反之，疾病就是陰陽失去平衡。中醫學從整體觀念出發，治療的目的主要是通過藥物、針灸、推拿等方法與技術來調動、發揮機體"陰陽自和"的自我調節機製，以期恢複陰平陽秘、內外和諧的生態平衡。

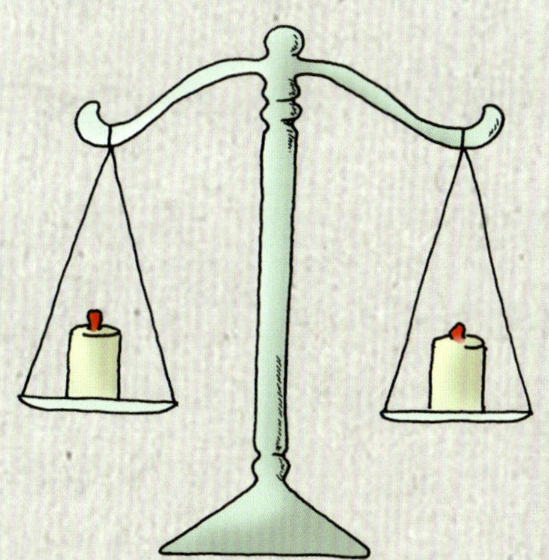

2) Preventing Disease Progression

If disease has already occurred, one should quickly diagnose and treat it, in order to prevent its progress and transmission.

(3) Treating the Spirit before Treating Diseases

Mental therapy, also called emotional therapy or psychological therapy, is often used in treating the spirit. It aims to affect the cognition, emotion and actions of the patients through speech, actions, emotions and so on. It can also be a treatment, to comfort patients, to regulate their health and mental functions and promote disease recovery.

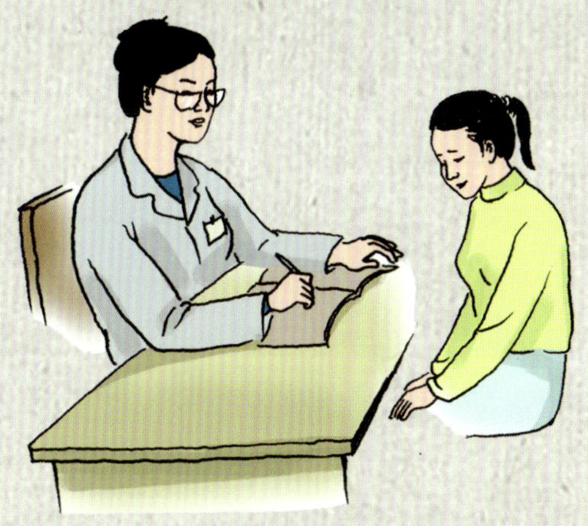

(4) Keeping Balance

Health is a result of balance between yin and yang, while disease is a state of imbalance between yin and yang. In light of the Chinese medical concept of viewing the body as a whole, medicinals, acupuncture and tui na are all techniques used to reach the treatment goal, which is balance yin and yang and to harmonize exterior and interior.

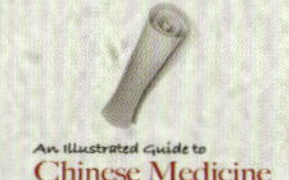

2. 基本治則

（1）祛邪扶正

疾病過程就是正氣與邪氣相互鬥爭的過程，邪勝正則病進，正勝邪則病退。

扶正，即扶助正氣，適用於以正虛爲主而邪氣不盛的虛性病證。例如氣虛、血虛或氣血兩虛的病人，應分別採取補氣、補血或氣血雙補的方法治療。

祛邪，即祛除邪氣，適用於邪氣盛而正氣未衰的病證。常用的發汗、攻下、清熱、消導、逐飲、化瘀等方法，就是在祛邪原則指導下，根據病人邪實的不同情況而製定的具體治法。

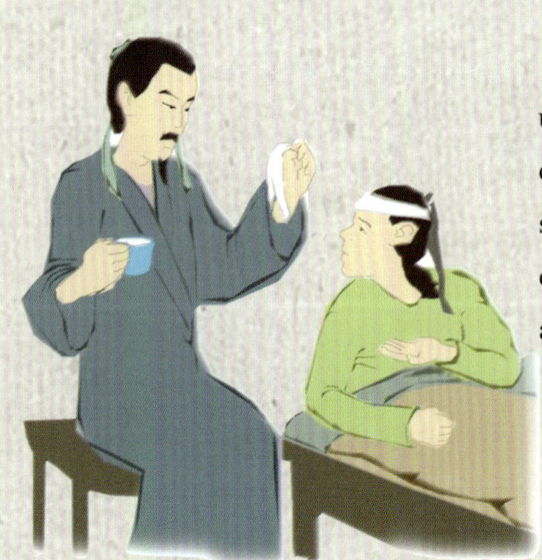

2. The Basic Treatment Principles

(1) Remove Evil Qi and Support Right Qi

The course of a disease is the struggle between right qi and evil qi. When evil qi suppresses the right qi, the disease prognosis is bad. When right qi suppresses the evil qi, the disease will decline.

Supporting right qi treats deficiency syndrome, where the right qi deficiency is the primary problem, while the evil qi is mild. For instance, tonifying qi and nourishing blood, or tonifying both of them, can treat a patient with deficiency of qi, blood or both.

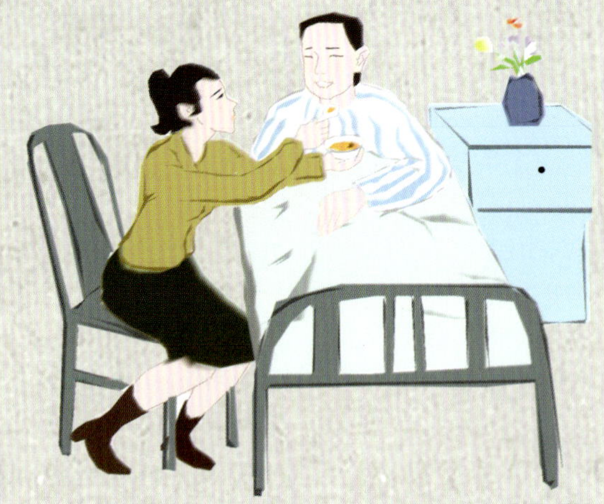

The method of removing the evil qi is mainly used when the evil qi is abundant and right qi is inadequate. Some common treatments such as inducing sweating, purgation, clearing heat, helping digestion, expelling fluids and transforming stasis are chosen according to the patients' different conditions.

（2）治標與治本

標和本是一個相對的概念。標本可以概括説明病變過程中多種矛盾的主次關係。從正邪雙方來説，正氣爲本，邪氣是標：以病因與癥狀來説，病因爲本，癥狀爲標；從疾病先後來説，舊病、原發病爲本，新病、繼發病爲標。

(2) Treating Branch and Root

Branch and root are two interconnected concepts. They explain the relationship of contradictions between the primary and secondary processes of disease changes. When discussing right qi and evil qi, the right qi is the root, and the evil qi is the branch; the cause of disease is the root and its symptoms is the branch, but in disease appearance times, chronic and primary diseases are the root, and new and secondary diseases are the branch.

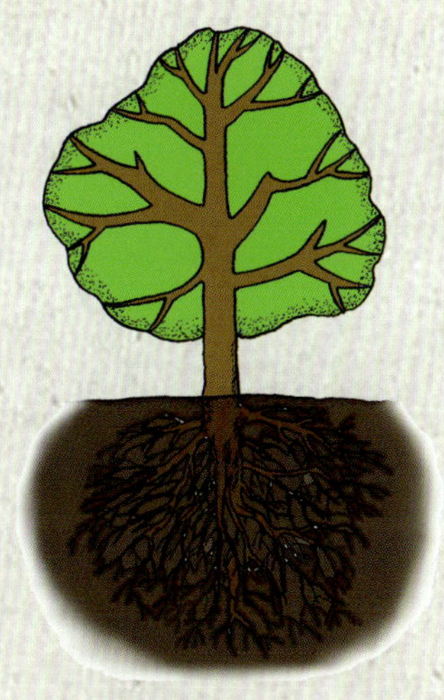

急則治標，標病危急，必須先治其標。如急性出血病人，血流不止，首先應將血止住，否則會引起嚴重後果、治標雖似一時權宜之計，但也是治本的必要環節。

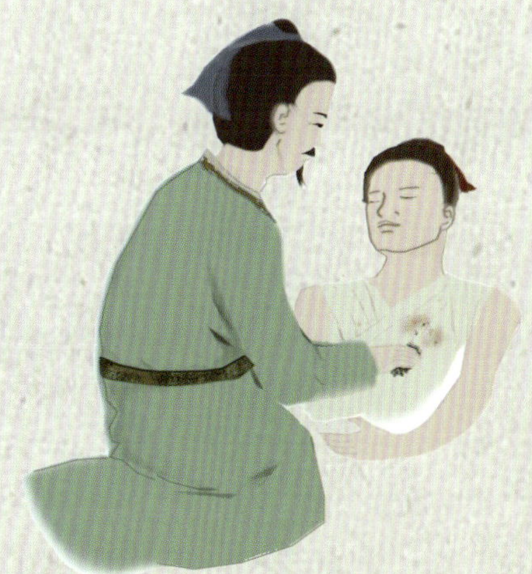

In emergency cases, the branch of the disease must be treated first. For example, in massive hemorrhage, emergency measures must be taken in order to stop the bleeding, otherwise, it will cause severe consequence. Although treating the branch in an emergency case is an expedient measure, it is also a necessary process for treating the root.

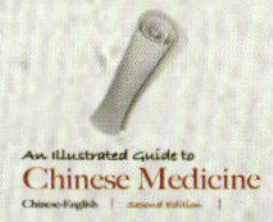

緩則治本：是指標癥不急，必須治其根本。因爲病本不去，則標癥不除。如慢性咳喘病人，如無急性發作，平時應健脾理氣，以杜生痰之源。

標本同治：在疾病標本並重的情況下，爲了提高療效，縮短療程，所採用標與本同時治療的原則。如氣虛感冒，多採用益氣兼以解表的標本兼顧治法。

In less urgent cases, the root of the disease must be first treated. If the root is not treated, the branch will not be eliminated. For example, with a non-emergency chronic bronchitis case, one should regulate the qi and strengthen the spleen in order to stop the source of phlegm generation.

During a disease, when both root and branch conditions are serious, one should treat them both simultaneously in order to shorten the course of disease and to improve the efficiency of the treatment. So, common cold with qi deficiency is treated by augmenting the qi and releasing the exterior, therefore both root and branch are being treated.

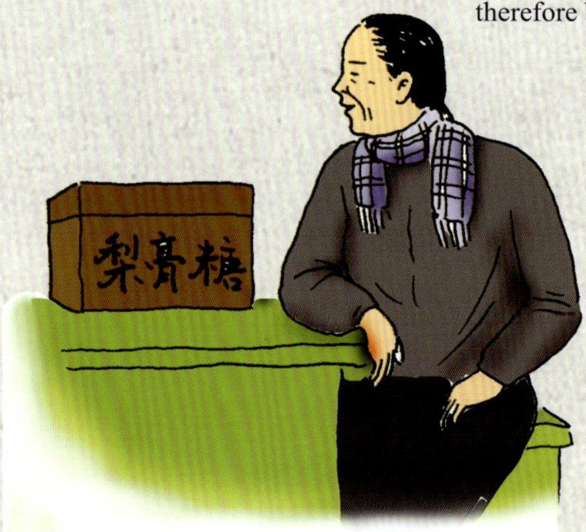

(3) 正治與反治

1) 正治

所謂正治，就是逆疾病癥狀而治的一種治療法則，故又稱爲“逆治”。適用於疾病的本質和癥狀相一致的病證。如寒證有寒象，熱證有熱象，虛證有虛象，實證有實象等。正治法有“寒者熱之”、“熱

(3) Straightforward Treatment and Contrary Treatment

1) Straightforward Treatment

Straightforward treatment refers to when clinicians use prescriptions which are opposite to the nature of the disease. This is also called opposition therapy. It is commonly used when the symptoms are identical with their nature. There are four kinds of routine treatments. Cold syndromes manifest cold symptoms,

者寒之"、"虛則補之"、"實則瀉之"之分。

寒者熱之，即寒證表現爲寒象，用溫熱藥治療。

熱者寒之，即熱證表現爲熱象，用寒涼藥治療。

虛則補之，即虛證表現爲虛象，用補益藥治療。

實則瀉之，即實證表現爲實象，用攻瀉祛邪藥進行治療。

2）反治

所謂反治，是順從疾病癥狀（假象）而治的一種治療法則，故又稱"從治"。適用於疾病的癥狀與本質不一致的病證。有些疾病較爲複雜嚴重，往往表現的證候與疾病的本質不相符合，出現一些假象，治療時就要透過假象，治其本質。反治法有"寒者寒用"、"熱因熱用"、"通因通用"、"塞因塞用"四種。

熱因熱用。即用熱性藥物治療有假熱癥狀的真寒假熱證。

寒因寒用。即是用寒性藥物治療具有假寒癥狀的真熱假寒證。

塞因塞用。即是用補益藥治療因虛而閉阻的真虛假實證。

通因通用。即用通利的藥物治療具有實性通泄癥狀的實證。

（4）三因製宜

"三因製宜"即論治時要因時、因地、因人製宜。疾病的發生發

therefore their suitable medicinals are warm in nature; heat syndromes manifest heat syndromes, therefore their suitable medicinals are cold in nature; deficiency syndromes manifest deficient symptoms, therefore their suitable medicinals are tonifying in nature; and excess syndromes manifest excess symptoms, therefore their suitable medicinals are draining in nature.

2) Contrary Treatment

Contrary treatment, also called inverse therapy, refers to the method of using medicinals with the same nature as the disease. It is commonly used when the symptoms are actually a false appearance of the disease's true nature, especially in complicated and serious cases. In order to treat successfully, clinicians must see through the false appearances to the disease's true nature. There are four kinds of contrary treatments. Using cold medicinals to treat false cold syndrome, using hot medicinals to treat false heat syndrome, using blocking medicinals for blockage and using tonifying medicinals for obstruction.

In a condition of false heat symptoms, when the disease's true nature is cold, warm medicinals should be used.

In a condition of false cold symptoms, when the disease's true nature is hot, cold medicinals should be used.

In a condition of false excess symptoms, when the disease's true nature is deficiency, tonifying medicinals should be used.

In a condition of false blockage symptoms, when the disease's true nature is excess, draining medicinals should be used.

(4) Treatments According to Different Conditions

The climate, local environment and different constitutions influence the occurrence and develop-

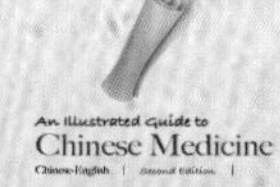

展，受多方面因素影響。如氣候變化、地理環境、個體的體質差異等，均對疾病有一定的影響。因此治療疾病時，必須把這些因素考慮進去，做到具體情況具體分析，以採取適宜的治療方法。

因時製宜，是根據四時氣候對人體生理、病理的影響而確立的治療原則。

一般説來，春夏氣候由溫漸熱，陽氣升發，人體腠理疏鬆開泄，即使患了外感風寒證，也不宜過用辛溫發散藥物，以免開泄太過，耗傷陰氣。而秋冬由涼變寒，陰盛陽衰，人體腠理致密，陽氣內斂，此時，若非大熱之證，當慎用寒涼藥物，以防傷陽。

因地製宜，是根據不同地區的地勢，氣候條件及生活習慣等，地理特點對疾病的影響，來考慮治療用藥的原則。

如中國西北地方，地勢高而寒冷少雨，故其病多燥寒，治宜辛潤。東南地區，地勢低而濕熱多雨，故其病多濕熱、治宜清化。

ment of diseases. Considering this, different treatments are suitable for different people. An objective analysis of the patient's condition is a precondition for treating on an individual basis.

The climate of the four seasons can influence the physiological functions and pathological changes of the body. Treatment according to seasons means to design treatment according to the characteristics of different climates.

In general, from spring to summer, the temperatures gradually change from warm to hot, the yang qi disperses and ascends, and the pores are more open and looser. Therefore, when treating exterior cold syndrome during spring and summer, medicinals that are warm and acrid should not be overused, in order to avoid too much draining and damage to yin qi. In autumn and winter, the weather is changing from cool to cold, yin is predominant, while yang is comparatively insufficient, the pores are more tightly closed, and yang qi is restrained. Therefore when treating very hot syndromes during autumn and winter, cold and cool medicinals should be cautiously used, in order to prevent damage to yang.

Different places have different topographic features, climate and life habits, which affect the choice of prescriptions.

The highlands in northwest China are cold and dry, with scanty amount of rainfall, many diseases have cold and dry features, therefore the flavors of the suitable medicinals are acrid and moistening. The lowlands of southeast China are hot and humid, with a lot of rainfall, many diseases have hot and damp features, therefore suitable medicinals are those that can clear and transform.

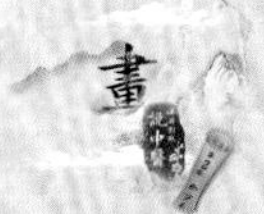

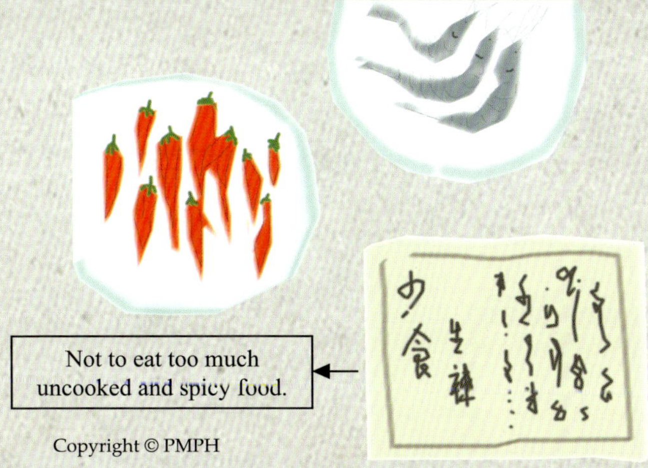

Not to eat too much uncooked and spicy food.

因人製宜，是根據病人的年齡、性別、體質、生活習慣等不同特點來考慮治療用藥的原則。

老年人生機減退、氣血虧虛，患病多虛證，應考慮顧護正氣，即使有實邪，需要攻伐，亦應慎重。

小兒生機旺盛，但氣血未充，臟腑嬌嫩、易寒易熱、易虛易實，病情變化迅速，故治小兒病應忌投峻攻，大補、藥量宜輕。

男女性別不同，生理特點亦有差異，婦女有經、帶、胎、產等情況，治療用藥應注譩。如在妊娠期，對峻下、破血、滑利、走竄、傷胎或有毒藥物，當禁用或慎閉；產後應考慮氣血虧虛及惡露情況。

During medicinal treatment, we should consider that people differ by age, sex, constitution and living habits.

Elderly people's qi and blood are deficient, their body functions are declining, so therefore deficiency syndromes are commonly seen in them. So, treatment is by strengthening right qi, and dispersing is only cautiously used.

Children's body functions are exuberant, yet their organs are tender and delicate, their qi and blood are not fully sufficient, disease conditions are easily and rapidly changing, and syndromes can easily transform from deficiency to excess, and from cold to heat, or from excess to deficiency, and from heat to cold. Therefore, while treating children, harsh and strong tonics medicinal should be avoided, and dosages should be low.

Men and women are physiologically different. Women experience menstruation, vaginal discharge, pregnancy, and delivery. Practitioners should pay attention to these special characteristics in clini-

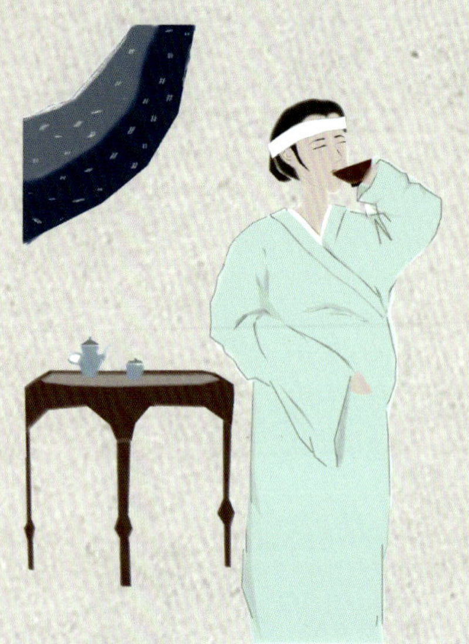

cal practice. Medicinals that are drastic purgatives, stasis-dispelling, slippery, moving and penetrate blockages, damaging to the fetus, and toxic, are prohibited or must be carefully used in pregnant patients. Patients who have lochia or are postpartum usually suffer from qi and blood deficiency.

在體質方面，每人的先天稟賦和後天調養不同，個體素質不但有强弱之别，而且還有偏寒偏熱以及素有某種慢性疾病等不同情况，所以雖患同樣的疾病，治療用藥亦當有所區别，如陽熱之體慎用溫熱，陰寒之體慎用寒涼。

Different people have different constitutions, some are stronger, weaker, colder or warmer due to chronic disease, or to different congenital and acquired essences. Therefore, different patients with the same disease should be treated according to their constitution. For example, warm or hot medicinals should be carefully used with yang-heat constitution patients, and cool or cold medicinals should be carefully used with yin-cold constitution patients.

四、治未病——中醫常見幾種保健方法

Preventive Treatment of Disease—Several Common Health Methods in Chinese Medicine

1. 中藥泡腳

中藥泡腳就是利用合適的中藥配方熬成中藥水來泡腳。在中藥泡腳的時候，其中有效的中藥成分在熱水的熱力作用幫助下，滲透

1. Foot Bath with Herbs

Foot bath with herbs is to soak feet in hot water with decocted herbs, whose effective ingredients would permeate the skin and enter into the

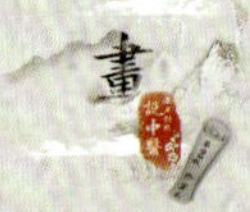

進皮膚，進入人體血液循環系統，從而達到改善體質、調理身體、治療疾病的效果。

民間則常以川芎、陳皮、石菖蒲、沉香或其他中藥配伍煎湯泡腳，藉以醒腦提神、消除疲勞；民間則常用菖蒲、艾葉等煮水給小孩泡腳，以達到防疫、保健作用。

blood system, owning to the heat of hot water, so as to improve the physique and cure diseases.

In folk, people usually do foot bath in decoction (composed of rhizome of chuanxiong, tangerine peel, eagle wood or other herbs) to refresh the mind and relieve fatigue. Children often have a foot bath in the water boiled with acorus (*chāng pú*, Rhizoma Acori Tatarinowii) and Chinese mugwort (*ài yè*, Folium Artemisiae Argyi) leaves to prevent diseases and stay healthy.

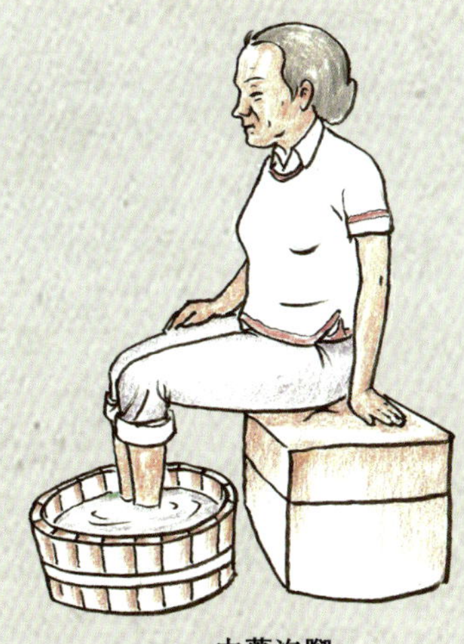

中藥泡腳
Foot Bath with Herbs

2. 穴位按摩

穴位按摩是以經絡腧穴學説爲基礎，以按摩爲主要施治，用來防病治病的一種手段。穴位按摩具有刺激人體特定的穴位，激發人的經絡之氣，以達到通經活血、調整人的機能、祛邪扶正的目的。

2. Point Massage

Point massage is a method of preventing diseases by applying massage on the acupoints as the main treatment method, based on TCM theories of channels and collaterals as well as acupuncture points. It can motivate qi of channels by stimulating specific points, so as to promote blood circulation, adjust human physical functions and remove evil qi and support right qi.

湧泉

位置：腳掌前面的三分之一的位置，彎曲腳趾出現的凹陷部位就是湧泉穴了。

功效：日常經常對湧泉穴進行按摩，能夠很好地促進腎臟健康，起到補腎、疏肝、明目等保健身體的作用。除此之外，還可以預防哮喘、高血壓等疾病，緩解失眠多夢、頭暈眼花等症狀。

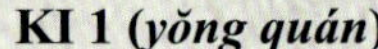

KI 1 (*yǒng quán*)

Position: This acupoint is found at the junction of anterior 1/3 and posterior 2/3 of the sole, and in the deepest depression when the toes are plantar-flexed.

Efficacy: Daily massage on this point has the function of promoting Kidney health, reinforcing the Kidney, soothing the Liver, improving eyesight, etc. Furthermore, it can prevent the diseases such as asthma and hypertension, and can alleviate the symptoms such as insomnia, dreaminess, dizziness, etc.

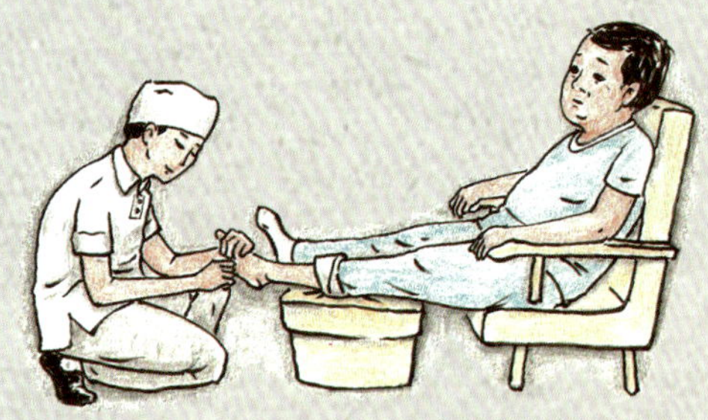

腳底按摩
Foot Massage

3. 三伏貼

又稱三伏天灸，以“冬病夏治”為原理，在一年中最炎熱的日子（即“三伏天”）將中藥敷貼在特定穴位上治療秋冬發作的疾病。

夏季人體氣血流通旺盛，藥物最容易吸收，而三伏期間是一年中陽氣最旺盛的時候，此時進行貼敷治療，最易恢復和扶助人體的陽氣，加強防衛功能，提高機體的抵抗力。進行三伏天灸時會使用辛

3. San Fu Tie

It is also known as dog-day moxibustion. According to the principle of “Treating Winter Diseases in Summer”, Chinese herbal medicine can be used as plasters for topical applicaiton on specific points in the three periods of greatest heat during the whole year to cure those diseases that occur during autumn and winter.

In summer, qi and blood circulate actively and medicine can be easily absorbed than in other seasons. As yang qi is most vigorous in the three

溫的外用藥材，如生薑、白芥子、麝香、細辛，敷貼於特定的身體穴位上，可防治過敏性哮喘、咳嗽、慢性支氣管炎、筋骨酸痛等秋冬易發作的疾病。這時，利用夏季陽氣旺盛，人體陽氣隨之生髮漸旺，體內凝寒之氣易解的狀態，運用補虛助陽藥或溫裡散寒藥物，天人合擊，最容易把冬病的病根拔除，這也是中醫強調"春夏養陽"的原因。

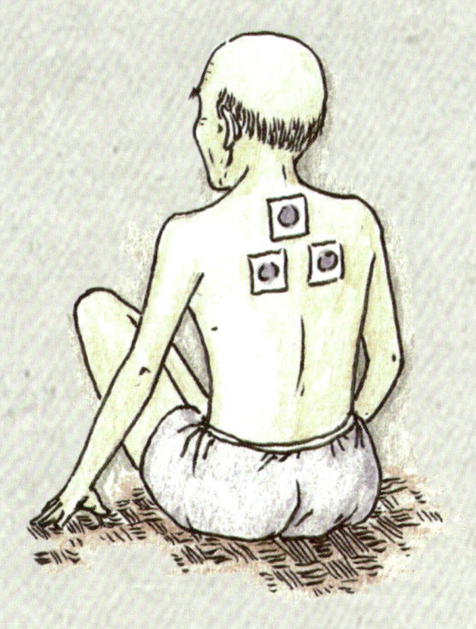

三伏貼
San Fu Tie

periods of greatest heat during the whole year, it is most easily to restore and support yang qi, strengthen body defense function and resistance by means of external application of Chinese herbal medicine. The pungent-warm external medicine like ginger (*shēng jiāng*, Rhizoma Zingiberis Recens), white mustard seed (*bái jiè zǐ*, Semen Sinapis), musk (*shè xiāng*, Moschus) and asarum (*xì xīn*, Radix et Rhizoma Asari) can be applied externally on specific points to prevent allergic asthma, cough, chronic bronchitis, aching tendons and bones and other diseases that easily occur during autumn and winter. At this time, owning to the most vigorous yang qi in summer, with yang qi in the body ascending and internal cold dissipating, the diseases that attack in winter can be easily eliminated by applying Chinese medicine with the effects of tonifying deficiency and reinforcing yang or warming the interior and dissipating cold. That's the reason why Chinese medicine emphasizes yang-preservation in spring and summer.

4. 拔罐

拔罐可以逐寒祛濕、疏通經絡、祛除瘀滯、行氣活血、消腫止痛、拔毒瀉熱，具有調整人體的陰陽平衡、解除疲勞、增強體質的功能，從而達到扶正祛邪、治癒疾病的目的。所以，許多疾病都可以採用拔罐療法進行治療。

4. Cupping

Cupping can eliminate cold and dampness, dredge channels and collaterals, dispel stasis, promote circulation of qi and blood, relieve swelling and pain, clear away heat and toxic substances and also balance yin and yang, relieve fatigue and enhance body. In this way, the purpose of removing evil qi and supporting right qi and curing diseases can be achieved. So, many diseases can be treated by cupping.

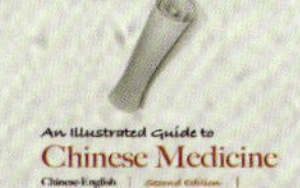

人到中年，筋骨疼常見，中醫認為多屬風濕入侵。拔火罐時罐口捂在患處，可以慢慢吸出病灶處的病氣，同時促進局部血液迴圈，達到止痛、恢復功能的目的，從而治療風濕“痹痛”、筋骨酸楚等不適。

When people are in middle age, it is common that tendons and bones ache, which is caused by invasion of wind-dampness according to the theory of Chinese medicine. When cupping, the jar is put on the affected area to suck pathogenic qi and promote local blood circulation to relieve the pain and regain function of the body, so as to cure disorders such as rheumatism, aches of tendons and bones, etc.

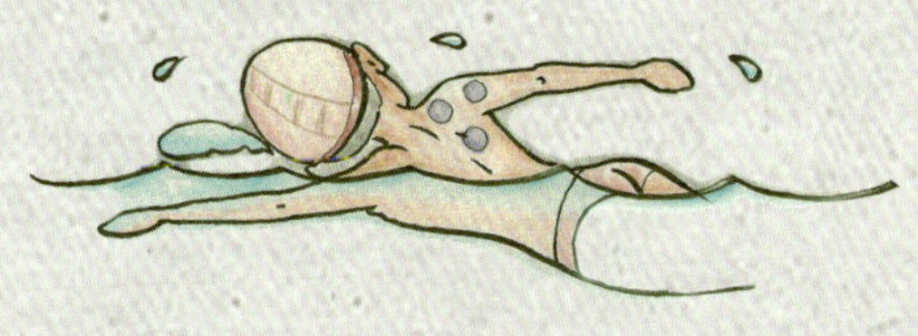

拔罐Cupping

5. 艾灸養生

足三裡位置：在小腿前外側，當犢鼻下 3 寸，距脛骨前緣一橫指（中指）。

足三裡是“足陽明胃經”的主要穴位之一，也是養生保健要穴之一。通過艾灸“足三裡”，可以促進氣血運行，起到溫中散寒、化瘀消腫的作用，並能健脾補胃，增強正氣，提高機體的免疫功能，從而發揮其防病強身、延年益壽的作用。

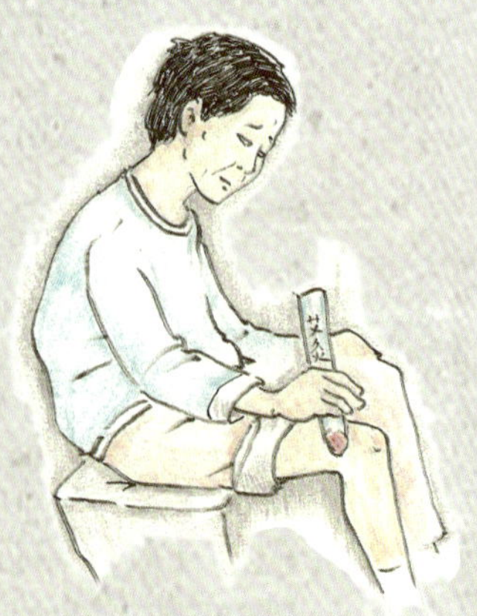

艾灸足三里
Moxibustion

5. Moxibustion

ST 36 (*zú sān lǐ*) acupoint: It is in the antero-lateral part of the leg, three inches under calf nose point, one finger (middle finger) wide to the anterior border of the tibia.

ST 36 (*zú sān lǐ*) is one of the main points of Stomach channel of foot yangming as well as one of the key points of health care. Through applying moxibustion on the point ST 36 (*zú sān lǐ*), the prevention of diseases, improvement of health and longer life can be achieved, as the movement of qi and blood can be promoted, coldness is scattered, stasis and swelling are reduced, the Spleen and Kidney are invigorated, the right qi is strengthened and the immune function is enhanced.

中文索引

H

J

K

L

M

N

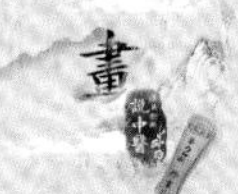

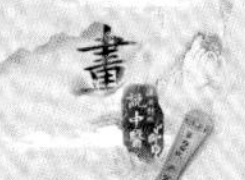

Z

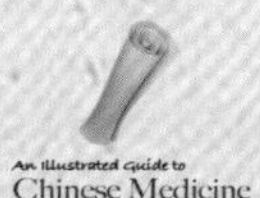

Index

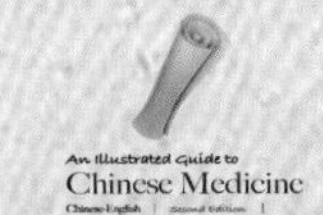

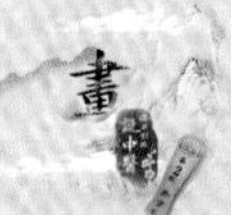

O

P

Q

R

S

T

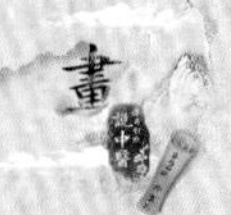

U

V

W

X

Y

Z

图书在版编目(CIP)数据

画说中医:汉英对照/徐宜兵,徐武,魏勤主编
.—2版.—北京:人民卫生出版社,2019
ISBN 978-7-117-28659-6

Ⅰ.①画… Ⅱ.①徐… ②徐… ③魏… Ⅲ.①中医学
—普及读物—汉、英 Ⅳ.①R2-49

中国版本图书馆CIP数据核字(2019)第134529号

画说中医(汉英对照)
第2版

主 编:徐宜兵 徐 武 魏 勤
出版发行:人民卫生出版社(中继线 010-59780011)
地 址:北京市朝阳区潘家园南里19号
邮 编:100021
E - mail:pmph @ pmph.com
购书热线:010-59787592 010-59787584 010-65264830
印 刷:北京顶佳世纪印刷有限公司
经 销:新华书店
开 本:710×1000 1/16 印张:16
字 数:286千字
版 次:2012年5月第1版 2019年12月第2版
2019年12月第2版第1次印刷(总第4次印刷)
标准书号:ISBN 978-7-117-28659-6
定 价:260.00元
打击盗版举报电话:010-59787491 E-mail:WQ @ pmph.com
质量问题联系电话:010-59787234 E-mail:zhiliang @ pmph.com

55检